TEACHING WRITING IN THE HEALTH PROFESSIONS

This collection provides a research-based guide to instructional practices for writing in the health professions, promoting faculty development and bringing together perspectives from writing studies, technical communication, and health humanities.

With employment in health-care sectors booming, writing instruction tailored for the health professions is in high demand. Writing instruction is critical in the health professions because health professionals, current and aspiring, need to communicate persuasively with patients, peers, mentors, and others. Writing instruction can also help cultivate professional identity, reflective practice, empathy, critical thinking, confidence, and organization, as well as research skills. This collection prepares faculty and administrators to meet this demand. It combines conceptual development of writing for the health professions as an emergent interdiscipline with evidence-based practices for instructors in academic, clinical, and community settings.

Teaching Writing in the Health Professions is an essential resource for instructors, scholars, and program administrators in health disciplines, professional and technical communication, health humanities, and interdisciplinary writing studies. It informs the teaching of writing in programs in medicine, nursing, pharmacy and allied health, public health, and other related professions.

Michael J. Madson is an Assistant Professor in the technical communication program at Arizona State University. He teaches courses related to health-care writing and user experience.

TEACHING WRITING IN THE HEALTH PROFESSIONS

Perspectives, Problems, and Practices

Edited by Michael J. Madson

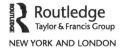

Routledge
Taylor & Francis Group

NEW YORK AND LONDON

First published 2022
by Routledge
605 Third Avenue, New York, NY 10158

and by Routledge
2 Park Square, Milton Park, Abingdon, Oxon, OX14 4RN

Routledge is an imprint of the Taylor & Francis Group, an informa business

Library of Congress Cataloging-in-Publication Data
Names: Madson, Michael J., editor.
Title: Teaching writing in the health professions : perspectives, problems, and practices / edited by Michael J. Madson.
Description: New York, NY : Routledge, 2022. | Includes bibliographical references and index.
Identifiers: LCCN 2021024198 (print) | LCCN 2021024199 (ebook) | ISBN 9780367755522 (hardback) | ISBN 9780367750886 (paperback) | ISBN 9781003162940 (ebook)
Subjects: LCSH: Medical writing. | Medical sciences.
Classification: LCC R119 .T423 2022 (print) | LCC R119 (ebook) | DDC 808.06/661--dc23
LC record available at https://lccn.loc.gov/2021024198
LC ebook record available at https://lccn.loc.gov/2021024199

ISBN: 978-0-367-75552-2 (hbk)
ISBN: 978-0-367-75088-6 (pbk)
ISBN: 978-1-003-16294-0 (ebk)

DOI: 10.4324/9781003162940

Typeset in Bembo
by SPi Technologies India Pvt Ltd (Straive)

CONTENTS

ILLUSTRATIONS

Figures

Tables

CONTRIBUTOR BIOGRAPHIES

Sarah Kosel Agnihotri is an Education Specialist at Wayne State University and was formerly the Writing Center Coordinator at Madonna University. She has an MA in Teaching English to Speakers of Other Languages, with experience teaching developmental and research writing. In addition, Sarah is a state-certified American Sign Language/English interpreter. Her research interests include second language acquisition, educational technology, and writing studies.

Elizabeth L. Angeli is an Associate Professor in Marquette University's English Department where she studies technical communication and writing education in health care. Liz is a leading expert in documentation practices and training for first responders, and her book, *Rhetorical Work in Emergency Medical Services* (Routledge), is the first book-length work to examine how first responders harness rhetoric's power to document patient care. Her work has also been published in academic and practitioner venues, including *Written Communication*, *Communication Design Quarterly*, *Rhetoric of Health and Medicine*, and *EMS1*.

Rebecca Day Babcock is the William and Ordelle Watts Professor at the University of Texas Permian Basin, where she teaches courses in writing and linguistics. She also serves as the Freshman English Coordinator and Director of Undergraduate Research. She has authored, coauthored, or edited several books on tutoring, writing centers, disability, and meta-research. Her latest book is *Theories and Methods of Writing Center Research*, edited with Jo Mackiewicz. *Researching the Writing Center*, written with Terese Thonus, has recently appeared in a revised edition. Babcock has also published research articles in *Writing Lab Newsletter*, *Linguistics and Education*, *Composition Forum*, *Praxis*, *The Peer Review*, and others. She won the International Writing Centers Association best article award in 2011 for her article on interpreted writing tutorials with deaf writers and the Council of Writing Program Administrators best article award this past summer for "Writing Center Directors and Diversity," written with Karen Keaton Jackson and Sarah Banschbach Valles.

Katharine Barnard practices and teaches family medicine at an urban community health center in Worcester, Massachusetts, affiliated with University of Massachusetts Medical School, where she is an Associate Professor in the Department of Family Medicine and Community Health. She received her medical degree from the University of Massachusetts Medical School and completed her residency at the same institution. Her personal and professional interests include integrating trauma-informed care and racial justice into the clinical workplace, providing high-quality care to vulnerable patients, and studying written and verbal narratives. She has received local awards for family medicine teaching and for the practice of community medicine.

Brian Callender is a Hospitalist and Assistant Professor of medicine at the University of Chicago. He is a fellow of the University's Academy of Distinguished Medical Educators, an associate junior faculty member of the Bucksbaum Institute for Clinical Excellence, and a faculty member of the MacLean Center for Clinical Medical Ethics and the Stevanovich Institute for the Formation of Knowledge. His academic interests focus on the intersection of the medical humanities, graphic medicine, and patient education. He regularly conducts graphic medicine workshops for patients and trainees. Courses that he teaches include The Body in Medicine and the Performing Arts, Graphic Medicine: Concepts and Practice, and The Art of Healing: Medical Aesthetics in Russia and the US, and the upcoming Death Panels: Exploring Death and Dying Through Comics. He has received funding to develop patient education materials that incorporate graphic medical narratives. His current funded activities with the Stevanovich Institute focus on graphic medicine and the formation of medical knowledge. He is coauthor of the chapter titled "Graphic Medicine" in the forthcoming Routledge Companion to the Health Humanities.

Lillian Campbell is an Assistant Professor of English at Marquette University, where she teaches academic and public writing and rhetorical theory. Her research focuses on the rhetorics of health and medicine, technical and professional communication, and feminist rhetorics. Her current project focuses on how clinical nursing simulations initiate students into the talk, writing, and action of the field and can be found in *Written Communication, Technical Communication Quarterly*, the *Journal of Writing Research*, and *Rhetoric of Health and Medicine*, as well as in the forthcoming collection *Gendered Pathologies*.

Lucy M. Candib, MD, is Professor Emerita of Family Medicine and Community Health at UMass Medical School. She practiced full-spectrum family medicine with obstetrics for over 40 years at the Family Health Center of Worcester, serving vulnerable low-income families including immigrants and refugees. After retiring from direct clinical care in 2016, Dr. Candib continues to precept resident and students and also performs and teaches asylum medical evaluations to clinicians wanting to learn this skill. Dr. Candib has written and lectured widely on topics of sexual abuse and violence against women and has drawn attention to the challenges facing women trainees. In her book *Medicine and the Family: A Feminist Perspective*, Dr. Candib offered a feminist approach to family issues in medical practice (Basic Books, 1995). Dr. Candib received a Fulbright scholarship in 1995 to teach family medicine in Ecuador, where she served as a visiting professor at the Pontificía Catholic University. Dr. Candib received the World Organization of Family Doctors (WONCA) Five Star Doctor Award in 2013. She initiated and continues actively in the Teacherless Writing Group within the University of Massachusetts Department of Family Medicine and Community Health.

Tracey Chan is an Adult Nurse Practitioner (NP) and current Chair of graduate nursing at Madonna University. She obtained her MSN with adult NP focus from Madonna University in May 2006. She worked in clinical practice as an NP until April 2012 when she transitioned to the academic setting, becoming a faculty member in the graduate nursing program at Madonna, teaching a variety of graduate nursing courses. During her time at Madonna University, she advanced from faculty member to NP program director and eventually chair of graduate nursing. In December 2019, she received her PhD in nursing from Duquesne University.

She has been involved with numerous research studies exploring student perceptions of clinical readiness and use of various modalities of simulation. She has published on the NP competencies in relation to NP practice and conducted a Delphi study revising the NP core competencies. During her tenure at Madonna University, she has remained active in clinical practice too.

Pilar Mirely Chois-Lenis is a Full Professor and Coordinator of the speech and language therapy major at Universidad del Cauca, Colombia. She founded and was the Director of the first Writing Center of her home university (2013–2015). She is completing her doctoral thesis in education, "Teaching Practices on Research Writing in Graduate Health Programs of Two Southwestern Colombian Universities," and has been granted a scholarship by Universidad del Cauca and Rudecolombia. She has been a researcher of reading and writing at school and university levels.

Barbara J. D'Angelo is a Clinical Professor of Technical Communication at Arizona State University. Barbara is the Graduate Advisor for the MS in technical communication, and she coordinates the Technical Communication Program's writing courses in collaboration with the Edson College of Nursing and Health Innovation. She is coeditor of *Information Literacy: Research and Collaboration Across the Disciplines*. Her publications include several book chapters and articles on the use of outcomes for curriculum development and assessment. She has presented on topics related to information literacy, health communication for nursing, technical communication, assessment, and curriculum development at the Council of Writing Program Administrators, Conference on College Composition and Communication, the Association for Business Communication annual conferences, and the International Writing Across the Disciplines conference.

Henry DelRosario is a Family Medicine Physician and Assistant Professor at the University of Massachusetts Medical School. He has clinical interests in adult and pediatric care, adult inpatient medicine, and obstetrics/maternity care. He received his medical degree from the Chicago Medical School at Rosalind Franklin University and then completed his residency at West Suburban Hospital Medical Center. His mission is to spread the full-spectrum joy of full-spectrum family medicine through teaching and life-long learning. Henry also has a passion for art and literature and through an online presence and social media hopes to share how humanities integrates with a medical career.

Kevin Dvorak is a Professor and Executive Director of the Write from the Start Writing and Communication Center at Nova Southeastern University (NSU). He is a past president of both the International Writing Centers Association and the Southeastern Writing Center Association (SWCA). He has cochaired two IWCA Summer Institutes, two SWCA Conferences, and one National Conference on Peer Tutoring in Writing. His book *Creative Approaches to Writing Center Work* (Hampton, 2008) won the 2009 IWCA Outstanding Scholarship Award for Best Book/Major Work. He has also published in *ESL Writers: A Guide for Writing Center Tutors, Tutoring Second Language Writers, The Writing Center Director's Resource Manual, The Successful High School Writing Center, Writing Studio Pedagogy: Space, Place, and Rhetoric in Collaborative Environments*, the *Journal of Faculty Development*, and the *Communication Center Journal*, as well as in *Praxis* and *The Writing Center Journal*. Dr. Dvorak earned the 2014 SWCA Achievement Award and the 2014 NSU Student Life Achievement Award for Professor of the Year.

Lisa S. Gussak is an Associate Professor of Family Medicine and Community Health at the University of Massachusetts Medical School. She practices family medicine in a clinical sites within Worcester County in Worcester, Massachusetts. In her clinical practice, she enjoys family-centered maternity care, family planning, women's health, and the care of children. Dr. Gussak has been involved in academic medicine and medical education since completing her residency. Her areas of academic interest include learners in academic difficulty, advanced communication skills, coaching, and mentoring. In 2014, she was awarded a Fulbright Scholarship to begin the development of a family medicine residency program in Leon Nicaragua. She moved to Nicaragua with her family for a six-month sabbatical in 2015. In 2015, Dr. Gussak's department recognized her teaching with an excellence in education award. In May of 2021, she completed an eight-month training program to become certified coach via the Gestalt International Study Center in Wellfleet, MA. She is the director of The Center for Clinical Communication and Professionalism and works with colleagues to enhance their communication skills and team function.

Neal Haldane has taught journalism, public relations, communication, and writing for more than three decades at Madonna University in Michigan. He currently serves as Writing Program Director and previously helmed the academic service-learning office at the university. Haldane's specialty areas include multimedia creation, academic service-learning, the first-year experience and learning communities, and writing across the curriculum. Prior to his teaching career, Haldane reported and edited news at community newspapers and also worked as a public relations specialist.

Chanaka Kahathuduwa is a faculty member at Texas Tech University Health Sciences Center at the Permian Basin, belonging to the Department of Human Development and Family Sciences. Dr. Kahathuduwa's research focuses primarily on studying neurophysiological mechanisms underlying human cognition and cognitive development. He is particularly interested in studying neurophysiological mechanisms affecting attention, concentration, learning, and development in populations with attention deficit hyperactivity disorder and autism. In addition to being an enthusiastic researcher, Dr. Kahathuduwa is very keen on creating an encouraging atmosphere for his trainees, and he tries his best to cultivate analytical skills and research ethics among his junior colleagues and trainees. At large, he strives to better understand the neurophysiological correlates of human diseases in order to explore sustainable therapeutic options for such conditions and to improve the quality of life of those individuals who are affected.

Jaanki Khandelwal was born and raised in Odessa, Texas. She graduated from Odessa High School with an International Baccalaureate degree. She then went on to Texas Tech University and majored in honors arts and letters with an emphasis in humanities. She graduated suma cum laude before she began medical school at Texas Tech School of Medicine. Jaanki is currently a medical student, and she enjoys reading, dancing, running, and singing in her free time. Her research endeavors include a paper entitled "Arginine Substitution of a Cysteine in Transmembrane Helix M8 Converts Na+,K+-ATPase to an Electroneutral Pump Similar to H+,K+-ATPase" published in 2017 in *PNAS*. Being a medical student who is actively involved in publishing research papers, she is passionate about how technology impacts the world of research and those involved.

Caleb Lalinsky graduated from Michigan State University in 2011 with a BA in English and a teaching certificate in secondary education. In 2014, he received his MFA in creative writing from Temple University. Today, he works as an Adjunct Writing Instructor at Madonna University, University of Detroit Mercy, and the College for Creative Studies, and as a specialist in the Madonna University Writing Center. He has presented at the Michigan Writing Centers Association conference and Corridors: The Great Lakes Writing and Rhetoric Conference. His previously published work is available for viewing online at the *Maudlin House* and *The Detroit Socialist*.

Daniel Lasser is Professor and Chair Emeritus of the University of Massachusetts (UMass) Medical School/UMass Memorial Department of Family Medicine and Community Health. Dr. Lasser also served as Interim President of the UMass Memorial Medical Group from 2007 to 2010 and led the medical school's Center for Advancement of Primary Care. As Senior Vice President for Primary Care, he led the UMass Memorial strategic initiative to create patient-centered medical homes across the system's primary care sites and was instrumental in the medical school ranking among the best medical schools for primary care, as well as leading a department that is among the largest and most respected departments of family medicine in the nation.

Emilie M. Ludeman is the Research, Education, and Outreach Librarian and Liaison to the School of Nursing at the University of Maryland Health Sciences and Human Services Library. As liaison since 2011, she instructs students on finding the best available evidence to support their writing and clinical practice. She is co-instructor of Library Resources and Scholarly Writing, a required course in the university's master of science in health science program.

Barry M. Maid is a Professor and Founding Head of the Technical Communication Program at Arizona State University. He was head of that program for ten years. He is the author of numerous articles and chapters primarily focusing on technology, independent writing programs, and program administration, including assessment. He and Barbara D'Angelo have written multiple articles on information literacy and writing. Maid and D'Angelo, along with Sandra Jamieson and Janice Walker, edited *Information Literacy: Research and Collaboration across Disciplines*. In addition, he is a coauthor, with Duane Roen and Greg Glau, of *The McGraw-Hill Guide: Writing for College, Writing for Life*.

Isabell C. May is the Director of the Writing Center at the University of Maryland, Baltimore (UMB), while also serving as a faculty member for UMB's Graduate School in the Science Communication Program (part of the master of science in health science). Dr. May was born in Germany and moved to the United States in 1999 to pursue her graduate education. She earned her PhD in American studies from the University of Maryland, College Park. Her publication record includes articles on American studies, as well as on learning and writing centers. Prior to her tenure at UMB, she headed the Writing Center at the University of Baltimore for two years. She also founded the Writing Center for Academic English at Leuphana University in northern Germany in 2012, which she directed for two years. Prior to her role at Leuphana, she worked for five years in a writing and learning center at the Universities at Shady Grove in Rockville, Maryland, a regional higher education center sponsored by the University System of Maryland. From November 2015 to April 2018, Dr. May served as the treasurer of the Mid-Atlantic Writing Center Association.

Janine Morris is an Assistant Professor in the Department of Writing and Communication in the College of Arts, Humanities, and Social Sciences at NSU. She is the Graduate Student Coordinator for the Write from the Start Writing and Communication Center and the Department of Writing and Communication's Alumni Relations Manager. She earned her PhD in English and comparative literature with a specialization in composition and rhetoric (along with a graduate certificate in women, gender, and sexuality studies) from the University of Cincinnati in 2016. She has presented at national and regional conferences, and her work has been published in *Pedagogy*, *The CEA Critic*, *Computers and Composition*, *Composition Studies*, and *Community Literacy Journal*. She was an editorial assistant for *Composition Studies* (2014–2016) and is a reviewer for *Composition Studies*, *Peitho*, and *Queen City Writers*. She is currently the Florida state representative for the SWCA.

Cynthia Moreau joined the faculty at NSU College of Pharmacy as an Assistant Professor of Pharmacy Practice in August 2016. Dr. Moreau received her doctor of pharmacy degree from the University of Florida College of Pharmacy in 2014. Following graduation, she completed a PGY1 pharmacy practice residency with an emphasis in ambulatory care at Florida Hospital Celebration Health and a PGY2 ambulatory care residency with a focus in academia at the University of Florida (UF) College of Pharmacy/UF Health Family Medicine. Dr. Moreau is part of the college's Accountable Care Organization Research Network, Services, and Education (ACORN SEED) team, which is working to expand clinical pharmacy services within accountable care organizations in the south Florida region. She currently maintains a clinical practice site within Accountable Care Options, LLC in Boynton Beach, Florida, providing chronic disease state management alongside primary care physicians.

Elizabeth Narváez-Cardona is an Associate Professor and Director of the Department of Education at Universidad Autónoma de Occidente (UAO), Colombia. She completed a PhD in education, with an emphasis in teaching and learning, and in writing studies at the University of California, Santa Barbara, USA, with a cooperative scholarship granted by Fulbright-Colombia, the Colombian Department of Science, Technology and Innovation (Colciencias), and UAO (2011–2016). She has been a writing instructor, researcher, and consultant about writing and university learning, academic writing and faculty development, and scientific publication and research education.

Stacy Potts is a Family Medicine Physician who practices broad spectrum family medicine with maternity care in a rural community. She is an associate professor and vice-chair of education in the University of Massachusetts Medical School Department of Family Medicine and Community Health. She completed her MD at the University of Vermont College of Medicine, then residency and faculty development fellowship at the University of Massachusetts Medical School. Among other venues, she has published in *Medical Education Online, Family Medicine,* and the *American Journal of Preventative Medicine.*

Cristina Reyes Smith is a graduate of the occupational therapy doctorate program at Thomas Jefferson University and the master of occupational therapy program at the Medical University of South Carolina (MUSC). She currently works as an Assistant Professor and Director of Admissions in the MUSC College of Health Professions Division of Occupational Therapy. Dr. Smith has served on the board of directors of the American Occupational Therapy Association since July 2020. She has also served on the editorial board of the *Journal of Occupational Therapy Education* since April 2020. She has over 15 years of experience in community health promotion, program development, and leadership development, with a focus on access to care for underserved communities. She has conducted presentations and published manuscripts about workforce diversity, cultural competence and sensitivity, and related topics for local, state, and international audiences.

Natalia Schlabritz-Loutsevitch is the Interim Chair of the Medical Center Hospital Institutional Review Board, Director of the Integration Seminar, and Associate Professor in the Department of Obstetrics and Gynecology and the Department of Pharmacology and Neurobiology at Texas Tech University Health Science Center School (TTUHSC) of Medicine and the Texas Tech University Health Sciences Center Graduate School of Biomedical Sciences. Upon transition of her laboratory onto the Permian Basin Campus of the Texas Tech University Health Science Center (Odessa, Texas), she contributed to the field of fetal programming by developing a human placental perfusion system.

Natalia enjoys mentoring medical students, residents, and fellows to develop them as well-rounded clinicians and researchers. Her mentees have received multiple awards, including travel awards from prestigious societies, the university president, and the dean for their scientific contributions. She is also proud to be a partner of the Ector County Independent School District (ECISD). They achieved the highest level of recognition by winning the NASA competition to perform a space flight experiment on mission 13 (July 2019). ECISD chose Natalia to receive a state award on behalf of TTUHSC "Stand up for public education."

Jill Tirabassi is a Clinical Assistant Professor at the University at Buffalo Department of Family Medicine. She earned her medical degree from SUNY Upstate Medical University and a master of public health degree at the University of Massachusetts-Amherst. She is dually boarded in family medicine and preventive medicine and has completed a fellowship in primary care sports medicine. She currently is performing research in chronic disease prevention as well as practicing clinically in an urban underserved residency training site. Her publications have appeared in the *Journal of Clinical Hypertension*, the *American Journal of Sports Medicine*, and *Sports Health*, among other venues.

Susan E. Thomas is the Founding Director of the Faculty of Arts and Social Sciences (FASS) Writing Hub and WRIT Program, both now housed in the Department of Writing Studies. She was previously Lecturer in English, Associate Dean Teaching and Learning (FASS), Director of Academic Writing in the former FASS Teaching and Learning Network, and Teaching Development Coordinator for Arts and Social Sciences, Education, and Social Work, Sydney College of the Arts and the Conservatorium of Music. She currently coordinates the Student Writing Fellows Program in the Writing Hub.

Susan's research focuses primarily on theories of writing, grounded in cognitive rhetoric, with a particular interest in affect and cognition. She is also interested in life writing, performative writing, feminist and global rhetorics, Native American rhetorics, writing across the curriculum, and writing centers.

Deborah E. Tyndall is an Assistant Professor in the Department of Nursing Science at East Carolina University. Her clinical practice experiences include behavioral health nursing, community nursing, and leadership. She has been in academia for over 13 years and has experience teaching in undergraduate, graduate, and doctoral programs. She is an educational scholar with a primary interest in advancing the science of nursing education. She has spent the last ten years examining writing development in nursing students and nurses in practice. Dr. Tyndall is collaborating with interdisciplinary colleagues within the University Writing Program and Writing Center to examine threshold concepts in writing.

Jennifer Weaver has an MA from Wayne State University and BA from Madonna University. She has taught college composition for various universities in the Detroit metro area for over 15 years, and she also works as a Writing Specialist at the Madonna University Writing Center.

Kathryn West is a Licensed Social Worker and Researcher with a background in medical humanities, poetry, and expressive therapies at the University of Chicago, where she works with ECHO-Chicago on capacity building for primary care providers in underserved communities. She also engages in graphic medicine and bioethics research projects across the university. Her work in graphic medicine has included the development and implementation of workshops for patients and providers across a variety of settings and has been copresented at multiple conferences. She received her AM from the University of Chicago's School of Social Service Administration with a certificate from the Graduate Program in Health Administration and Policy (GPHAP); while there, she was the recipient of GPHAP's Bugbee Award. She completed her undergraduate studies at Northwestern University, where she studied creative writing and philosophy and completed independent research, which used poetry to examine philosophical and ethical issues. Kathryn's poetry has been presented and published, including a reading at the Poetry Foundation.

C. Erik Wilkinson is the Regional Library Director for the Libraries of the Health Sciences at the Permian Basin and holds the title Faculty Associate. He attended Hardin-Simmons University, receiving his bachelor's in 1992. He then went on to attend the University of North Texas, completing a master's in library science in 1998. Over the course of his professional career, he served a myriad of public libraries before moving into academia in 2011. During a break from librarianship, he served as program manager for the Amarillo Breast Center of Excellence (2011–2012), affiliated with Texas Tech University Health Sciences Center. He currently is a member of the Medical Library Association (MLA), South Central Chapter of MLA. He serves on the board of the Permian Basin Adult Literacy Center, plus various campus committees.

Sarah Yonder is an Assistant Professor of Family Medicine at Central Michigan University's College of Medicine. She has been the Course Director of the pre-clerkship clinical skills course since 2016, both administering the course and serving as an instructor. She is board certified in family medicine and is in clinical practice. Originally from Buffalo, New York, she earned her bachelor's degree from Cornell University and her medical degree from St. George's University School of Medicine in Grenada. She completed a family medicine residency at the University of Massachusetts Medical School Worcester.

EDITOR BIOGRAPHY

Michael J. Madson is an Assistant Professor in the technical communication program at Arizona State University. He teaches courses related to health-care writing and user experience.

His research explores how communication practices can contribute to health and wellness, focusing on three key areas: the training of health professionals, drug safety (especially opioids and cannabis), and wayfinding in health-care facilities. His scholarship has recently appeared in *HERD: Health Environments Research and Design*, *Medical Teacher*, *Journal of Continuing Education in Nursing*, and *Nurse Educator*. He also serves on the editorial boards of two journals dedicated to online learning: *Online Literacies Open Resource* and *Research in Online Literacy Education*.

Before coming to Arizona State, Michael was a full-time faculty member at the Medical University of South Carolina, teaching writing to students across the health professions. He remains an Adjunct Associate Professor there, running a writing course for the online Bachelor of Health-Care Studies program. He has also taught at the University of Minnesota, Utah State University, the Harvard Extension School, Yonsei University, and Far East University.

ACKNOWLEDGMENTS

This collection has left me indebted to a great many people. Yet, I owe special thanks to my colleagues at the Center for Academic Excellence at MUSC: Jennie Ariail, Tom Smith, Lisa Kerr, Shannon Richards-Slaughter, John Dinolfo, Christy Huggins, Casey O'Neill, and Michelle Cohen. Without their mentorship over the years, an undertaking like this would not have been possible.

I owe extra special thanks to Christina, Alice, and Nico, who moved with me across the country in the middle of a pandemic. Their encouragement and good humor were invaluable throughout the cycles of imagining, proposing, compiling, and (re)drafting.

—Michael J. Madson

Introduction

WRITING IN THE HEALTH PROFESSIONS

An Emergent Interdiscipline for Teachers

Michael J. Madson

Demand for the health professions has perhaps never been greater. As burdens on health-care systems grow heavier, countries around the globe face alarming shortages of physicians, nurses, pharmacists, and allied health professionals, who include physician assistants, occupational therapists, and emergency medical technicians. On the whole, the world is facing a shortfall of 18 million health professionals, with rural regions and low- and middle-income countries hit the hardest.[1] As a partial response, workforce challenges have been repeatedly highlighted by the World Health Assembly, the decision-making arm of the World Health Organization. Among other actions, the Assembly instituted the International Year of the Nurse and Midwife in 2020 and the International Year of Health and Care Workers in 2021, calling greater attention to the training of health professionals.[2,3]

In health professions training, students complete exercises in classrooms ("didactic" instruction) and health-care workplaces ("clinical" instruction), gaining the knowledge, skills, and attitudes they need to excel in their chosen specialties as members of a team. These basic trajectories are well-known. What is often unacknowledged, however, is the prominent place of writing: health professionals need to learn a variety of written genres while in the classroom or on the job—and often produce them under tight constraints. There have been several foundational studies in this area.

Surveying medical schools in the United States, Yanoff and Burg[4] cataloged the genres considered the most important to teach. At the top of the list were write-ups of patient histories and physician examinations, progress notes and discharge summaries, peer-reviewed publications, and grant proposals. Other important genres included letters to referring doctors, outpatient records, consultation reports, and admitting notes.

Nursing education has made extensive use of writing. A curricular review found that, in one nursing program, writing assignments were required in 86% of the courses.[5] In another study, Gimenez[6] explored the writing assignments of more than 100 nursing and midwifery students at a London university, listing out common genres. These included care plans, case studies, article reviews, portfolios, reflective essays, argumentative essays, and culminating theses.

Hobson et al.[7] analyzed the writing tasks that pharmacy students performed during clerkships. The researchers identified 28 genres, and the most prevalent were in-service presentations, patient case write-ups, formulary reviews, and newsletter articles. Others included patient education materials, drug information inquiries, procedures, market analyses, research reviews, research method comparisons, informed consent documents, and adverse drug reaction reports. Discussing their findings, the researchers took aim at the common belief that "pharmacists don't write."[7(p61)]

DOI: 10.4324/9781003162940-1

A more recent study was conducted in public health. August et al.[8] surveyed the number and type of writing assignments taught in accredited public health programs. According to the findings, nearly all of the courses in epidemiology had writing assignments, some of which were specific to the practice of public health: original research articles, surveillance systems evaluations, annotated bibliographies, and issue briefs, to name only a few. Some assignments were more general and academic, such as term papers, critiques, short-answer essay questions, research summaries, and presentations of an epidemiological method. At one school of public health, students have additionally been asked to write health alerts, health promotion brochures, health status reports, letters to the editor, tweets, website content, and more.[9]

These foundational studies, though limited geographically, provide a sense of the prevalence and variety of writing tasks in health professions training. In short, the studies show that students and trainees need to write in order to complete their academic requirements (although general essays and summary documents may have little instructional value[6,7]), as well as to do the work of health care and health promotion. Indeed, the success of a health organization relies largely on the writing done within it.[10]

Importantly, writing in the health professions is not just about the *writing*, meaning the textual artifact and its process of production. It is also about the *writer*, and the benefits to the writer are legion. For starters, writing can facilitate professional identity formation: the psychological development of health professionals, along with their socialization into their organizational roles, behaviors, relationships, and values that inspire public trust.[11] More particularly, writing can help future and current health professionals cultivate

- empathy and reflective practice;[12–17]
- critical thinking and collaborative learning;[18–20]
- research skills;[21–23]
- greater knowledge of their chosen specialty, including concepts that can be challenging to teach;[24–26]
- patient education skills;[27]
- leadership;[28,29]
- cultural competence, awareness, and humility;[29–32]
- self-expression, organizational abilities, along with observational and descriptive skills;[33]
- clinical judgment;[34,35] and
- partnerships with community organizations, when used in conjunction with service learning.[36]

Some evidence suggests that writing can also assuage burnout, a major challenge in the health professions.[16,37,38] Accordingly, accrediting agencies have affirmed the need to develop student competencies in and through writing.[e.g., 39–47]

Approaches to Writing Instruction

Writing instruction in the health professions is not a recent innovation, of course. As early as 1953, an international congress resolved that writing instruction should be included in the medical curriculum.[48] In English language publications, journal articles in this area began to appear regularly around the same time, exploring topics like prescription writing,[49] history writing,[50] the humanities,[51] the proper use of medical libraries,[48] innovative course and workshop designs,[52–54] and what we now call "writing to learn."[55,56] Some of this work was quite colorful. To spotlight only one example, Walter R. Bett, a research librarian working in London, advised writers to avoid dedications. Imagine the awkwardness, he stated, of dedicating a medical article to your parents, "as a token of my undying gratitude," when the article subject is "On general paralysis in the young in relation to hereditary syphilis."[48(p26)] Unintended assumptions may be made.

During those early years, many teachers of "writing in the health professions" may have had little awareness of each other, given that they rarely built on each other's scholarship. This could certainly have contributed to the impression that "like the weather, medical writing is eternally the subject of criticism, but, also like the weather, nothing is done about it."[52(p481)] Based on citations, it appears that, at least in health professions journals, few instructional articles on writing attracted much interest until the 1980s and later, when authors began to ground their writing-related studies more consistently in theory and/or empirical data. This history would be a fruitful topic for future research.

How is writing in the health professions taught today? Reviewing the literature from nursing, Oermann et al. identified several overlapping strategies.[57] One was "writing across the curriculum," which rests on the assumption that the whole academic community, not just the English department, should support students' growth as writers. Thus, writing instruction is integrated throughout a program of study, typically with additional supports, such as peer tutoring programs and faculty development seminars.[58]

A second strategy to teach writing was stand-alone writing courses. These can be taught by nursing faculty alone or in collaboration with colleagues in English or technical communication. A third was assignments in nursing courses, such as blogs, reflections, and clinical writings. A fourth was faculty behaviors, such as feedback on student work, the creation of assignment guidelines, partnerships with students, and enlisting volunteers to serve as writing tutors. A fifth was workshops, retreats, and self-directed activities, which, for practicing nurses, were used most frequently to facilitate papers for publication. Oermann et al. noted that only one-third of the strategies they found in the literature had been evaluated for effectiveness, a clear need.[57]

Barriers to Writing Instruction

There are numerous barriers to teaching and learning writing in the health professions. Many programs, especially at graduate and professional levels, do not offer systematic instruction in writing,[4,22,59] expecting students to "sink or swim."[60(p109)] As Sasson et al. lamented, it is still common for trainees (in radiology, specifically) to receive little if any writing instruction, even though they are expected to participate actively in research and publication.[60] An underlying assumption may be that trainees will master unfamiliar genres quickly or that they will learn to write somewhere else.

No question, there are health professions educators who teach writing with considerable skill and effectiveness. Some hold degrees in writing-intensive fields, such as literature, communications, or journalism. Yet many have had little experience or training in writing instruction,[59,61-65] considering it an "afterthought" or an "unwelcome challenge."[66] Some struggle to design effective assignments,[7,8] supervise writers,[67] or return constructive feedback, focusing excessively on grammar, mechanics, citation styles, and "thou shalt nots."[22,68] A common concern is the time needed to teach writing.[58,68,69] Subsequently, health professions educators may defer to writing specialists. True, instructors from the humanities, composition studies, technical communication, library science, and adjacent fields have long played roles in health professions training.[e.g., 48,52] These writing specialists do good work, though their knowledge of students' course content and chosen specialty is typically limited. Students often prefer to receive feedback from health professions educators as well, as they are the gatekeepers of the discipline, have subject matter expertise, and will be the ones assigning a grade.[68]

Entering their programs with varying levels of preparedness, students and trainees may already feel jaded toward writing based on their past experiences. They may initially question the value of writing, unaware of its benefits in learning and in their future careers.[69] They may fear that no matter what they write, their instructors will "tear it apart."[70(p1350)] At any level, students and trainees (as well as faculty) may struggle with writing because of its cognitive, linguistic, and sociolinguistic demands.[6] For instance, they may struggle to articulate a clear position, support their reasoning with persuasive evidence, evaluate the quality of a source, or maintain an appropriate tone.[6] They may also need to write in a diversity of voices. As one scholar put it, "So pity the poor nursing student, who is required to write at times like a sociologist, at others like a philosopher, yet again like a scientist and finally as a reflective practitioner!"[71(p188)] Completing the circle, some students and trainees will one day serve as faculty members, when they will be expected to publish[72,73] and, potentially, even teach writing themselves. They will need to be prepared.[63]

Barriers like these can be significant indeed, and numerous handbooks have been written for health professions students and trainees. For teachers, instructional knowledge tends to be shared in a highly segmented way, scattered across scholarly journals and course syllabi. There are surprisingly few accessible "middle-range" resources to support health professions educators who want to improve how they teach writing, writing specialists who want to better understand health professions training, and others seeking professional development and a broader community of colleagues. To be sure, surveys of faculty development needs in the health professions have recurrently stressed writing and teaching,[74–76] and calls have sounded for the creation of additional resources.[e.g., 77,78]

Why This Collection?

As a step forward, we consider "writing in the health professions" not only as a set of program- and industry-specific practices but also as an emergent interdiscipline: a growing body of knowledge and professional connections that cut across disciplines. Current trends suggest that writing in the health professions, as an emergent interdiscipline, is expanding steadily and becoming more visible: studies on the writing done by health professionals appear in many scholarly venues, including those dedicated to the humanities, applied linguistics, technical communication, health communication, rhetoric, composition studies, and education, among other fields. Health-care discourse is being (re) emphasized in professional organizations, among them the Society for Technical Communication,[79] in addition to the accrediting agencies over health professions training. In the field of writing studies, job advertisements have regularly requested candidates who can teach medical writing, the rhetoric of health and medicine, and other practices intertwined with writing in the health professions. Since some of the first were established at the University of Toronto[80] and the Medical University of South Carolina,[81,82] the number of writing centers dedicated to the health professions has risen significantly.

These trends are promising, and it seems clear that many instructors and scholars are working in this emergent interdiscipline already. Yet we need ongoing dialogue to both deepen and broaden our instructional efforts.

This edited collection, therefore, has a twofold purpose:

First, to strengthen "writing in the health professions" practically, sharing evidence-based instructional practices from academic, clinical, and community settings. This first purpose invokes the long tradition of promoting faculty development through exemplary models.

Second, to advance "writing in the health professions" conceptually, exploring how this emergent interdiscipline does—or can—draw on social psychology, writing across the curriculum, writing in the disciplines, literacy studies, sociocultural theory, ethnography, graphic medicine, and related scholarly discourses.

The collection was compiled in the spirit of interprofessional education, a robust movement in the health professions internationally. According to Bridges and colleagues, interprofessional education involves members of different professions "learning with, from, and about each other."[83(p2)] The intended result is to share knowledge and skills, as well as to strengthen mutual understanding, shared values, and respect.[83] In the long term, we hope to foster a "culture of solidarity" across fields, encouraging "consistent writing support and a collective message of the significance of good writing."[84(p195)]

This is not to minimize the importance of disciplinary approaches to writing instruction.[6,78,85] Health professionals need to learn the genres deployed in their workplaces and training programs, and scholarship has cast serious doubt on the effectiveness of overly general writing pedagogy. Still, we maintain that instructors from different disciplines can learn with, from, and about each other, and interdisciplinary collaboration is already common. Furthermore, many health professions have not yet established their own lines of scholarship on teaching writing, and it would be hasty to assume that findings from other traditions cannot be tested and adapted in new contexts. Nursing scholarship on writing, in particular, exemplifies the power of cross-field synergies. We, therefore, encourage readers to approach the teaching of writing from both angles: *inter*professionally and *intra*professionally.

How This Collection Is Organized

In the collection, the four parts are generally divided by health profession, with the chapters arranged from lower to higher educational levels. In other cases, they are arranged in an order intended to instill a sense of progression or conceptual unity.

The first part is *writing in medicine and public health*. In Chapter 1, Sarah Yonder shares how she teaches clinical notes to pre-clerkship medical students, drawing on expectancy-value theory and colleague assessments. In Chapter 2, Elizabeth Narváez-Cardona and Pilar Mirely Chois-Lenis parse the literacy expectations in two health professions programs (a master's degree in public health and a specialization in pediatrics), grounding their mixed methods in sociocultural theory. Rebecca Day Babcock and her colleagues, in Chapter 3, present findings from a broad survey of medical writing, foregrounding influences from the "fourth industrial revolution" and language globalization.

The second part is *writing in nursing*. In Chapter 4, Barbara J. D'Angelo and Barry M. Maid trace how they (re)designed a course for an online RN to BSN program, emphasizing the value of institutional ethnography. In Chapter 5, Lillian Campbell explores how "intermediary genres" can help nursing students connect classroom and clinical experiences, sharing data from interviews and classroom observations. In Chapter 6, Sarah Kosel Agnihotri and her colleagues describe how they "semi-embedded" writing tutors in an online course for master's students, navigating unanticipated challenges from the COVID-19 global pandemic. Deborah E. Tyndall, in Chapter 7, illustrates how she has applied "threshold concepts" to guide doctoral students through a particularly difficult genre: the literature review. Selecting from five years of data, she shares insights from students' reflective writings.

The third part is *writing in allied health and pharmacy*. In Chapter 8, Elizabeth L. Angeli summarizes her ongoing curriculum development efforts for emergency medical and fire services, synthesizing several years of ethnographic data. In Chapter 9, Isabell C. May and Emilie M. Ludeman describe how they improved an online course for physician assistant students, blending graduate writing instruction with information literacy and online learning. In Chapter 10, Janine Morris and her colleagues detail a partnership between a college of pharmacy and a writing center, which generated workshops to support the existing curriculum.

The fourth part, perhaps the most eclectic, is *writing in interprofessional contexts*. In Chapter 11, Cristina Reyes Smith explains how she has incorporated reflective writing in an elective course on culturally sensitive care, which she teaches at an academic health sciences center. In Chapter 12, Susan E. Thomas investigates patient-centered care at a cancer treatment center in Australia and provides a detailed analysis of communication practices that she has reshaped for case-based learning. In Chapter 13, Kathryn West and Brian Callender, an interprofessional teaching team, illustrate graphic medicine workshops that they created for patients and health professionals, viewing their work through an autoethnographic lens. Finally, in Chapter 14, Lucy M. Candib and her colleagues reflect on their teacherless writing group that, at various points, has included not only family physicians and a medical geneticist but also professionals in behavioral health, social work, and pharmacy.

The 34 contributors, who represent a range of health professions, thus capture a rich diversity of instructional contexts, strategies, and needs. Yet readers should also notice conceptual and methodological confluences that create streams of internal dialogue within the collection. I have marked some of these confluences with cross-references, referring readers to corresponding chapters.

While they were drafting, I asked the contributors to follow several guidelines: each chapter should be 5,000 to 7,000 words in length, cite peer-reviewed literature related to "writing in the health professions," be grounded in empirical data of some kind, propose practical takeaways for instructors or administrators, and use as much nonspecialist language as possible. That last guideline was a challenge for us all, as disciplinary knowledge is often bound up in disciplinary language. Even so, we hope readers across fields will find the collection accessible.

References

1. World Health Organization. *Global Strategy on Human Resources for Health: Workforce 2030*. Geneva, Switzerland: World Health Organization; 2016. https://www.who.int/hrh/resources/global_strategy_workforce2030_14_print.pdf. Accessed April 14, 2021.
2. World Health Organization. *State of the World's Nursing 2020: Investing in Education, Jobs and Leadership*. Geneva, Switzerland: World Health Organization; 2020: https://www.who.int/publications-detail/nursing-report-2020. Accessed April 14, 2021.
3. World Health Organization. *Year of Health and Care Workers 2021*. World Health Organization. https://www.who.int/campaigns/annual-theme/year-of-health-and-care-workers-2021. Published 2021. Accessed April 14, 2021.
4. Yanoff KL, Burg FD. Types of medical writing and teaching of writing in US medical schools. *J Med Educ*. 1988;63(1):30–37.
5. Graves R. Writing assignments across five academic programs. In: Graves R., Hyland T, eds. *Writing Assignments across University Disciplines*. Bloomington, IN: Trafford Publishing; 2017: 1–30.
6. Gimenez J. Beyond the academic essay: discipline-specific writing in nursing and midwifery. *J English Acad Purp*. 2008;7(3):151–164.
7. Hobson EH, Waite NM, Briceland LL. Writing tasks performed by doctor of pharmacy students during clerkship rotations. *Am J Health Syst Pharm*. 2002;59(1):58–62.
8. August E, Burke K, Fleischer C, Trostle JA. Writing assignments in epidemiology courses: how many and how good?. *Public Health Rep*. 2019;134(4):441–446.
9. Mackenzie SL. Writing for public health: strategies for teaching writing in a school or program of public health. *Public Health Rep*. 2018;133(5):614–618.
10. Opel DS, Hart-Davidson W. The primary care clinic as writing space. *Written Commun*. 2019;36(3):348–378.
11. Cruess RL, Cruess SR, Boudreau JD, Snell L, Steinert Y. Reframing medical education to support professional identity formation. *Acad Med*. 2014;89(11):1446–1451.
12. Chen I, Forbes C. Reflective writing and its impact on empathy in medical education: systematic review. *J Educ Eval Health Prof*. 2014;11:20.
13. Lemay M, Encandela J, Sanders L, Reisman A. Writing well: the long-term effect on empathy, observa-

tion, and physician writing through a residency writers' workshop. *J. Grad. Med. Educ.* 2017;9(3):357.

14. Deen SR, Mangurian C, Cabaniss DL. Points of contact: using first-person narratives to help foster empathy in psychiatric residents. *Acad. Psychiatry.* 2010;34(6):438–441.

15. Tsingos C, Bosnic-Anticevich S, Smith L. Reflective practice and its implications for pharmacy education. *Am J Pharm Educ.* 2014;78(1). Article 18.

16. Schoonover KL, Hall-Flavin D, Whitford K, Lussier M, Essary A, Lapid MI. Impact of poetry on empathy and professional burnout of health-care workers: a systematic review. *J Palliat Care.* 2020;35(2):127–132.

17. Charon R. Narrative medicine: a model for empathy, reflection, profession, and trust. *JAMA.* 2001;286(15):1897–1902.

18. Sahoo S, Mohammed CA. Fostering critical thinking and collaborative learning skills among medical students through a research protocol writing activity in the curriculum. *Korean J Med Educ.* 2018;30(2):109–118.

19. Woldt JL, Nenad MW. Reflective writing in dental education to improve critical thinking and learning: a systematic review. *J Dent Educ.* 2021. doi.:10.1002/jdd.12561.

20. McMichael MA, Ferguson DC, Allender MC, Cope W, Kalantzis M, Haniya S, Searsmith D, Montebello M. Use of a multimodal, peer-to-peer learning management system for introduction of critical clinical thinking to first-year veterinary students. *J Vet Med Educ.* 2021;11:e20190029.

21. Lundgren SM, Halvarsson M. Students' expectations, concerns and comprehensions when writing theses as part of their nursing education. *Nurse Educ Today.* 2009;29(5):527–532.

22. Aguayo-González M, Leyva-Moral JM, San Rafael S, Fernandez MI, Gómez-Ibáñez R. Graduated nurses' experiences with baccalaureate thesis writing: a qualitative study. *Nurs Health Sci.* 2020;22(3):563–569.

23. Tyndall DE, Forbes III TH, Avery JJ, Powell SB. Fostering scholarship in doctoral education: using a social capital framework to support PhD student writing groups. *J Prof Nurs.* 2019;35(4):300–304.

24. Poirrier GP. *Writing-to-Learn: Curricular Strategies for Nursing and Other Disciplines.* New York, NY: Jones & Bartlett Learning; 1997.

25. Brown EA, White BM, Gregory A. Approaches to teaching social determinants of health to undergraduate health care students. *J. Allied Health.* 2021;50(1):31E–36E.

26. Steinhardt SJ, Kelly WN, Clark JE, Hill AM. An artistic active-learning approach to teaching a substance use disorder elective course. *Am J Pharm Educ.* 2020;84(4):498–503.

27. Ness SM. Reflections on writing an engaging patient blog. *J of Cancer Educ.* 2017;32(4):933–934.

28. Stucky CH. Advancing nursing leadership through writing: strategies for publishing success. *J Contin Educ Nurs.* 2020;51(10):447–449.

29. Quaye B, Weismuller P. Nurse leader stories reveal themes in US and Cuban cross-cultural experience. *Nurse Lead.* 2018;16(5):308–314.

30. Kripalani S, Bussey-Jones J, Katz MG, Genao I. A prescription for cultural competence in medical education. *J Gen Intern Med.* 2006;21(10):1116–1120.

31. Poirier TI, Butler LM, Devraj R, Gupchup GV, Santanello C, Lynch JC. A cultural competency course for pharmacy students. *Am J Pharm Educ.* 2009;73(5):Article 81.

32. Sanchez N, Norka A, Corbin M, Peters C. Use of experiential learning, reflective writing, and metacognition to develop cultural humility among undergraduate students. *J Soc. Work Educ.* 2019;55(1):75–88.

33. Cowen VS, Kaufman D, Schoenherr L. A review of creative and expressive writing as a pedagogical tool in medical education. *Med Educ.* 2016;50(3):311–319.

34. Christensen N, Black L, Furze J, Huhn K, Vendrely A, Wainwright S. Clinical reasoning: survey of teaching methods, integration, and assessment in entry-level physical therapist academic education. *Phys Ther.* 2017;97(2):175–186.

35. Smith T. Guided reflective writing as a teaching strategy to develop nursing student clinical judgment. *Nurs Forum.* 2020;2020:1–8. doi: 10.1111/nuf.12528.

36. Anderson OS, August E. The Real-World Writing Project for public health students: a description and evaluation. *Pedagogy Health Promot.* 2020:doi: 10.1177/2373379920928094.

37. Wald HS, Haramati A, Bachner YG, Urkin J. Promoting resiliency for interprofessional faculty and senior medical students: outcomes of a workshop using mind-body medicine and interactive reflective writing. *Med Teach.* 2016;38(5):525–528.

38. Winkel AF, Feldman N, Moss H, Jakalow H, Simon J, Blank S. Narrative medicine workshops for obstetrics and gynecology residents and association with burnout measures. *Obstet Gynecol.* 2016;128:27S–33S.

39. Council on Social Work Education. *Educational Policy and Accreditation Standards for Baccalaureate and Master's Social Work Programs.* Council on Social Work Education; 2015. https://www.cswe.org/getattachment/Accreditation/Accreditation-Process/2015-EPAS/2015EPAS_Web_FINAL.pdf.aspx. Accessed April 15, 2021.

40. American Veterinary Medical Association. *Accreditation Policies and Procedures of the AVMA Council on Education.* American Veterinary Medical Association; 2020. https://www.avma.org/sites/default/files/2021-02/coe_pp.pdf. Accessed April 15, 2021.

41. Association of Faculties of Pharmacy of Canada. *Educational Outcomes for First Professional Degree Programs in Pharmacy in Canada.* Association of Faculties of Pharmacy of Canada; 2017. https://www.afpc.info/system/files/public/AFPC-Educational%20Outcomes%202017_final%20Jun2017.pdf. Accessed April 15, 2021.

42. Accreditation Council for Pharmacy Education. *Accreditation Standards and Key Elements for the Professional Program in Pharmacy Leading to the Doctor of Pharmacy Degree.* Canada: Accreditation Council for Pharmacy Education; 2015. https://www.acpe-accredit.org/pdf/Standards2016FINAL.pdf. Accessed April 15, 2021.

43. Council on Education for Public Health. *Accreditation Criteria: Schools of Public Health & Public Health Programs.* Canada: Council on Education for Public Health; 2016. https://media.ceph.org/wp_assets/2016.Criteria.pdf. Accessed April 15, 2021.

44. General Medical Council. *Outcomes 2- Professional Skills.* United Kingdon: General Medical Council; 2019. https://www.gmc-uk.org/education/standards-guidance-and-curricula/standards-and-outcomes/outcomes-for-graduates/outcomes-for-graduates/outcomes-2---professional-skills. Accessed April 15, 2021.

45. American Association of Colleges of Nursing. *The Essentials of Baccalaureate Education for Professional Nursing Practice.* American Association of Colleges of Nursing; October 20, 2008. https://www.aacnnursing.org/Portals/42/Publications/BaccEssentials08.pdf. Accessed April 15, 2021.

46. American Association of Colleges of Nursing. *The Essentials of Master's Education in Nursing.* American Association of Colleges of Nursing; 2011. https://www.aacnnursing.org/Portals/42/Publications/MastersEssentials11.pdf. Accessed April 15, 2021.

47. American Association of Colleges of Nursing. *The Essentials of Doctoral Education for Advanced Nursing Practice.* American Association of Colleges of Nursing. https://www.aacnnursing.org/Portals/42/Publications/DNPEssentials.pdf. Accessed April 15, 2021.

48. Bett WR. Desirability and methods of teaching medical writing to senior medical students. *Miss Valley Med J.* 1954;76(1):24–26.

49. Carr CJ. The teaching of prescription writing in medical schools. *J Assoc Am Med Coll.* 1941;16(1):42–44.

50. Hines LE. The use of a large clinic to teach history writing to the sophomore students. *J Assoc Am Med Coll.* 1944;19(4):229–230.

51. McHenry L. Medical writing as seen by an undergraduate medical student. *Miss Valley Med J.* 1954;76(1):41–42.

52. Zisowitz ML. Teaching medical students and physicians to write. *J Med Educ.* 1964;39(5):481–484.

53. DeBakey L. Instruction in scientific communications. *J Med Educ.* 1965;40(10):928–930.

54. Froelich RE, Kimpton RS. An experience in improving medical writing: a staff and student workshop-seminar. *Mo Med.* 1967;64(4):325–327.

55. Barloon MJ. How to teach students to write clearly in courses other than English. *J Med Educ.* 1954;29(3):30–34.

56. Craig J. Essay-writing as a teaching technique. *Lancet.* 1955;266(6887):420–421.

57. Oermann MH, Leonardelli AK, Turner KM, Hawks SJ, Derouin AL, Hueckel RM. Systematic review of educational programs and strategies for developing students' and nurses' writing skills. *J Nurs Educ.* 2015;54(1):28–34.

58. Luthy KE, Peterson NE, Lassetter JH, Callister LC. Successfully incorporating writing across the curriculum with advanced writing in nursing. *J Nurs Educ.* 2009;48(1):54–59.

59. Marušic A, Marušic M. Teaching students how to read and write science: a mandatory course on scientific research and communication in medicine. *Acad Med.* 2003;78(12):1235–1239.

60. Sasson A, Okojie O, Verano R, Moshiri M, Patlas MN, Hoffmann JC, Hines JJ, Katz DS. How to read, write, and review the imaging literature. *Curr Probl Diagn Radiol.* 2020;50(2):109–114.

61. Hegmann TE, Axelson RD. Benchmarking the scholarly productivity of physician assistant educators: an update. *J Physician Assist Educ.* 2012;23(2):16–23.

62. Lang TA. Who me? Ideas for faculty who never expected to be teaching public health students to write. *Public Health Rep.* 2019;134(2):206–214.

63. Jackson A. The scholarship of writing. *Nurse Educ.* 2016;41(5):238.

64. Troxler H, Vann JC, Oermann MH. How baccalaureate nursing programs teach writing. *Nurs Forum.* 2011; 46(4):280–288.

65. Whitehead D. The academic writing experiences of a group of student nurses: a phenomenological study. *J Adv Nurs.* 2002;38(5):498–506.

66. Mandleco BL, Bohn C, Callister LC, Lassetter J, Carlton T. Integrating advanced writing content into a scholarly inquiry in nursing course. *Int J Nurs Educ Scholarsh.* 2012;9(1). Article 4.

67. Friberg F, Lyckhage ED. Changing essay writing in undergraduate nursing education through action research: a Swedish example. *Nurs Educ Perspect.* 2013;34(4):226–232.

68. Mitchell KM. Constructing writing practices in nursing. *J of Nurs Educ.* 2018;57(7):399–407.

69. Mitchell KM, McMillan DE, Lobchuk MM, Nickel NC. Writing activities and the hidden curriculum in nursing education. *Nurs Inq.* 2021;26:e12407.

70. Diekelmann N, Magnussen Ironside P. Preserving writing in doctoral education: exploring the concernful practices of schooling learning teaching. *J Adv Nurs.* 1998;28(6):1347–1355.

71. Baynham M. Academic writing in new and emergent discipline areas. In: Clarke J, Hanson A, Harrison R, Reeve F, eds. *Supporting Lifelong Learning: Volume I: Perspectives on Learning.* Routledge; 2001: 188–202.

72. Kumar DV. The oppressive pressure to publish. *Indian J Med Ethics.* 2018;3:344–345.

73. Pololi L, Knight S, Dunn K. Facilitating scholarly writing in academic medicine. *J Gen Intern Med.* 2004;19(1):64–68.

74. Haden NK, Chaddock M, Hoffsis GF, Lloyd JW, Reed WM, Ranney RR, Weinstein GJ. Preparing faculty for the future: AAVMC members' perceptions of professional development needs. *J Vet Med Educ.* 2010;37(3):220–232.

75. Smith A, Hardinger K. Perceptions of faculty development needs based on faculty characteristics. *Curr Pharm Teach Learn.* 2012;4(4):232–239.

76. Behar-Horenstein LS, Beck DE, Su Y. Perceptions of pharmacy faculty need for development in educational research. *Curr Pharm Teach Learn.* 2018;10(1):34–40.

77. Riley E. Exploring strategies to enhance scholarly writing for RN-BSN students using an online tutorial. *Teach Learn Nurs.* 2019;14(2):128–134.

78. Hawks SJ, Turner KM, Derouin AL, Hueckel RM, Leonardelli AK, Oermann MH. Writing across the curriculum: strategies to improve the writing skills of nursing students. *Nurs Forum.* 2016; 51(4): 261–267.

79. STC health and medicine SIG. *Society for Technical Communication.* https://www.stchealthmed.org/. Accessed April 16, 2021.

80. University of Toronto Health Sciences Writing Centre. *Welcome to the Health Sciences Writing Center: We Are Celebrating 25 Years of the Health Sciences Writing Centre!* University of Toronto Health Sciences Writing Centre. https://www.hswriting.ca/ Accessed April 16, 2021.

81. Smith TG, Ariail J, Richards-Slaughter S, Kerr L. Teaching professional writing in an academic health sciences center: the writing center model at the Medical University of South Carolina. *Teach Learn Med.* 2011;23(3):298–300.

82. Ariail J, Thomas S, Smith T, Kerr L, Richards-Slaughter S, Shaw D. The value of a writing center at a medical university. *Teach Learn Med.* 2013;25(2):129–133.

83. Bridges D, Davidson RA, Soule Odegard P, Maki IV, Tomkowiak J. Interprofessional collaboration: three best practice models of interprofessional education. *Med Educ Online.* 2011;16(1):6035. doi:10.3402/meo.v16i0.6035.

84. Capous-Desyllas M, Bromfield NF, Nava A, Barnes B. Teaching note—strategies for enhancing writing among first-generation social work students: reflections on the use of peer writing mentors. *J Soc Work Educ.* 2021;57(1):189–196.

85. Rawson RE, Quinlan KM, Cooper BJ, Fewtrell C, Matlow JR. Writing-skills development in the health professions. *Teach Learn Med.* 2005;17(3):233–238.

PART I

Writing in Medicine and Public Health

1

TEACHING MEDICAL STUDENTS TO WRITE PROPER CLINICAL NOTES USING EXPECTANCY-VALUE THEORY

Sarah Yonder

Teaching clinical skills to pre-clerkship medical students is both rewarding and challenging. Students are excited to learn history taking and physical exams as they begin to feel more like doctors in training. It is surprising, though, how often students are taken aback by the extent of writing involved. After one of my teaching sessions, a student remarked, "I did not realize how much writing there is in medicine." This statement was a wake-up call, motivating me to emphasize the importance of good writing.

The clinical note assignments and debriefs in my two-year clinical skills course illustrate how writing, especially quality writing, is essential to medicine. Even in the era of electronic medical records (EMRs), if you cannot write well, your notes will not translate to a good clinical record. Many students have an ill-conceived notion that they can just click boxes and copy and paste. Yet typing or recording notes in EMRs still requires all parts of basic organization, including subjective, objective, assessment, and plan. Free text and comment boxes allow clinicians to clinically reason, describing, supporting, refuting, and creating a plan to manage patients, in addition to clicking boxes. I believe that more focus needs to be placed on this important form of "writing in the health professions" early in training, helping students meet the communication standards set by medical education organizations.[1,2] But how can clinical notes be taught effectively?

In this chapter, I look at some of the literature about note-writing instruction for pre-clerkship medical students. Next, I outline how I use expectancy-value theory to help students see how integral writing is to the medical profession, with examples of how to put it into practice. Results from a small peer review of student notes produced from this approach will be shared, as well as some practical takeaways.

Literature Review

While not historically known for its focus on writing, undergraduate medical education (the time when students are in medical school rather than, say, a residency or fellowship) has incorporated more writing instruction into the curriculum recently. Courses have focused on reflective writing, narrative medicine, and health humanities, but not typically the quality of clinical notes.[3,4] While preparing this chapter, I found more literature on clinical note instruction aimed at clerkship or transition to clerkship training, rather than pre-clerkship training—the first two years. Yet there may be numerous advantages to honing this skill earlier in a medical student's training, such as making

DOI: 10.4324/9781003162940-3

students aware that well-written notes support good patient care and that the health-care team relies on quality notes to function effectively. Consequently, this skill is something students need throughout their careers, not just in training.

Medical school faculty teach note writing in multiple ways to first- and second-year medical students. Many draw from what they learned and practice, as well as rely on medical textbooks that outline the basic clinical note, combined with how to begin to elicit patient history.[5] There have also been more creative approaches to teaching clinical notes. One approach I found involved a faculty-created student guide, a videotaped clinical encounter, a sample write-up, and a faculty grading rubric. In a writing workshop, students first viewed the encounter and then created a note. Afterward, a group session was held with faculty to assist with editing the notes to enhance the quality.[6]

Another approach involved pre-clerkship and clerkship students volunteering at a free clinic. The students were able to practice many aspects of patient care, including clinical note documentation. All work, including note documentation, was reviewed and signed off by a clinical attending.[7]

In my review, I also found authors describing the use of templates to teach clinical note writing. However, I found more usage of templates in clerkship and residency training than in undergraduate medical education.[8,9]

Expectancy-Value Framework for Teaching Clinical Notes

Being unable to find a model or framework specifically used to instruct first- and second-year students about the basics of clinical note writing, I have developed my own over the years. The framework that I use involves expectancy-value theory.

Expectancy-value theory has been studied at various instructional levels, from the past decades into recent times.[10–12] The theory has been shown to be effective in the field of education, as well as other fields, including economics, marketing, and communication. In medical education, similar theories of motivation, notably expectancy theory, have been applied to improve residency training.[13] It does not seem unreasonable, then, to look at expectancy-value theory in the context of undergraduate medical education.

Broadly, expectancy-value theory holds that doing well on a task is affected by two key factors: a person's feeling of (1) the value they place on the task and (2) how well they can perform it. Thus, in order for future physicians to understand the value of well-written notes, instructors should demonstrate that good note-writing skills are important in medical practice. In addition, we must give learners confidence that they have the knowledge and skills to be successful.[14]

The two aforementioned key factors are not unrelated. Expectancy-value theory supports that if one *values* a task (such as well-written clinical notes), one will *want* to perform well on this task. Thus, pre-clerkship medical students should understand the potential impact of their notes. For example, notes not only influence patient care but also the patients' own understanding of personal health matters.[15] Moreover, if we are not writing well in the record, there may be financial consequences. If notes contain an incomplete history of present illness (HPI) or exam findings, or if plans and patient instructions are missing or not well clarified, they can affect billing and reimbursement.[16] Students do not always appreciate this early on. However, as they progress, they will see for themselves the effects of their documentation, especially in residency training and afterward. Instructors should therefore stress the importance of writing in students' future practice, as well as their own, using real-world examples. In short, there is value in a quality note, and that is what we are trying to convey in our process of teaching and learning.

To build students' confidence in writing clinical notes, instructors can utilize templates, which help students manage the complexity of the task, including idea development and organization. Over time, as instructors "take off the training wheels," students become more independent with the writing, determining what goes where, as well as the amount of information needed to tell the patient's story in an effective, clinically relevant manner. Along the way, faculty debriefing and review of student work, similar to the approaches mentioned earlier, can be very helpful.

Again, the two key factors in this learning process, according to expectancy-value theory, are demonstrating that good note-writing skills are important to quality patient care and giving learners confidence that they have the knowledge and skills to be successful. (An interesting cross-reference, Chapter 6 also explores how students' perceptions of value influence their behavior, focusing on a writing center and master's program in nursing.)

How We Put It into Practice

I teach a longitudinal, clinical skills course to the first- and second-year pre-clerkship medical students at an allopathic medical school. There are approximately 104 students enrolled in all courses for their specified year. Our course begins with the basics of patient history taking and communication skills. Then we build by introducing exam skills for different organ systems. With the time and emphasis placed on writing, our summative course exams ask students to both read/interpret notes and compose sections of notes on their own.

Our course integrates with students' other courses, so they take a foundations course when I teach the basic history taking and communications. Then I begin to focus on exam skills, complementing the organ system courses students take after they complete their foundations course.

Over our two-year course, we include a broad introduction to different note categories that students will encounter over their training and career. For example, the daily progress note details the story of the patient's inpatient stay or outpatient course over months and years and continuity of care from one provider to another if care is taken over or shared among providers. If the patient's usual provider is absent, a colleague should be able to read a chart note and get a good sense of how the patient was doing when last seen, what test results showed, and how management of the condition is progressing. Referrals to specialists share just what is going on and why a provider needs the specialist to see a patient. Admitting notes in a hospital need to be easy to get through during a busy shift but also detailed, giving a full picture as to why the patient was admitted, as well as what plans are in place. Likewise, a discharge note weaves together the entire hospital course, which should give the reader a sound understanding of the patient's care, outcomes, and plans going forward. This broad introduction demonstrates the value of a well-written note and impresses its importance upon students, who hopefully want to produce quality notes of their own, aligning with expectancy-value theory.

From the beginning of the first semester, the course incorporates standardized patient (SP) sessions as part of students' learning. SPs are people trained to interact with students, taking on the role of a patient in a clinical encounter. This allows students to practice skills, as well as be assessed on their performance.[17]

When students finish an SP session, we debrief the case and explain how the elicited information can develop into a note. Students are responsible for submitting a clinical note assignment for every SP session. Having faculty with clinical experience helps us bring the everyday work of clinical writing to life. The main faculty in the course, a part-time colleague and I, are both physicians and draw multiple examples from practice to highlight how integral writing is to our daily work.

Also important in our teaching is keeping the focus on the patient, and with time, helping students create notes that are easier to read and comprehend.[18] To guide students, we utilize the SOAP note template (see Appendix 1), which is commonly utilized in medicine and allied health. The SOAP note was developed by Dr. Lawrence Weed, professor of medicine and pharmacology at Yale University.[19,20]

SOAP stands for subjective, objective, assessment, and plan,[21,22] providing a basic organization for a clinical note. However, general variations have also been suggested over the years,[21,22] and there can be adaptations to the SOAP note depending on the needs of the specific user. In this chapter, I focus on the template's basic utility to help pre-clerkship students organize clinical information. (For additional perspectives on SOAP notes, see Chapters 5 and 8.) It may appear simple to teach a clinical note and follow the main organization. However, organizing and plugging in the information does not necessarily make the note well written.[18]

I use the word "practice" often in my two-year clinical skills course. If asked, students may say I am quite repetitive with its use, not only for physical exam skills but also for note writing. As I often tell students, if you do not practice a skill, you will not improve. Just as a musician or athlete must practice, so too must future physicians.[23]

Let me share more about how our course unfolds, semester by semester.

Year 1, Semester 1

As suggested earlier, we begin with teaching how to elicit a patient's medical history, which is a comprehensive recording; it covers everything from present concern to already diagnosed medical conditions, surgeries, medications, and allergies, as well as family and social history.

The patient's medical history is written in the subjective area of the SOAP note template, which we break down into several sections. The first of those sections is the chief concern and HPI. Unlike most other parts of a clinical note, the HPI is often written out in a paragraph. A well-written paragraph is important because it provides a thorough record, including details of the chief concerns, and supports development of the differential diagnoses. It also will help students to develop an oral presentation of the case. In our class, we begin listing the elements of the HPI, but within 3 to 4 weeks, we require the students to write out these elements in paragraph form. It takes one set of skills to obtain and list the proper information. It takes another set of skills to sew the details of the HPI material together and create a well-constructed narrative.[5,8,21,24]

Students are next taught to obtain the past medical history, which includes any diagnosed medical conditions and medications (prescription and over-the-counter), as well as allergies to medications, food, indoor and outdoor allergens, and other agents. Following are the surgical history and hospitalizations, as well as health maintenance items, such as a patient's current vaccine status and health screening tests he/she has had. The next sections are family history and social history, including sexual health history. A full history in these sections includes the record of three generations of family members, including their ages and health conditions. Social history encompasses occupation, past and current; alcohol, tobacco/vaping, and illicit drug use, past and current; exposures to occupational hazards; and education level achieved, to name just some of the information gathered.[5,8,21,24] Even from this early time of collecting and recording information, we emphasize the importance of comprehensively writing out the history since others will rely on this written record.

As we teach more of the clinical note, we add on sections, including the objective or physical exam, the assessment, and the plan. We thereby create a more complete note, having students practice this note-building so that they feel more comfortable and confident in their skills. In line with expectancy-value theory, giving students the sense they can write notes well can increase their desire to perform well on this task.

Year 1, Semester 2

As we move into organ systems, which begins in the second semester of the first year, we teach physical exam skills for each system. This involves hands-on skill sessions where faculty and the SP team demonstrate exam skills to students, which students then perform under our observation. Students are expected to add their exam findings to the notes under the objective section.[5,8,21,24] For example, in the cardiopulmonary organ system, they learn to inspect, percuss, and auscultate the posterior, lateral, and anterior chest. They have SP sessions that involve a focused history and a focused exam. Their exam findings then need to be documented in their notes for that session.

Even when students write the objective section, faculty stress well-composed findings. Using the term "normal" is discouraged, as we want new learners to describe what they do or do not observe. For example, stating that a patient's throat exam is normal is not correct. Rather, students should state that a patient's throat is without erythema or inflammation. If the throat is red or erythematous, adding a description such as "posterior pharynx is erythematous with tonsils +1 and exudates present bilaterally" can give readers a clearer understanding.

We also teach students that well-written descriptions can help capture findings that vary from day to day. Imagine that a rash is noted one day as "erythematous streaks on right anterior forearm measuring 8 cm," and treatment is given. The provider who sees the patient in the next few days will have an idea of how the initial concern presented, and they can record how it has changed. For example, "right anterior forearm with fading erythematous streaks, measuring 4 cm."

Again, all SP sessions in the course are followed by debrief sessions with clinical faculty. In these sessions, students are expected to discuss the information they elicited, as well as exam findings. Faculty assist with the note development, and this offers a great opportunity to emphasize eloquent and organized writing. These sessions also allow us to share real-world clinical examples.

Clinical examples are brought in, first and foremost, to drive home the point that good note writing really does translate into quality patient care.[25] In class, we have stressed that not only does the provider writing the note need it as a reference but also other physicians and health-care professionals will use it to provide follow-up care, including referrals to specialists. For example, we need to give specialists a detailed reason why we are sending the patient to them.

Moreover, for years, we have seen how poorly written clinical documentation can contribute to medical errors.[16,26,27] Given the intricacies of health-care systems, as well as human errors, the breakdown of communication has resulted in putting patients at unintended risk and causing harm.[28] Students often comment in our course evaluation that they appreciate the clinical relevance we bring to the sessions.

Next is the assessment section, which follows the objective exam findings. This section is where diagnoses are listed, including the acute or presenting concern, followed by a list of possible diagnoses or differentials.[5,8,21,24] The patient's previously confirmed chronic diagnoses are also listed here. Potential diagnoses for the presenting health concern are listed with supporting or refuting data from the history (subjective) and physical (objective) sections in order of the most likely. This section also calls for quality writing to strengthen the argument for or against diagnoses listed. We look at our history and exam findings to point us to a diagnosis, but assessment needs to be put together in a succinct and well-crafted manner. The student's clinical reasoning comes out in this section, so the better it is written, the better their reasoning can be translated to readers.

The assessment section often starts with a summary statement before the possible diagnoses are listed. The summary statement ties key history and exam findings together to lay the foundation for, hopefully, a great presentation of the differential diagnoses. If poorly put together, the "train goes off the tracks." For example, if we have ascertained through history and exam findings that the patient is a "42-year-old female smoker with asthma presenting with a cough for 5 days, and on exam was found to be febrile with expiratory wheezes noted in her right upper lung field," these pertinent items should go in the statement. The student needs to take all the findings elicited and develop a sentence that highlights the most important aspects, setting up a potential diagnosis. This, like other components of the note, takes practice. Clinical reasoning takes practice as well. Thus, in our course, we marry good writing with clinical reasoning to really capture the patient's problem in this section.

An example of the differential diagnoses following the previous summary statement could be as follows:

4-year-old female asthmatic smoker presenting with a cough for 5 days, on exam found to be febrile with expiratory wheezes noted in her right upper lung field, most consistent with the following:

1) *Asthma exacerbation with upper respiratory infection (URI)*
2) *Bronchitis*
3) *Pneumonia*

From here, the student needs to describe pertinent material from the history and exam that support and/or refute each diagnosis presented. For asthma exacerbation with URI, support data may be written as "the patient's presenting history of cough, asthma, and tobacco use supports this diagnosis." There may be other factors in the HPI (not listed previously) that could be used, including, "other evidence supporting the diagnosis include recent exposure to an ill coworker, and poor compliance with her asthma medications, as well as expiratory wheezes on exam." The items that support or refute the diagnoses should be well composed. There can be several sentences written out for each differential diagnosis.

The plan, our last section of the note, is also vital and demands clarity and completeness in writing. The plan outlines how the writer will narrow the list of differential diagnoses for the presenting concern through testing and/or possible treatments if needed. This section should also comment on plans to manage each chronic medical condition. Again, same basic note organization. While some notes are not as detailed as others and may focus on one concern, the plan still needs to tell the reader the next steps. Plans typically cover the main elements of testing, treatment or therapeutics, patient education, and follow-up.[5,8,21,24]

To continue the previous clinical example of the patient with a cough for 5 days, an example of testing may include a simple test in the office, and treatments may include administering a nebulized medication. This could be written out as follows:

Plan

Testing: Pulse oximetry was done in the office pre- and posttreatment. Rapid flu testing was conducted and was negative. Blood work and a chest X-ray are not needed at this time.

Treatment: In-office nebulized albuterol was given and improved both the patient's breathing and posttreatment pulse oximetry. Her regular medications will be continued, and we will prescribe nebulized albuterol to use as needed. Acetaminophen or ibuprofen may be used for fever control, and we advised staying well hydrated with water.

Patient Education: We discussed a likely diagnosis of a viral URI exacerbating her asthma. The patient was advised that tobacco use will hinder recovery and worsen symptoms.

Follow Up: Advised the patient to return in 48 hours or sooner as needed if worsening. If symptoms are worsening, we will need to consider labs and a chest X-ray. If we are closed and the patient is worsening, she is advised to go to urgent care or the Emergency Room. Once symptoms have resolved, there is a need to discuss tobacco cessation and medication compliance with the patient.

The note plan reflects what the provider has done and discussed with the patient, underlining the importance of good communication with the patient. Relaying this information to the patient in a clear manner, as well as answering any questions and concerns, is vital to the physician-patient relationship.

The student is writing both the assessment and plan sections in their notes from early in the second semester of their first year in our course. With early introduction and multiple opportunities for practice over time, we support learners' confidence that they have the skills to be successful with note-writing basics.

Year 2, Semester 1

Our course continues to integrate with the organ systems being taught. Students write notes with all the aforementioned elements for the SP cases that they complete for each system, including neuroscience, behavior, and the gastrointestinal system. Previous systems, including reproduction, human development, cardiopulmonary and ears, nose, and throat, as well as renal-endocrine, were covered in Year 1, Semester 1.

Year 2, Semester 2

After the students finish their musculoskeletal dermatology course, which rounds out all the organ systems, a full physical exam formative session with an SP takes place. Students are then expected to produce a complete history and physical exam note using the SOAP format.

All the while, my colleague and I help construct the note in the debrief sessions with students. Since we want students to gain reliance on their skills of writing and clinical reasoning, they finish the remainder of the note after our sessions, hand them in, and a correction sheet is then shared with them to fill in gaps. We aim to build confidence with this exercise, again using expectancy-value theory: showing if students begin to feel more secure in their skills, they will feel more able to perform the task well. Between our debrief sessions and the correction sheet, students should gain a better understanding of how well their notes were written.

In addition, the first note of each organ system is reviewed by one of us. We make comments and record them in a student curricular platform, which is an online system for courses that students and faculty are able to access. Usefully, the platform provides another means of communication with students, helping us comment on areas of growth and areas where more assistance is needed. We recognize that quality feedback at this stage, as at all stages of clinical training, helps improve students' skills.[6,29]

Although our course finishes up at the end of Year 2 in medical school, writing continues to be integral in students' third and fourth years. In clerkships, students will be introduced to writing applied in all specialties, with them coming to understand how the notes of psychiatrists differ from surgeons', which differ from family physicians', for instance. The template is the same and the quality needs to be consistently high as students become residents, when expectations increase.

In our class, then, we try to lay the foundation, so clerkships and residency programs can build upon it for all clinical skills. Our aim is for the initial confidence to have taken root, and we expect it will continue to grow as students progress. Drawing on a framework of expectancy-value theory, we explain the importance and relevance of quality notes, equip students with tools such as templates, demonstrate how they can apply the knowledge they learned through ongoing practice, and encourage them to make all this part of their approach to quality patient care.

But how well does our approach work? We wanted to know in greater detail.

Evaluation of the Framework

To assess our process using expectancy-value theory, I conducted an external note review. Ten pairs of student notes (note pairs A to J) were pulled randomly, one from first-year students in the early spring semester of 2019 and one from their second year in the mid-fall semester. Since students would be receiving more instruction on the note-writing process in the time between early spring and mid-fall, the hypothesis was that the second note should show improvement over the first note. All student names and identification were removed prior to the review.

A survey was created that asked reviewers to rate the quality of the earlier note with the later note in each pair based on quality indicators. The reviewers (reviewer "A" and "B") utilized a Likert scale from 1 through 7, with 1 being "strongly disagree" and 7 being "strongly agree" for each indicator. The quality indicators used to compare the early and later notes were (1) well-organized, has formal clinical note format (subjective, objective, assessment, plan); (2) sufficiency of information, enough information to list diagnoses, develop plan; (3) improved readability (understandable, clear, fluent); and (4) shows overall improvement.

A medical colleague outside our institution was asked to pilot the survey with a small selection of notes. She reported the survey was easy to read and understand. Two faculty members who work in our institution, but do not teach in the course, agreed to be reviewers and were sent the 10 pairs of notes and survey. Each faculty member was given 3 weeks to evaluate the student notes and complete the survey. Their scores are shown in Tables 1.1 and 1.2.

Improvement between notes was seen in eight out of ten note pairs for reviewer A and eight out of ten for reviewer B. Improvement here is defined as Likert scores of 5 or greater on three out of

TABLE 1.1 Scores from reviewer A

		Note Pairs									
		A	B	C	D	E	F	G	H	I	J
Quality criteria for November notes	Better organized, follows SOAP format	6	7	5	5	4	4	7	6	6	6
	Greater sufficiency	7	7	5	4	3	4	6	7	6	5
	Improved readability	6	6	5	5	3	4	7	5	7	7
	Overall improvement	7	7	5	5	3	4	7	6	6	6

1 = strongly disagree, 2 = disagree, 3 = somewhat agree, 4 = neutral, 5 = somewhat agree, 6 = agree, 7 = strongly agree

TABLE 1.2 Scores from reviewer B

		Note Pairs									
		A	B	C	D	E	F	G	H	I	J
Quality criteria for November notes	Better organized, follows SOAP format	5	5	3	5	5	4	7	5	6	5
	Greater sufficiency	6	7	4	7	5	4	4	6	4	6
	Improved readability	5	6	5	6	4	4	6	3	6	5
	Overall improvement	5	6	5	6	5	4	6	5	6	5

1 = strongly disagree, 2 = disagree, 3 = somewhat agree, 4 = neutral, 5 = somewhat agree, 6 = agree, 7 = strongly agree

the four quality indicators. This finding shows there has been some improvement in the quality of notes with our teaching method.

Even though the majority of notes improved according to the reviewers, two pairs did not. For reviewer A, it was note pairs E and F and for reviewer B, it was note pairs C and F. Both reviewers gave note pair F a score of "4" on all four quality indicators. Reviewer A commented, "Both notes were good and of the same caliber; I'm not convinced the November (later) note is better. Review B commented, "Note does not seem to show improvement in November, but largely because January note is also very strong."

On note pair E, reviewer A commented, "Jan note actually read better than the Nov note." On note pair C, reviewer B commented, "readability improved, but not very much."

As I reviewed their scores and comments for these specific note pairs (C, E, and F), I found that, overall, the earlier note was stronger than the later note. The writing of the earlier notes takes place soon after students finish Year 1 Semester 1, which emphasizes good history taking and basic note structure. It also takes place early in Year 1 Semester 2, when we add the remainder of the note sections, the assessment and plan. This greater emphasis and fresh instruction on these components may have led to stronger notes in January versus later in the year, when I rely more on students to practice and review these fundamentals first taught in Year 1. Even though I review some of these fundamentals throughout the course, these findings may show the need for a greater in-depth review or refresher each semester.

Discussion and Implications for Practice

Writing this chapter has helped me review and reflect. The external peer-review results have led me to begin reexamining some elements of my instruction, as well as to consider conducting more note reviews at different times during the two years of the course. To be sure, the external reviewer helped me see potential weaknesses in my instruction. I suggest other faculty, if not already doing this, consider an external review of their teaching.

Since I see students through the early part of training, I lose touch and do not always know how the course impacted their later writing and clinic note development. As a future follow-up, I may consider surveying students in clerkships to assess their view on the importance of writing clinical notes, as well as the impact of notes on patient care.

For all those teaching clinical note writing, I believe in emphasizing quality writing to students early and throughout their instruction. Indeed, writing should be a defined skill embedded in a medical curriculum because it is an integral part of clinical practice—whether a note is used to record a medical encounter, liaise with others on the care team, refer the patient to a specialist, sew together the patient's story from hospital admission to discharge, or establish care of a new patient. Using examples of well-written notes from our own work can be very helpful. In our course, students appreciate the clinical relevance we bring to the classroom.

To encourage students, faculty who teach clinical notes should consider using templates or other organizational "blueprints." Faculty should also provide observation and generous feedback on students' practice notes. Doing so helps improve students' performance,[6,29] as well as build their confidence, in harmony with expectancy-value theory.

I hope that the importance of good writing stays with our students and that they continue to hone their writing as expectancies and values meld to create further success.[30] From this review, I see opportunities for faculty to apply other educational psychology theories to undergraduate and graduate medical education, as well as "writing in the health professions" more broadly. Expectancy-value theory may be just a start.

Appendix 1

SOAP Note Template for Case 1
Subjective
    Patient identifying information
    Chief complaint/agenda
    HPI
    Past Medical History and Health Maintenance
    General state of health
    Significant medical diseases/conditions
    Patient Health Questionnaire-9 (PHQ9)
    Prescription medications
    Nonprescription medications
    Allergies
    Hospitalizations/surgeries
    Ob-gyn history (if applicable)
    Health maintenance
    Immunization status
    Family History
    Relatives with similar illness
    Family medical history
    Diseases that run in the family
    Personal and Social History
    Education
    Marital status/living situation
    Occupations/hazards/military
    Financial resources
    Nicotine (tobacco) use
    Alcohol use
    Recreational drug use
    Sexual history
    Dietary practices
    Support system
    Safety practices
    Review of Systems
    OBJECTIVE
    Vital signs
    General observations
    Head, eyes, ears, nose, throat (HEENT)
    Chest and lungs
    Cardiac
    Gastrointestinal
    Musculoskeletal
    Neurologic
    ASSESSMENT (Add Summary Statement)
    Differential Diagnosis #1
    Subjective elements that support/refute
    Objective elements that support/refute

Differential Diagnosis #2
Subjective elements that support/refute
Objective elements that support/refute
Differential Diagnosis #3
Subjective elements that support/refute
Objective elements that support/refute
PLAN
Further testing/investigation
Treatment/therapeutics
Patient education
Follow up

References

1. Liaison Committee on Medical Education. *Functions and Structure of a Medical School: Standards for Accreditation of Medical Education Programs Leading to the Md Degree.* LCME. https://www.lcme.org/publications. Published March 2020. Accessed January 10, 2019.
2. Medical Schools Council. *Medical Schools Council. Statement on the Core Values and Attributes Needed to Study Medicine.* Medical Schools Council. http://www.medschools.ac.uk/SiteCollectionDoucments/Statement-on-core-values-and-attributes.pdf. Published 2014. Accessed January 10, 2019.
3. Feigelson S, Muller D "Writing about medicine": an exercise in reflection at Mount Sinai (with five samples of student writing). *Mt Sinai J Med.* 2005;72(5):322–332.
4. Cowen VS, Kaufman D, Schoenherr L. A review of creative and expressive writing as a pedagogical tool in medical education. *Med Educ.* 2016;50(3):311–319. doi:10.1111/medu.12878.
5. Bickley L, Szilagyi P, Hoffman R, Soriano R. *Bate' Guide to Physical Examination and History Taking.* 13 ed. Philadelphia: Wolters Kluwer;2017.
6. Bynum D, Colford C, Royal K. Teaching medical students the art of the " write-up." *Clin Teach.* 2015; 12(4):246–249. doi:10.1111/tct.12304.
7. Nakamura M, Altshuler D, Chadwell M, Binienda J. Clinical skills development in student-run free clinic volunteers: a multi-trait, multi-measure study. *BMC Med Educ.* 2014;14(1):250–250. doi:10.1186/s12909-014-0250-9.
8. Hadvani T, Hubenthal E, Chase L. Transitions to inpatient medicine clerkship—SOAP: notes and presenting on rounds. *MedEdPORTAL.* 2016;12:10366. https://doi.org/10.15766/mep_2374-8265.10366.
9. Nackers KAM, Shadman KA, Kelly MM, et al. Resident workshop to improve inpatient documentation using the Progress Note Assessment and Plan Evaluation (PNAPE) tool. *MedEdPORTAL.* 2020;16:11040. https://doi.org/10.15766/mep_2374-8265.11040.
10. Yahata S, Takeshima T, Kenzaka T, Okayama M. Fostering student motivation towards community healthcare: a qualitative study. *BMJ Open.* 2021;11(1). doi:http://dx.doi.org/10.1136/bmjopen-2020-039344.
11. Mak-van der Vossen M, Teherani A, van Mook WN, Croiset G, Kusurkar RA. Investigating US medical students' motivation to respond to lapses in professionalism. *Med Educ.* 2018;52(8):838–850. doi:10.1111/medu.13617.
12. Eccles J. Expectancies, values, and academic behaviors. In: J. T. Spence, ed. *Achievement and Achievement Motives: Psychological and Sociological Approaches.* San Francisco, CA: W. H. Freeman; 1983: 75–146.
13. Shweiki E, Martin ND, Beekley AC, et al. Applying expectancy theory to residency training: proposing opportunities to understand resident motivation and enhance residency training. *Adv Med Educ Pract.* 2015;6:339–346. doi:10.2147/AMEP.S76587.
14. Wigfield A. Expectancy-value theory of achievement motivation: a developmental perspective. *Educ Psychol Rev.* 1994;6(1):49–78.
15. Malick B. The value of writing skills as an addition to the medical school curriculum. *Adv Med Educ Pract.* 2017;8:525–526. doi:10.2147/AMEP.S140585.
16. Schaeffer J. *Poor documentation: why it happens and how to fix it. For the record.* https://www.fortherecord-mag.com/archives/0516p12.shtml. Published May 2016. Accessed February 20, 2020.

17. Karkowsky, CE, Chazotte, C. Simulation: improving communication with patients. *Semin Perinatol.* 2013;37(3):157–160. doi:10.1053/j.semperi.2013.02.006.

18. Robey T. The art of writing patient record notes. *Virtual Mentor.* 2011;13(7):482–484. doi:10.1001/virtualmentor.2011.13.7.cprl1-1107.

19. Weed LL. Medical records that guide and teach. *N Engl J ed.* 1968;278(11):593–600. doi:10.1056/NEJM196803142781105.

20. Jaroudi S, Payne, D. Remembering Lawrence Weed: a pioneer of the SOAP note. *Acad Med.* 2019;94(1):11. doi:10.1097/ACM.0000000000002483.

21. Gossman W, Lew V, Ghassemzadeh S. SOAP notes. *StatPearls* [Internet]. 2020 Jan. https://www.ncbi.nlm.nih.gov/books/NBK482263/.

22. Dolan R, Broadbent P A quality improvement project using a problem based post take ward round proforma based on the SOAP acronym to improve documentation in acute surgical receiving. *Ann Med Surg.* 2016;5:45–48. doi:10.1016/j.amsu.2015.11.011.

23. Ericsson KA. Acquisition and maintenance of medical expertise: a perspective from the expert-performance approach with deliberate practice. *Acad Med.* 2015;90(11):1471–1486. doi:10.1097/ACM.0000000000000939.

24. Tierney LM, Smetana GW. *The Patient History: An Evidence-Based Approach to Differential Diagnosis.* New York, NY: McGraw-Hill Medical; 2012.

25. Mathioudakis A, Rousalova I, Gagnat AA, et al. How to keep good clinical records. *Breathe* 2016;12:369–373. doi:10.1183/20734735.018016.

26. Elkbuli S, Godelman S, Miller A, et al. Improved clinical documentation leads to superior reportable outcomes: an accurate representation of patient's clinical status. *Int J Surg.* 2018;53:288–291. doi:10.1016/j.ijsu.2018.03.081.

27. Russo R, Fitzgerald S, Eveland JD, Fuchs B, Redmon D. Improving physician clinical documentation quality: evaluating two self-efficacy-based training programs. *Health Care Manage Rev.* 2013;38(1):29–39. doi:10.1097/HMR.0b013e31824c4c61.

28. Leonard M, Graham S, Bonacum D. The human factor: the critical importance of effective teamwork and communication in providing safe care. *BMJ Quality & Safety* 2004;13(suppl 1):i85–i90. doi:10.1136/qshc.2004.01003.

29. Bienstock JL, Katz NT, Cox SM, Hueppchen N, Erickson S, Puscheck EE. To the point: medical education reviews—providing feedback. *Am J Obstet Gynecol* 2007;196(6):508–513. doi:10.1016/j.ajog.2006.08.021.

30. Trautwein U, Marsh HW, Nagengast B, Lüdtke O, Nagy G, Jonkmann K. Probing for the multiplicative term in modern expectancy–value theory: a latent interaction modeling study. *J Educ Psychol.* 2012;104(3):763–777. doi:10.1037/a0027470.

2

WHAT CAN WE LEARN ABOUT "ADVANCED LITERACY FOR RESEARCH" IN TWO COLOMBIAN GRADUATE PROGRAMS?

Elizabeth Narváez-Cardona and Pilar Mirely Chois-Lenis

Incorporating "writing in the health professions" into medical education may have multipurpose benefits. For instance, writing instruction can help medical students and trainees learn discipline-specific concepts, form professional identities, and strengthen their grant writing and research skills.[1–3] These skills may include reading and producing reviews of the literature,[4] case reports,[5] and other genres that are important for scholarship in their fields, supporting evidence-based practice.[6] Writing in the health professions can also support health literacy: medical professionals may write to educate patients, peers, or their local communities.[7] These roles and curriculum opportunities have barely been explored in Latin America.

Since the '90s, Latin American scholarship has increasingly studied reading and writing in higher education. Yet the focus has been on undergraduate levels.[8] Studies related to scientific or professional writing are scattered, and many of the publications in this area are essays rather than empirical studies, which mainly take linguistic perspectives.[9–20] When they do appear in scholarship, empirical studies highlight writing to learn: "writing as a means of acquiring information, understanding concepts, and appreciating significance in any discipline." Writing to learn is different from learning to write: "acquiring the socially-mediated communication skills and genre knowledge appropriate to a specific discipline."[21]

Within this Latin American context, our chapter presents data from a study on two health sciences programs in southwest Colombia: one a master's degree in public health and one a specialization in pediatrics. In Latin America, a specialization is a graduate program in which professional knowledge is updated and deepened.[22]

We have organized our chapter into six sections. The first one provides additional insights from Latin American scholarship on postsecondary reading and writing. The second section presents our theoretical framework, and we explain why the concept of "literate activity" may fittingly capture what health practitioners do. The third section describes the institutions where we collected data, as well as our methods: content analysis, time analyses, and participant observations. The fourth and fifth sections share a small part of our data analysis that supports our empirical conclusions. In the sixth section, we draw implications for graduate writing curricula in the health professions.

DOI: 10.4324/9781003162940-4

The State of Latin American Scholarship on Postsecondary Reading and Writing

As suggested previously, writing in the health professions as an interdiscipline is barely emerging in Latin America, where scholarship has primarily focused on undergraduate and academic writing.[8] Narváez and Moritz conducted an analysis, currently under review, of 104 Latin American publications (2004–2019) on postsecondary reading and writing in Spanish (n = 60) and Portuguese (n = 44). The results showed that for the Spanish-speaking countries and Brazil, the publications were research papers, literature reviews, or essays. Most of these publications present undergraduate pedagogical experiences, with the intention to support learning or analyze teaching practices.

Empirical studies on teaching graduate writing in Spanish are limited, and a literature review of 52 Latin American publications (2014–2016) revealed several interesting patterns: About two-thirds of the publications explored master's levels (64.3%) rather than doctoral (28.6%) levels or specializations (7.1%). About 70% covered the "final stretch" of graduate experiences, such as the writing of the senior thesis or dissertation (71.42%). Most analyzed student experiences (82%) rather than curriculum or faculty practices (20.5%). About two-thirds focused on the social sciences and humanities (66.7%) rather than the natural sciences (20.5%). About a quarter considered writing ease or difficulty as a textual process (23%).[23]

Therefore, studies analyzing writing in the health professions are important not only to advance Latin American scholarship generally. They are also important to advance writing curricula in fields other than the social sciences or humanities, including pediatrics and public health—the focus of this chapter.

Sociocultural Approaches to Writing in the Health Professions

To study writing in the health professions, it is useful to conceptualize writing socioculturally or, in other words, as social practices. In this approach, writing is more than a process of generating a text that is full of sentences and paragraphs. Writing is a "situated activity": it takes place in discontinuous moments in which writers and readers have diverse materials (paper, pencils, computers), "semiotic tools" (language systems, images, numbers), and flows of activity (reading, speaking, observing, acting, processing, thinking, and feeling).[24]

For this reason, writing is limited as a unit of analysis if we consider it simply an alphabetic, textual thing done by a single writer in a fixed period of time. It is more productive to acknowledge that writing in the health professions involves many social practices, some of which have established names: laboratory writing, scientific writing, health literacy, grant writing, and writing for evidence-based practice. We suggest that the concept of "literate activity" might be well suited to embrace these and other practices in the health professions. With the concept of literate activity, we can more clearly see writing as an interactive social process that weaves—and not always harmoniously—minds, actions, times, and spaces.[24]

If we consider writing as a literate activity, we must acknowledge the relationship between language and power. We should welcome inherent contradictions and tensions that emerge from interprofessional communication, interactions between health workers and patients, and institutional regulations, among other fields of power. There are also influences from the hierarchies in organizations and cultures, differences in communication styles, and varying motives of writers and readers.[25–27]

How might a sociocultural approach like this apply to teaching and learning? In general, we learn to write by participating in "literacy events." That is to say, we write to fulfill social goals that are relevant and meaningful to us.[28] Since we write with multiple social goals and in diverse spaces, instructors should recognize that there is not one kind of literacy, but many.[29–34] For example, there are academic literacies used in school settings, particularly across subjects, and mostly for teaching and learning purposes. Academic literacies are part of the everyday practices of academics, including faculty members who work with master's and doctoral students. (See Chapter 9, which applies an academic literacies model in an online course for physician assistants.) There are also literacies that are specific to the health professions, such as pediatrics and public health. However, because these literacies have become intuitive for faculty members, they may struggle to explain and teach them to their students.[33]

In Latin America, there are two main ways to help graduate students learn to write, and the first one centers on deliberate instruction, which often occurs through curricula and other formal training.[35-37] Some of the most common forms of deliberate instruction are workshops that demystify genres for students. These genres may be academic (such as a thesis proposal) or scientific (such as a paper for publication).

The second way centers on enculturation, which involves natural encounters with real-world writing and communication situations.[24,31,38] Students learn literate activity by participating in a "disciplinary community" consisting of their peers and other professionals in their discipline. Mentors provide feedback that helps students explore and understand tacit rules of the community. Meanwhile, students negotiate meanings and identities; therefore, coming to know the "rules of the game" is not automatic and requires more than obedience to authority. The process of enculturation is well described by the theory of "communities of practice."[39]

It seems clear that learning advanced literacy at the graduate level depends not only on deliberate instruction. Enculturation is needed as well, and this is reflected in scholarship from Latin America and elsewhere. Several studies have confirmed that research groups and lab projects are beneficial sources of mentorship, particularly since students are able to interact and share resources and ideas.[38,40-42] In the health professions specifically, one initiative involved textual feedback provided by a team: a faculty member in the students' field, peers, and a writing expert.[42] Another initiative introduced medical narrative writing to improve decision-making in health care since medical records are based primarily on narratives.[43] There is also a writing program aimed at helping students master scientific and professional genres related to their fields.[44]

To teach research skills, online instruction has been offered on writing master's theses in public health.[45] There has also been an analysis of how using research articles as exemplary cases can help graduate students formulate research questions.[46] In another master's program in public health, writing instructors were invited onto the teaching team.[47,48]

As suggested by this literature, there are numerous ways to integrate deliberate instruction and enculturation (which, again, are not mutually exclusive), and doing so effectively can be a challenge in any graduate program. Public health and pediatrics are no exceptions, and we sought to better understand how students in these disciplines learn "advanced literacy for research."

Institutional Context of the Two Graduate Programs

We collected data from two Colombian graduate programs. The pediatrics specialization program was founded in the 1970s and aims to help pediatricians master key knowledge, skills, and attitudes of their profession. These include advocating for children's health and acknowledging the biological, psychological, and social dimensions of child development. The specialization requires students to attend full time and participate in diverse learning activities. These include medical rotations at local facilities, community work, case study groups, topic reviews, and journal clubs.

The public health master's program was founded in the 1960s and aims to prepare public health practitioners to be researchers and university teachers. To this end, students should be able to articulate key knowledge and methodologies in the field, as well as advocate for transformative policies. Both of the graduate programs that we studied are recognized nationwide for their teaching and research accomplishments, especially those involving partnerships with other universities locally and abroad. Both programs are delivered face-to-face.

Eight students from the public health master's program participated in our study. They were 32 years old, on average, and were working in a variety of fields, including medicine. Two faculty members participated as well: one holds a PhD in epidemiology, and the other holds a PhD in environmental sciences. The latter was the lead instructor of a research methods course.

Two students (31 and 36 years old) in the pediatrics specialization, both physicians, participated in this study. So did three faculty members, who joined as mentors: one faculty member who holds a PhD in public health and two others who were pursuing doctoral studies in epidemiology.

To get a wider perspective on deliberate instruction and enculturation, we also collected data in Spanish from national public policies on Colombian graduate education, institutional documents associated with the two graduate programs, and observations of a research course and thesis mentoring sessions. The study was initiated as part of the second author's doctoral thesis (Institutional Review Board approval 4620).

What Do the Policies and Institutional Document State?

The first part of our study explored the learning expectations reflected in several sets of documents:

- Public policies from the Ministry of Education, which regulates Colombian graduate education. This includes the standards set for medical and surgical degrees (Decrees 80, 1001, and 1665)
- Graduate student regulations from the two programs we studied
- Curriculum documents available at the websites of the two selected graduate programs

We applied content analysis to these documents based on Bengtsson,[49] who describes four stages: decontextualization, recontextualization, categorization, and compilation. We used diverse techniques to identify the sections of the documents that needed in-depth analysis.

First, we did exploratory reading of the documents by focusing on titles and subtitles, and searching for key words in Spanish for PDF and Word documents. The key words in Spanish were as follows: *posgrado, formación posgraduada, maestría, doctorado, especialización, especialización médico quirúrgica/investigación, trabajo de grado, tesis, publicación, investigación, científico (a), escritura, escribir, escrito, publicación, producción científica.*

Afterward, we analyzed, paragraph by paragraph, sections that include the key words. We assigned codes by inductive and deductive procedures based on multiple readings of the selected sections. The final codes we grouped into two categories: features of the research training curriculum and expectations for graduate students' research writing.

We will share some direct quotations from the documents that we translated into English. Original quotations in Spanish appear below the English translations.

We use acronyms to identify each document or the name of the study participants.

Features of the Research Training Curriculum

Our content analysis suggested that in pediatrics, research training is intended primarily to support clinical practice. In both programs, it is intended to foster skills in decision-making. Thus, in both, research training helps cultivate the students' professional identities.

In the pediatrics program, the official documents we analyzed state that physicians must be able to conduct research or make decisions based on scientific evidence. For example,

> physician residents must benefit from daily practice to conduct decision making in health care. To this aim, research, self-reflection, and peer evaluation are necessary.

> Los residentes deben beneficiarse de su práctica diaria y usufructuar de ella con el apreciable fin de mejorar en forma permanente e integral para optimizar las prácticas de la atención médica. La investigación, la autoevaluación y la heteroevaluación les ayudarán en este propósito.

In the public health program, the documents make a similar point: graduate students might work not only as researchers, and they must make decisions based on scientific findings:

> Learning of research in Public Health is paramount for students to master it…, since they are called to actively contribute in knowledge production and evidence-based decision making.

> La formación en investigación en el campo de la salud pública es fundamental para los estudiantes de las Maestrías en Salud Pública…, quienes se espera que contribuyan activamente en la gestión del conocimiento y en la toma de decisiones basadas en evidencia.

We made time-scale comparisons of research courses and mentoring in the two graduate programs. In pediatrics, students complete a sequence of research courses during the first year, and they are mentored over the whole 3-year program. Students may have the opportunity to work with two types of mentors: a research mentor and an "area of specialization" mentor (Figure 2.1).

In public health, students take research courses between their second and fourth semesters, and they can have a mentor during that time. Students are expected to complete their master's thesis no later than four semesters from their first year.

In pediatrics, the research course involves 168 hours of face-to-face instruction. Of these, 110 (66%) focus on epidemiology and research methods. Other subjects that receive less time include communication (5.0%), pedagogy (5.0%) bioethics (7.0%), and physical formative education (17.0%).

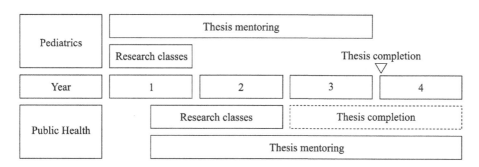

FIGURE 2.1 Time-scale comparison of curriculum experiences

Faculty Teams

According to the documents analyzed, there are multidisciplinary teams supporting the resource courses in both graduate programs. The undergraduate majors of the faculty were speech therapy, health sciences, physical therapy, nursing, sociology, communication, and geography. The specialized fields of affiliation are pediatrics, anesthesiology, gynecology, family medicine, pedagogy, and social management. The graduate-level fields of affiliation are public health, epidemiology, environmental sciences, education, and linguistics.

In both programs, the instructors leading courses on academic reading and writing are professionals in speech therapy who have completed graduate studies in literacy pedagogy. In the public health master's program, the instructor in this area carries up to a 17.5-hour course that, according to the course syllabus, is intended to help students experience and analyze disciplinary reading and writing. Ultimately, the aim is to support the writing of a thesis proposal. In the pediatrics program, the speech therapist leads a 4-hour course on the textual formats of scientific articles in the health sciences.

Literacy Expectations

The official documents we analyzed mention genres that students should be able to read and write during their time in the program. In the pediatrics specialization, students must write and submit a research proposal by the midpoint of their first year, while public health graduates must submit the proposal at the end of their second year. Both programs expect students to complete and defend a final research report in their final semester. In pediatrics, students must additionally work on a research publication. Thus, the last two semesters in pediatrics are focused on article revision and publication.

As for genres to read, our analysis revealed that students in pediatrics are expected to read biomedical literature, in particular clinical trials since they inform clinical practice (Figure 2.2).

Dashed boxes indicate genres that students need to read. Solid boxes indicate genres that students need to write.

Students in public health must notice differences among scientific publications, especially to develop their research proposals. The documents also mention other types of writing that might help them complete their theses. For instance, the documents mention a poster of the research

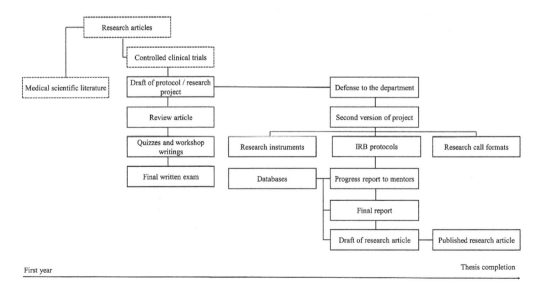

FIGURE 2.2 Major genres to read and write in the pediatrics specialization

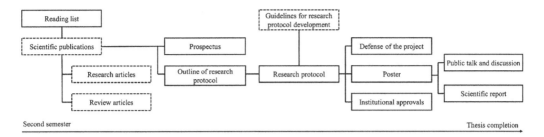

FIGURE 2.3 Major genres to read and write in the public health master's program

proposal in the third semester, other academic genres such as reading planners and templates for research proposals, and administrative-academic genres, such as notes from mentoring meetings. Although the institutional documents state that students must be able to write scientific publications, we did not detect that particular expectation across the curriculum (Figure 2.3).

Dashed boxes indicate genres that students need to read. Solid boxes indicate genres that students need to write.

It is important to note the differences between utilizing advanced literacy to support practice (e.g., research knowledge is necessary to make decisions in public health and to treat patients in pediatrics) and to support further research (e.g., all graduate students in Colombia are expected to communicate research findings). Our data confirm that what is read and written can vary depending on the program's emphasis, which might be focused more on professional performance or academic identity. To further support this claim, the next section describes our analysis of how faculty interacted with students during curricular experiences in both programs.

Navigating between Research Courses and Mentoring

Complying with human subject approvals, we collected data through participant observation, including audio and video recordings. We were participant observers in six mentoring sessions in the last year of the pediatric specialization (August 2017 to June 2018) and 16 sessions of a research methods course in the second semester of the public health master's program (February to June 2018).

We used grounded theory[50] to code (open, axial, and selective coding) the transcriptions of the records that resulted. Our coding categories were *genres, purposes, tools, interactions, writing knowledge,* and *knowledge about teaching.* To characterize what participants did and what they talked about, we created "thematic threads" based on semantic and pragmatic coherence—that is, patterns in their language that we could identify based on uses, meanings, and contexts.[51] We share some examples from our data in the next section.

Writing a Research Article: A Shared Task

In the pediatrics specialization, data from our participant observations allowed us to group activities carried out by faculty and students across mentoring sessions. All of the participants we observed, three mentors and two students, were engaged in preparing, revising, editing, and literature searching. Moreover, one of the faculty members, "the methodological mentor," was an active participant across diverse thematic threads (e.g., instrument design, fieldwork, research article, and proposal submission). The other participants took part in at least one learning activity aimed at producing the coauthored research article.

Our analysis of the conversation between the three mentors and two students allowed us to identify several types of exchanges during the research article writing experience: planning cooperatively, writing together, writing by yourself, and reviewing/rewriting together.

In *planning cooperatively*, the mentors and two students asked themselves questions such as "When could we start?" Before starting the actual writing, the participants anticipated what they would write, how they would write, what resources they would use, and in what moments.

> MENTOR But, we have still time. I mean, a year, nine, eight months. [The mentor emphasizes the time available students have to complete their graduation requirements].
>
> STUDENT Yes, but we have not started the actual writing.
>
> MENTOR We have to start writing to keep a record…actually, we could record audios, record the memories and then start writing from them, what do you think?

In this example, the mentor is estimating how much time is needed to complete the tasks, such as the data analysis and research article writing. He is also proposing to record information as a way to start the research article writing later.

In *writing together*, the participants ask themselves questions such as "Should we write this?" For example, one student talked about a particular section of the article while another typed the ideas in a Microsoft Word document. This snippet of recorded conversation illustrates the case.

> STUDENT 1 Ok, then, if you want, could you write down there, something like phase one titled: research instrument development.
>
> STUDENT 2 Ah, phase one? No, I mean, this was the first decision, I'm gonna write this, but we will revise this later. We will change this since we won't put it…ok, let's say "assessing mother knowledge and research instrument development. The idea is to make…" [the student reads what s/he wrote]. This is just to have the idea in mind; the initial purpose of the research work.

Unlike the previous exchange, the students here, without any mentor intervention, discuss what to write about and how. These exchanges associated with *writing together* also reveal a variety of negotiation strategies and cooperative decision-making between mentor and students.

Writing by yourself could sound like the snippet of dialogue that follows.

> MENTOR Everybody, in a different place, can reread what we have done since right now because of the noise, one can't see the details…then, the material will be uploaded in Dropbox.

As the mentor points out, it was expected that each of the participants (mentors and students) contribute to the article writing. The contributions could occur not only in physical writing spaces, such as the classroom, but also through online cooperative work tools.

Finally, *review and rewrite together* involves responding to a mentor's request to review and reorganize. Here, the participants read aloud a specific part written by one of the writers of the team and then feedback is provided for the next version, as in this snippet of conversation.

> MENTOR, **reading aloud** Delaying introducing complementary feeding is not advised…
>
> STUDENT …or delaying to introduce complementary feeding is not advised…
>
> MENTOR Where?
>
> STUDENT For instance, instead of saying "delaying" it might be said "delaying of."

This exchange illustrates how students can raise ideas and objections to the mentor's writing ideas.

Ultimately, this section reveals that writing a research article is actively embraced by the mentors and the students as a shared task.

Writing a Research Proposal: Nobody Can Write Your Proposal but You!

In this section, we summarize the amount of time utilized in the five thematic threads that we identified. Next, we present the thematic threads from the highest to lowest time investment, based on our records:

The student research proposals: Students present, revise, and give feedback to their proposals, or work individually in their own texts. (18h:54m:04s)

Research projects: Instructors present expectations and features of research proposals based on guidelines of the national research agency and national health public agencies. (08h:51m:36s)

Research practitioners: Instructors present research abilities graduate students must master as researchers in public health (i.e., reference management software, search and analysis of datasets, and analysis of research articles). (03h:53m:43s)

Research education: Instructors argue the importance of the course and present learning expectations, deliverables, and course timeline. (02:21:09)

Fostering of teamwork: Instructors present activities to foster teamwork and interpersonal engagement (00h:53m:21s).

Similar to the previous section, analyzing the conversations between the faculty and students allowed us to identify the *types* of exchanges used to support the development of the students' research proposals. These exchanges demonstrate the pedagogical goal of the instructors, one of whom declared that "nobody can write your proposal but you!" The types of exchanges were an *explanation of what and how to write*, *writing practice*, *providing and receiving feedback*, and *live writing in the classroom*.

Explanation of what and how to write is well captured by the faculty member who said, "I will tell you the process," since the instructors explain writing expectations regarding texts and procedures. Additionally, an instructor said,

> We saw an exemplary research question from a Colciencias project [The Colombian Department of Science, Technology, and Innovation]; so, when I read a research statement, the first thing I look for is this…[The instructor draws questions marks on the board].

In *writing practice*, the students start the actual writing, saying "let's do it" when instructors proposed to present simulations, hypothetical situations that allow students to apply their research-writing procedures and skills.

INSTRUCTOR The first group will select a research question from the list, that we utilized at the last Colciencias research call [Colciencias is the Colombian Department of Science, Technology, and Innovation, which is the national sponsor for research calls]; we just need to identify which question from the list might be the best option for the call.

The learning activity is presenting a hypothetical research-writing situation to help students think about their own research questions.

In *providing and receiving feedback*, instructors encourage cooperative learning. They may encourage students to submit drafts or present their proposals orally to peers, faculty, or invited researchers.

INSTRUCTOR OK guys, we listen and provide brief feedback, and [the name of two researchers invited] will freely ask and provide positive comments. And let's get started, now! [The instructor turns on the timer.]

The instructor was explaining the rules of a learning activity in which the students would prepare an "elevator speech" of their proposals within a minute. Students would receive feedback from two researchers invited to the class.

Finally, *live writing in the classroom* means "get the ball rolling" when students have time in class to write. This was clearly stated in the first class session.

INSTRUCTOR You all are not here to "see the class," you are here to write, and if you feel better writing in the coffee shop at the mall, feel free to go there! The point is you all have to be dedicated and disciplined with writing.... The research proposal will not get written by itself, right?

Our prior analysis of exchanges between the instructors and the students (in the master's in public health program) showed that although learning support was available, students were primarily responsible for the writing. As one instructor said, "Nobody can write your proposal but you!"

As mentioned earlier, students in the public health program must write a thesis in order to graduate. Students in the pediatrics specialization must go a step further: they must utilize advanced literacy to both meet a graduation requirement and learn about research publication. According to our findings, the latter literate practice (research publication) involves teams in which members hold diverse levels of control and autonomy over collecting data, analyzing data, and writing sections of the research article. For example, first- and second-year students in pediatrics work individually to collect data, while more senior students take charge of data analysis.

We have only presented a small part of our data in this chapter. Yet we believe our data can support several key conclusions. First, there is a difference between utilizing advanced literacy for clinical practice, such as decision-making, and research publication. Second, advanced literacy for research publication involves teams in which members hold diverse levels of control and autonomy over collecting data, analyzing data, and writing a research manuscript. Third, if students are expected to do research, literate activity may be focused on designing and justifying research methods. For example, students in the public health program must write research problem statements that display the relationships between two or more variables. If research knowledge is additionally expected to lead to publishing, as in the pediatrics program, literate activity may focus more on authorship development.

Our chapter may thus have implications for teaching "writing in the health professions."

Implications for Graduate Literacy Curricula

This chapter offers data that can inform curriculum development in literacy at the graduate level. Based on our study, it seems clear that graduate students learning "advanced literacy for research" will be able to complete some learning activities on their own (e.g., conduct searches in online databases), whereas other learning activities might require networks of collaboration (e.g., deciding which authors to read based on the students' disciplines). To help students acquire the needed competencies, we recommend that instructors emphasize both enculturation and deliberate instruction in their teaching. For instance, instructors can hold formal workshops or class sessions on key genres that students need to learn, "telling students the process." Meanwhile, they should provide mentorship through additional team activities, one-on-one coaching, and other meaningful participation in the students' disciplinary communities, helping students develop their own professional identities.

Of course, instructors should also strive to align their curricula with the literacy expectations of the students' disciplines. Our study showed that research training in different disciplines does not necessarily involve the same strategies or have the same purposes. For example, some students may be expected to gain research knowledge primarily to inform everyday practice and others to produce further research. Yet, as our study found, some of these expectations may be hidden or taken for granted. Thus, it can be useful to apply a sociocultural approach that considers writing as a literate activity, employing methods such as content analysis of policy documents, time analyses of curricular content, and participant observations of teaching and learning in action. This kind of approach can provide a fuller picture of what students need to learn, how they learn it, and how well the curriculum aligns. Instructors can then make adjustments as needed.

In the future, sociocultural approaches can be used to explore "writing in the health professions" in disciplines other than pediatrics and public health. They can also be applied to areas of practice that are critical across specialties, such as public policy and health literacy, and in geographical regions where empirical scholarship is limited. These are just a few possibilities as writing in the health professions, as an interdiscipline, continues to emerge in Latin America and beyond.

References

1. Kim S, Yang JW, Lim J, Lee S, Ihm J, Park J. The impact of writing on academic performance for medical students. *BMC Med Educ.* 2021;21(1):1–8.
2. Kostenko VG, Solohor IM. How to incorporate writing pedagogy in undergraduate and postgraduate medical education. *Wiadomosci Iekarskie.* 2018;1(2):79–86.
3. Nasab S, Rushing JS, Segars JH, et al. A mentorship program for academic obstetrician gynecologists that improved publication and overall confidence for success. *Semin Reprod Med.* 2019;37(5–6):257–264.
4. Pieper D, Müller D, Stock S. Challenges in teaching systematic reviews to non-clinicians. *Zeitschrift für Evidenz, Fortbildung und Qualität im Gesundheitswesen.* 2019;147:1–6.
5. Vaughan B, Fleischmann M. A guide to writing a case report of an osteopathic patient. *In J Osteopath Med.* 2020;37:34–9.
6. Skela-Savič B, Gotlib J, Panczyk M, et al. Teaching evidence-based practice (EBP) in nursing curricula in six European countries—a descriptive study. *Nurse Educ Today.* 2020;94:104561.
7. Samerski S. Health literacy as a social practice: social and empirical dimensions of knowledge on health and healthcare. *Soc Sci Med.* 2019;226:1–8.
8. Navarro F, Ávila N, Tapia M, et al. Panorama histórico y contrastivo de los estudios sobre lectura y escritura en educación superior publicados en América Latina. *Revista Signos.* 2016;49:78–99
9. López F. El análisis de contenido como método de investigación. *Revista Educación.* 2002;4:167–179. http://rabida.uhu.es/dspace/bitstream/handle/10272/1912/b15150434.pdf?sequence1
10. Cassany D. La lectura y escritura de géneros profesionales en EpFE. In: *Español para fines específicos: actas del II CIEFE: II congreso internacional de español para fines específicos. Congreso internacional de español para fines específicos.* Amsterdam; noviembre de 2003. [Madrid];[Utrecht]: Ministerio de Educación y Ciencia; Instituto Cervantes; 2004. ISBN 90-806886-3-0 2004.
11. Morales OA. Enseñanza de la escritura académica con base en el análisis del género: del resumen a la tesis. *Legenda.* 2014;18(8):35–65.
12. González de la Torre Y. Configuraciones de las prácticas lectoras en contextos sociales: la lectura situada en la escuela y el trabajo. *Perfiles Educativos.* 2011;33(133):30–50.
13. Bach C, López C. De la academia a la profesión: análisis y contraste de prácticas discursivas en contextos plurilingües y multiculturales. *Cuadernillo Comillas.* 2011;1:142–153.
14. Álvarez A, Perlaza D, Rivera D, Suárez A. *Análisis discursivo de los textos que escriben los profesionales en fonoaudiología en diferentes ámbitos laborales (Tesis de pregrado).* Cali, Colombia: Universidad del Valle; 2012.

15. González B, Vega V. Lectura y escritura en la educación superior colombiana: herencia y construcción. *Pontificia Universidad Javeriana, Revista Interacción.* 2012;12(13):196–201.

16. Vásquez A, Jakob II, Rosales PA, Pelizza L. Prácticas de escritura profesional: los psicopedagogos en el ámbito educativo. *Innovación Educativa.* 2014;14(65):17–42.

17. Narváez E. Exploración del desarrollo de la escritura de dos egresados de medios y comunicación a propósito de una prueba de escritura a gran escala en Colombia. *Espaço pedagógico.* 2015;22(1):51–78.

18. Sánchez F. The roles of technical communication researchers in design scholarship. *J Tech Writ Commun.* 2016;47(3):359–391. doi:10.1177/0047281616641929

19. Arnoux EN, di Stefano M, Pereira MC Las escrituras profesionales: dispositivos argumentativos y estrategias retóricas/Professional writings: argumentative devices and rhetorical strategies. *Revista Signos.* 2016;49(suppl 1):78–99.

20. Mateos LS, Dietz G, Mendoza RG. Saberes-haceres interculturales? Experiencias profesionales y comunitarias de egresados de la educación superior intercultural veracruzana. *Revista Mexicana de Investigación Educativa.* 2016;21(70):809–835.

21. Carter M, Ferzli M, Wiebe EN Writing to learn by learning to write in the disciplines. *J Bus Tech Commun.* 2007;21(3):278–302.

22. MEN. (2006). *Decreto 1001.* http://www.mineducacion.gov.co/1621/articles-96961_archivo_pdf.pdf

23. Chois P, Jaramillo L. La investigación sobre la escritura en posgrado: estado del arte. *Lenguaje.* 2016;44:227–259.

24. Prior PA. *Writing/Disciplinarity: A Sociohistoric Account of Literate Activity in the Academy.* New York, NY: Lawrence Erlbaum Associates, Inc; 1998.

25. Barton D, Hamilton M. *Local Literacies: Reading and Writing in One Community.* London, UK: Psychology Press; 1998.

26. Cassany D. *Tras las Líneas. Sobre la Lectura Contemporánea.* Barcelona: Anagrama; 2006.

27. Perry K. What is literacy?—a critical overview of sociocultural perspectives. *J Lang Lit.* 2012;8:50–71.

28. Ivanic, R. Discourses of writing and learning to write. *Lang Educ.* 2004;18:220–245.

29. Carlino P. Escribir y leer en la universidad: responsabilidad compartida entre alumnos, docentes e instituciones. In: Carlino, P. (coord.) *Textos en Contexto Núm. 6. Leer y Escribir en la Universidad.* Buenos Aires: Asociación Internacional de Lectura; 2004.

30. Lea MR, Street BV The "academic literacies" model: theory and applications. *Theory Into Practice.* 2006;45:368–377.

31. Prior P, Bilbro R. Academic enculturation: developing literate practice and disciplinary identities. In: Castelló M, Donahue C eds. *University Writing: Selves and Text in Academic Societies.* Bradford, UK: Emerald; 2012;24:19–32.

32. Rose M, McClafferty KA. Call for the teaching of writing in graduate education. *Educ Res.* 2001;30:27–33.

33. Simpson S. The problem of graduate-level writing support: building a cross-campus graduate writing initiative. *Writing Program Adm.* 2012;36:95–118.

34. Zavala V. La literacidad o lo que la gente hace con la lectura y la escritura. *Textos de Didáctica de la Lengua y la Literatura.* 2008;47:71–79.

35. Mendoza A Las prácticas de evaluación docente y las habilidades de escritura requeridas en el nivel posgrado. *Innovación Educativa, México* 2014;14:147–175.

36. Ainciburu MC. *El plagio en la escritura académica de posgrado y su influencia en la práctica ELE: Herramientas antiplagio y su uso en ámbito universitario.* Italia: Universidad degli Studi di Siena; 2014:33–42.

37. Espino S. La enseñanza de estrategias de escritura y comunicación de textos científicos y académicos a estudiantes de posgrado. *Revista Mexicana de Investigación Educativa.* 2015;20:959–976.

38. Delamont S, Atkinson P. Doctoring uncertainty: mastering craft knowledge. *Soc Stud Sci.* 2001;3(1):87–107. doi: https://doi.org/10.1177/030631201031001005.

39. Lave J, Wenger E. *Situated Learning: Legitimate Peripheral Participation.* Cambridge, UK: Cambridge University Press; 1991.

40. Carrasco A, Kent R. Leer y escribir en el doctorado o el reto de formarse como autor de ciencias. *Revista Mexicana de Investigación Educativa.* 2011;16(51):1227–1251.

41. Carrasco A, Kent R, Keranen N Learning careers and enculturation: production of scientific papers by PhD students in a Mexican physiology laboratory: an exploratory case study. In: Bazerman C, Dean C, Early J, Lunsford K, Null S, Rogers P, and Stansell A, eds. *International Advances in Writing Research: Cultures, Places and Measures*. Fort Collins, CO: The WAC Clearinghouse and Parlor Press; 2012: 335–351.

42. Carrasco A, Kent R, Díaz L, Palacios P. La escritura disciplinar en el doctorado científico: aprendizaje social situado, roles e identidades. En: González Y, Ponce A. (coord.). *Lectura, Escritura y Matemáticas. Una Mirada Desde los Estudios de Literacidad*. México: Universidad de Guadalajara; 2018.

43. Liao J, Secemsky B. The value of narrative medical writing in internal medicine residency. *J Gen Intern Med*. 2015; 30(11):1707–1710.

44. Clemmons A, Hoge S, Cribb A, Manasco K. Development and implementation of a writing program to improve resident authorship rates. *Am J Health-Syst Pharm*. 2015;1(72):S53–S57, doi:10.2146/ajhp150159.

45. Harrison R, Gemmell I, Reed K. Student satisfaction with a web-based dissertation course: Findings from an international distance learning master's programme in public health. *Int Rev Res Open Dis*. 2014;15(1):182–202. doi:10.19173/irrodl.v15i1.1665.

46. Padilla M, Solórzano W, Pacheco V. Efectos del análisis de textos sobre la elaboración y justificación de preguntas de investigación. *Electro J Res Educ Psychol*. 2009; 17:77–102.

47. Narváez E. Escritura académica en un programa de formación en epidemiología: reflexiones sobre prácticas de enseñanza. *Revista de la Maestría en Salud Pública*. 2009;7(13):13.

48. Chois P, Hernández K, Arias A, Becerra J. Apoyar la escritura del proyecto de tesis en salud. *Magis, Revista Internacional de Investigación en Educación*. 2020;12(25):39–58. doi:10.11144/Javeriana.m12-25.aept

49. Bengtsson M. How to plan and perform a qualitative study using content analysis. *NursingPlus Open*. 2016;2:8–14.

50. Strauss A, Corbin J. *Bases de la Investigación Cualitativa. Técnicas y Procedimientos para Desarrollar la Teoría Fundamentada*. Medellín: Editorial Universidad de Antioquia; 2002.

51. Kerbrat-Orecchioni C. *Les Interactions Verbales: Approche Interactionnelle et Structure des Conversations*. Tome I. Troisiéme Èdition. Armand Colin. (Primera Edición francesa: 1990). Paris, France. 1998.

3

SUPPORTING MEDICAL WRITERS IN THE TWENTY-FIRST CENTURY

Rebecca Day Babcock, Jaanki Khandelwal, C. Erik Wilkinson, Chanaka Kahathuduwa, and Natalia Schlabritz-Loutsevitch

Humanity is balancing on the edge of the fourth and arguably most exciting industrial revolution.[1-3] This revolution is paralleled by the rapid development of biosensors and novel methods of diagnosing and treating patients. Patients and medical consumers need to be informed in order to benefit from these technologies. Thus, the global future is making it more and more important to communicate in English in all reputable medical information outlets. The writing done in the field of medicine, in particular, may become more challenging and require nonstandard approaches, accommodating students and professionals with varying levels of English language proficiency. (See Chapter 11 for insights into cultural competence.)

This chapter attempts to describe the challenges of supporting medical writers as they prepare their writing for publication, an important part of professional advancement and evidence-based practice.[4-6] We wanted to investigate the challenges that medical writers face and some possible supports to offer them. For data, we first provide an "environmental scan" of the extant literature, summarizing relevant studies. We then report our survey of journal editors and technical editors who work in a university medical writing center, medical students, residents, and faculty writers. Our conclusion offers recommendations to improve the writing process of both native and nonnative speakers for academic and professional writing in medicine. We emphasize that twenty-first-century medical communication requires technical literacy, English competency, and an ability to communicate in nontraditional ways.

Forms of Medical Writing Education and Support

While scanning the literature, we identified several key forms of medical writing education and support, which we summarize in the following sections. Some of the literature we summarize is specific to writing in medicine, and other literature is drawn from adjacent fields that can inform medical writing more generally.

Research/Writing Group (RWG). Fleming et al. described an RWG at the University of Mississippi intended to increase scholarly productivity and efficiency among pharmacy faculty.[7] Faculty members met for 1 hour per month, discussing their scholarly activity and assessing their own progress. The purpose was primarily to provide motivation, accountability, and interim deadlines rather than formal instruction on writing. The effectiveness of this model was quantified by comparing scholarly activity from participants in the RWG to a matched cohort of clinical faculty

DOI: 10.4324/9781003162940-5

not participating in the group. After the third year, scholarly activity in the RWG was greater than the comparison group in manuscripts and posters. In addition, participants strongly agreed that the RWG provided helpful feedback on their manuscripts, kept them accountable for their work, and kept them on task.

Writer's Circle. In a writer's circle, members exchange manuscripts, edit them online, and then meet for face-to-face discussion. Brandon et al. described the creation of a writer's circle to increase scholarly productivity by collegially revising previously rejected manuscripts and resubmitting them for publication.[8] The writer's circle consisted of five members who were clinical faculty in radiology for more than 6 years, and of these, two had training in writing and reviewing for academic journals. At the start of the study, each member had more than 20 publications, with a total number of 233. The group started with 10 previously rejected articles. After feedback from group members and resubmission, within 6 months after the start of the group, four of those articles were accepted and five were undergoing active revision. Data showed that participating in the writers' circle increased confidence and motivation, and the writers appreciated colleagues' support. (For a discussion of "teacherless writing groups," which resemble a writer's circle in some ways, see Chapter 14.)

Residential Retreat. Jackson described an innovative leadership strategy to help novice writers (clinical staff, faculty, and higher degree students) develop their skills in scholarly writing and submitting papers for publication. A residential retreat of 3 days and 2 nights was developed and run on three separate occasions.[9] After the first retreat, 16 papers were submitted to peer-reviewed journals and 15 were published. After the second retreat, 12 papers were submitted, 2 were accepted, and 10 were under review. After the third retreat, nine papers were submitted, and two book chapters were completed and submitted.

Andresen, Laursen, and Rosenberg conducted a study about writing biomedical journal articles and investigated the efficacy of using outlining and dictation to write articles. "The dictation usually takes place during a writing retreat, where all participants dictate their manuscripts in a 'disturbance free' environment."[10(p2)] Researchers conducted focus groups of three to six participants to find out how the writing retreat affected their writing processes. One participant explained that the "monk-like" atmosphere of the writing retreat enabled them to focus and be without distractions for the dictation. All of the participants were successful with the dictation process. Each of the participants involved in the study was Danish, and none were native speakers of English.

Franks[11] described a faculty program called Writers Block that supported writers with monthly meetings. Pharmacy faculty participated in the group that was designed to assist them with producing a manuscript for a peer-reviewed journal. Specific activities included setting goals and reporting on progress, group feedback and advice on papers, and discussing specific aspects of the writing and publishing process. The facilitator uploaded resources to a shared folder, scheduled guest speakers on relevant topics of interest, and suggested writing plans to meet the time line of the program. Participants were expected to complete a manuscript by the end of the program and were paid a small stipend for their time and participation.

Writing Courses. Keen explored the barriers to medical writing, along with resources to help academic and clinical nursing staff publish more.[6] Academic writing courses were identified as being helpful to the overall writing experience. The course focused on three central themes: confidence, writing, and publishing. The results of the course showed that formal education helped 65% of the students to be published within a year of course completion.

Rickard et al. described a Writing for Publication course, which was combined with a monthly writers' support group to increase publication rates.[12] The course included instruction on writing for publication, writing support and discussion among participants, focused writing time, and feedback from a consultant. Two-year pre- and post-submissions increased from 9 to 33 articles in peer-reviewed journals. Overall, publications per person increased from a baseline of 0.5–1.2 per year.

Barroga and Mitoma[13] developed a 3-week course to enhance critical thinking, logical reasoning, and communication skills in Japanese medical students writing in English. Students followed a 3-week research course in which they learned to identify a research topic; create a slide presentation on the topic featuring medical research; after receiving feedback, create educational materials based on the presentation; and, finally, present the materials. Students struggled most with discussing and understanding the material in English. They also were weak in presentation skills and revision practices. Strengths included adaptability and enthusiasm. The researchers recommended that medical educators develop better teaching approaches, help students to develop higher-order thinking skills, develop critical-thinking-oriented classes with an emphasis on research and publishing, use evidence-based teaching methods, and teach students a variety of learning methods and study skills.

Writing Workshops. Kramer and Libhaber described writing workshops that were set up at Wits Faculty of Health Sciences in South Africa.[14] Workshops centered on topics such as how to write an abstract, introduction, and discussion. Special annual workshops were also included to help critique articles that were introduced in previous workshops. Upon surveying the participants, assessment of the writing courses was positive, and many found the retreats helpful in decreasing anxiety regarding the difficulty of medical writing, viewing the course as being a "very helpful guide to this wilderness of writing."

Kulage and Larson described another faculty-based, peer-review manuscript writing workshop model.[15] The workshop focused on the peer review of manuscripts dealing with macrolevel issues, such as "clarity, organization, meaning, understanding, and flow"[15(p263)] rather than lower-level issues, such as grammar and punctuation. Sessions were 1 hour with 4 to 7 participants, including faculty members, postdoctoral fellows, and predoctoral students, all from nursing. The sessions took place over a semester with 7 live sessions, including one orientation and 8 hours of preparation time. Participants were offered tips for effective writing at the orientation session. The workshop sessions themselves were very structured with a manuscript assessment form used for focused attention. Post workshop, researchers surveyed participants to learn their satisfaction with the workshops. Participants rated the workshops, and their effectiveness was overwhelmingly positive. All but one of the 17 manuscripts that were workshopped were published or in the review process.

Hosseini and colleagues[16] conducted a writing workshop for physicians where they learned to create high-quality research proposals and to avoid plagiarism when writing in languages other than their native language, English in particular. In addition to education on plagiarism, including specific warnings, use of plagiarism detection software, sharing of knowledge, and efforts to improve academic writing skills, the authors suggested the use of a discussion forum moderated by a native English speaker where young authors could share ideas and get support. This was a descriptive article, so the authors did not provide evidence that the intervention worked. They did express reservations about the capability of the researchers to avoid plagiarism in the future since their reported self-efficacy with English was low.

Salamonson and colleagues[17] developed an approach to assisting low-to-medium English proficiency first-year nursing students by developing a 4-day writing workshop. Out of 106 students, 59 were randomized to attend the workshop, but only 28 attended. The control group was not scheduled to attend the workshop, which covered instruction on medical writing through feedback and written suggestions. Workshop attendees outperformed both the control group and nonattendees on the assessment measures of a wound-care essay and the final examination of a bioscience course.

Faculty Development Programs. Pololi, Knight, and Dunn described a writing and faculty development program, which consisted of seven monthly 25-minute sessions embedded in a collaborative mentoring program.[18] This was conducted twice over two academic years. The writing project helped students gain knowledge and skills in such areas as deciding authorship, identifying a topic and target audience, using strategies to overcome common barriers to writing, writing good lead-in paragraphs and abstracts, and deciding what should be included in each segment of a medical/scientific article. Participants of the first program published 16 manuscripts, while those in the second program published 11.

Franks[11] described a faculty program called "Writers Block" that supported writers with monthly meetings. Faculty participated in the group that was designed to assist them with producing a manuscript for a peer-reviewed journal. Specific activities included setting goals and reporting on progress, receiving group feedback and advice on papers, and discussing specific aspects of the writing and publishing process. The facilitator uploaded resources to a shared folder, scheduled guest speakers on relevant topics of interest, and suggested writing plans to meet the time line of the program. Participants were expected to complete a manuscript by the end of the program and were paid a small stipend for their time and participation. Participants were satisfied with the program. Out of 20 manuscripts, 12 were submitted, and out of the 12, 10 were accepted for publication, with 1 undergoing peer review. The participants also developed camaraderie and served as a support system for each other.

University Editing System. Barroga and Mitoma proposed a university editing system and writing program for medical writers. The system would consist of an editing system featuring online submission and expert editors and an educational component featuring internships, courses, lectures, seminars, mentoring, networking, and resources about topics in medical writing, predatory publishing, preparing and submitting articles, and similar topics.[19]

Barroga and Vardaman[20] proposed an educational program on biomedical writing, editing, and publishing in English for non-English speakers. The program activities included basics such as instruction on English grammar, writing style, and sentence structure and then went on to presentations, workshops, and lectures on biomedical writing such as the peer-review and submission process. Finally, the program covered topics related to publishing, internships, and statistics. The authors recommend that the participants in this program have experience with biomedical writing and the nomenclature of medical terminology. By the end of the program, "biomedical professionals, graduate students, and researchers [will] publish their papers in the best target journals indexed by MEDLINE, Scopus, and Web of Science with high impact factors (IFs)."[20(p1382)]

Use of Outside Writing and Editing Services. Marchington and Burd[21] surveyed 76 authors of medical articles about their attitudes toward professional medical writers who provide services to writers of industry-sponsored research. According to the survey results, the use of professional medical writers was deemed ethical following these guidelines: the professional medical writer (PMW) should be acknowledged. Failure to acknowledge the PMW is ghostwriting. Naming the PWD as the author is gift authorship.[21] Both of these are unethical practices according to the International Council of Medical Journal Editors.

Many of the previously described studies are small scale, with relatively low levels of evidence, and they generally pay little attention to the potential impacts of "new" media, which we had expected to find but did not. Thus, we believe that, while these studies are a useful foundation, there is much more work to be done in these areas.

Research Questions

Building on our scan of the literature, our survey questions were as follows.

- In our professional communities, what kinds of documents are medical writers producing?
- What kinds of support do medical writers believe they need?
- What is the writing process that medical writers go through, and what is the role of feedback and other input to that process?

Methods

In order to begin answering these questions, the research team developed a survey using Qualtrics software. The survey itself is made up of a combination of both Likert and free-text questions. Institutional Review Board (IRB) approval (exempt) was obtained from boards at the University of Texas at the Permian Basin (UTPB) and Texas Tech University Health Sciences Center (TTUHSC) (#2020-015 and #L20-159, respectively). We have included a copy of the survey in the Appendix.

Researchers sent the survey via email to students, residents, and faculty of TTUHSC and the UTPB nursing faculty and through relevant LISTSERVs such as WCenter for writing center professionals and the Consortium for Graduate Communication. To ensure consistency and fidelity to best practices, seminal works on survey research methods were consulted.[22,23]

Specifically, Cowles and Nelson assert,

> question content, design, and format serve as the fundamental elements in building and executing good surveys. Research has provided some guidance on best practices. For example, some general design and question order recommendations have emerged from research: (a) order questions from easy to difficult, (b) place general questions before specific questions, (c) do not place sensitive questions at the beginning of the survey, and (d) place demographics at the end of the questionnaire to prevent boredom and to engage the participant early in the survey.[22(p27)]

This project utilized purposive sampling, defined as a

> common nonprobability method. The researcher selects the sample based on judgment. This is usually an extension of convenience sampling. For example, a researcher may decide to draw the entire sample from one "representative" city, even though the population includes all cities. When using this method, the researcher must be confident that the chosen sample is truly representative of the entire population.[24]

In our case, we targeted those individuals in an academic environment likely to be involved in medical writing and publishing.

Data of participants who answered at least one question in the survey besides the demographic questions were included in the analyses. All statistical analyses were performed using the R statistical software (version 3.6.2). Means and standard deviations were computed for continuous variables, and the proportions and percentages were computed for categorical variables. Responses of native English speakers were compared with English as a second-language (ESL) participants. The continuous variables were compared in a series of students' t-tests applying Welch-Satterthwaite correction. Proportions were compared using chi-square tests of independence with the Yate's continuity correction.

Results

Ninety-three participants answered at least one question on the survey besides the demographic questions. English was the primary language in 77 of the respondents (English as a primary language [EPL]) (82.7%). The remaining 16 (17.3%) respondents reported ESL with their primary languages, including Spanish, German, Russian, Arabic, Gujarati, French, and Hindi. The sample characteristics are summarized in Table 3.1. There were no differences in the gender of participants in ESL and EPL groups.

When asked about their writing and editing experience, some people wrote about the genres they had written, and others answered with the amount or type of professional experience they had. Out of 93 who answered this question, some had more than one answer. A total of 42 people answered the question with some type of genre they were writing (abstracts, posters, research papers). For those who answered with a level of experience, it was about mixed, with 21 people having little experience, 12 having moderate experience, and 13 having extensive experience. Nine people had unconventional experience, such as being self-taught or participating in a health humanities session in New Jersey. As for the roles they assumed, 17 worked in writing support, such as editing or working in a writing center; 12 were reviewers for peer-reviewed journal articles; 7 were writing teachers; 4 were journal editors or on the editorial boards of journals; and 1 answer was not easily categorized ("I feel pretty comfortable").

The majority of respondents either published more than 4 manuscripts per year or had never published an article; this was similar in ESL and EPL groups. Both groups had experience with multiauthored papers, and the majority of the groups of coauthors comprised 2 to 4 members. The most important genres for career advancement were abstracts, journal articles, research proposals, IRB/QI protocols, and reviews. For the ESL group, grant proposals were more important for career advancement compared to the EPL group (Table 3.2). These data were in line with the publication types expected to be produced (Table 3.3).

TABLE 3.1 Characteristics of the survey respondents

Variable	Overall[a] (n = 93)	EPL[a] (n = 77)	ESL[b] (n = 16)	Statistic[b]	P-value
Age (years)	42.96 ± 16.08	43.47 ± 16.78	40.50 ± 12.36	−0.817 (28.047)	0.421
Sex				0.161 (1)	0.689
Male	51 (54.8%)	41 (53.2%)	10 (62.5%)		
Female	42 (45.2%)	36 (46.8%)	6 (37.5%)		
Profession				12.989 (3)	0.005
Medical faculty	41 (44.1%)	36 (46.7%)	5 (31.2%)		
Medical students	19 (20.4%)	18 (23.4%)	1 (6.2%)		
Medical residents	21 (22.6%)	12 (15.6%)	9 (56.2%)		
Medical writing staff	12 (12.9%)	11 (14.3%)	1 (6.2%)		
Education				10.422(4)	0.034
Bachelor's	13 (14.0%)	12 (15.6%)	1 (6.2%)		
Master's	11 (11.8%)	11 (14.3%)	0 (0.0%)		
PhD	13 (14.0%)	12 (15.6%)	1 (6.2%)		
MD/DO	48 (51.6%)	38 (49.3%)	10 (62.5%)		
MD, PhD	8 (8.6%)	4 (5.2%)	4 (25.00%)		

a Mean ± SD for continuous variables, n (%) for categorical variables

b T-statistic (df) derived from students' t-tests with Welch-Satterthwaite correction for continuous variables, chi-square statistic (df) with Yate's continuity correction for categorical variables

EPL – English as a primary language, ESL – English as a secondary language

TABLE 3.2 Experience of the respondents with medical writing

Variable	Overall[a]	EPL[a]	ESL[a]	Statistic[b]	P-value
Number of articles published (n = 92; English = 76; ESL = 16)				3.475 (4)	0.482
0	22 (23.9%)	20 (26.3%)	2 (12.5%)		
1	5 (5.4%)	3 (3.9%)	2 (12.5%)		
2	10 (10.9%)	8 (10.5%)	2 (12.5%)		
3	10 (10.9%)	9 (11.8%)	1 (6.2%)		
≥ 4	45 (48.9%)	36 (47.4%)	9 (56.2%)		
Number of coauthors on average (n = 75; EPL = 60; ESL = 15)				6.336 (3)	0.096
1	2 (2.7%)	2 (3.3%)	0 (0.0%)		
2–4	52 (69.3%)	45 (75.0%)	7 (46.7%)		
5–7	14 (18.7%)	9 ((15.0%)	5 (33.3%)		
≥ 8	7 (9.3%)	4 (6.7%)	3 (20%)		
Format of work (n = 74; EPL = 60; ESL = 14)				0.878 (2)	0.645
Print	9 (12.2%)	8 (13.3%)	1 (7.1%)		
Online	20 (27.0%)	15 (25.0%)	5 (35.7%)		
Both	45 (60.8%)	37 (61.7%)	8 (57.2%)		
Perceived importance for career (n = 73; EPL = 59; ESL = 14)					
Abstracts	6.16 ± 3.09	6.21 ± 30.3	5.93 ± 3.41	0.285 (18.204)	0.779
Journal articles	6.16 ± 3.09	6.21 ± 30.3	5.93 ± 3.41	0.285 (18.204)	0.779
Blog posts	2.12 ± 2.07	1.94 ± 2.01	2.85 ± 2.23	−1.332 (17.222)	0.200
Patient communications	4.77 ± 3.48	4.36 ± 3.37	6.46 ± 3.55	−1.933 (17.688)	0.0694
Research proposals	6.57 ± 2.87	6.30 ± 2.90	7.77 ± 2.52	−1.833 (20.073)	0.082
IRB/QI protocols	6.10 ± 2.97	5.91 ± 3.06	6.92 ± 2.53	−1.247 (20.836)	0.226
Grant proposals	6.04 ± 3.22	5.48 ± 3.27	8.38 ± 1.56	−4.681 (40.686)	<0.001
Pamphlets	2.77 ± 2.47	2.52 ± 2.24	3.77 ± 3.11	−1.358 (15.388)	0.194
Booklets	2.59 ± 2.44	2.36 ± 2.17	3.46 ± 3.23	−1.163 (14.941)	0.263
Editorials	4.17 ± 3.07	3.83 ± 3.09	5.54 ± 2.73	−1.970 (20.267)	0.063
Reviews	5.49 ± 2.87	5.30 ± 3.00	6.31 ± 2.10	−1.421 (24.909)	0.168
Proceeding papers	3.81 ± 2.94	3.61 ± 2.97	4.67 ± 2.77	−1.174 (17.439)	0.256
Catalogues	2.07 ± 2.10	2.04 ± 2.13	2.08 ± 2.17	−0.185 (17.257)	0.855
Encyclopedias	2.80 ± 2.80	2.50 ± 2.60	4.00 ± 3.36	−1.443 (14.473)	0.170

a Mean ± SD for continuous variables, n (%) for categorical variables
b T-statistic (df) derived from students' t-tests with Welch-Satterthwaite correction for continuous variables, chi-square statistic (df) with Yate's continuity correction for categorical variables
EPL – English as a primary language, ESL – English as a secondary language

Finally, a majority of participants (over 90%) felt that editing and statistical services are beneficial (Table 3.4).

Out of the 37 people who answered Question 17 ("If you had the opportunity to have technology-specific training for medical writing [e.g., AI, crowdsourcing, etc.] what would it be?"), nine would like training on artificial intelligence, six would like general training on all the platforms we mentioned in Questions 14 and 15 or to have someone "walking them through for the first time." Another five people wanted training on crowdsourcing. Five did not know what kinds of training they needed. Three wanted training on editing. Two wanted training on statistics. One each listed specific things they wanted training on like "grant proposals," "[L]atex," "reference managers software," and "fundraising."

TABLE 3.3 Types of documents the respondents are expected to produce

Document	Number of Participants (%)[a]
Abstracts	65 (84.4)
Journal articles	61 (79.2)
Blog posts	8 (10.4)
Patient communications	24 (31.2)
Popular articles/editorials	14 (18.2)
Research proposals	47 (61.0)
IRB/QI protocols	43 (55.8)
Grant proposals	32 (41.6)
Pamphlets	10 (13.0)
Booklets	5 (6.5)
Editorials	17 (22.1)
Reviews	34 (44.2)
Proceeding papers	8 (10.4)
Catalogues	2 (2.6)
Encyclopedias	3 (3.9)
Other	11 (14.3)

a Percentages are expressed from the number of participants who responded (N = 77)

TABLE 3.4 Types of writing support preferred by faculty, residents, and students

Type of Support (Please Refer to the Questionnaire)	n (%)
1. One-on-one tutorial	37 (60.6)
2. Editing services	55 (90.2)
3. Statistical services	55 (90.2)
4. Writing retreats and boot camps	17 (27.9)
5. Ghostwriting	6 (9.8)
6. Grants	32 (52.5)
7. Computer spelling and grammar checkers	29 (47.5)
8. Bibliographic assistance (library)	43 (70.5)
9. Training on the new collaborative publishing platforms	38 (62.3)
10. Other	1 (1.6)

Discussion

Information ecology around health care is changing such that (a) patients can get information without guidance and (b) as a result, medical writers and communicators have to be particularly more careful with methods of writing and communication. ESL writers are also a rapidly growing community in the world of global communication and as such need special support.

The results presented here clearly demonstrate future targets of education for medical writers, such as writing groups and courses for students, residents, and faculty members new to publishing, especially non-native English speakers. The focus should be on abstracts, journal articles, and research proposals, as these are the most commonly required genres in our data. Medical writers in our study almost unanimously desire editing and statistical services. A high percentage also want library support, training on new publishing platforms, and one-on-one tutorials.

While our study demonstrated no differences between EPL and ESL writers, there are specifics that should be taken into consideration in the education of ESL writers. Our findings support those of Kostenko and Soloho,[25] who emphasized that "writing in genres other than original research articles seems to be quite demanding and is often associated with the lack of self-confidence and language anxiety."

Implications for Practice

As we wrote in the intro, twenty-first-century medical communication requires technical literacy, English competency, and the ability to communicate. Our conclusion includes recommendations to improve the writing process of both native and non-native speakers for academic and professional writing in medicine. Based on our findings and previous studies, offering classes,[6] retreats,[9] or workshops[14] that set aside dedicated time for writing would be helpful. These classes could focus on providing participants with the knowledge that many felt they lacked, including challenges with editing and grammar and how to properly compose a research paper. Information or classes could also be offered to help participants navigate how to get their work published; widely offered and easily accessible ones would be the most beneficial.

Libraries/librarians could be a great resource for organizing this information and redirecting people to places where information on how to use these resources is available. Surprisingly enough, the second most needed and requested service was bibliographic/library assistance. Since academic and public libraries already offer these services, the need or suggestion would be for them to do more with outreach and promotion.

Some other treatments we might suggest are writing groups, retreats, and boot camps, although only 28% of respondents said they were interested in such things. We feel perhaps they fear that these events will take up too much of their precious time. This may also help participants overcome psychological anxieties and stressors associated with writing, as dedicated time often helps overcome issues with motivation. Since the #1 most requested services are editing and statistical services, institutions may investigate offering these services, without charge, to both students and faculty.[19] As it is now, most people will have to pay for these services. Other suggestions are for faculty and students to form writers' circles,[8] RWGs,[7] or a collaborative mentoring program[18] Kostenko and Soloho[25] suggested that in order to support second-language medical writers of English, we should "focus on the basic elements of academic writing, characteristics of written genres across the disciplines, providing a framework in which expert and practical knowledge is internally organized." Regarding systematic reviews and meta-analyses,[26] a number of students, residents, and faculty members who responded to our survey were unaware of the writing support services available to them.

Many health science libraries help with comprehensive literature searches. Including a librarian means that an author has a competent helper throughout the entire process—covering the areas of planning a strategy, navigating the myriad databases and other resources, and reporting the results. Libraries can even help authors choose a publication venue. A number of institutions also provide writing centers, which can help review a manuscript for syntax, grammar, and formatting in addition to organization and content—many of the issues that our survey respondents, who are writing in health professions, wanted assistance with (see Chapters 6, 9, and 10 for models of collaboration with writing centers; Chapter 9 additionally covers "information literacy."). Future studies should explore additional forms of support in "writing in the health professions," an emergent interdiscipline.

Acknowledgments

The authors wish to acknowledge the help of students, faculty, and residents of TTUHSC and UTPB in the completion of this survey and participation in this research. Special thanks to Karen Douglas (TTUHSC) for her guidance in human subject protection questions. The authors are grateful to Mikayla Rodriguez for her contribution to the manuscript editing. The writers also acknowledge each other for their support, contributions, and collegiality through a difficult year.

Appendix: Our Survey

Q1   Before we start the main survey questions, we would first like to ask you a few questions about yourself. Please note that these questions will not be connected with your identity in any way, but they will help us get a broad sense of the different types of people who are participating in this research.

   Age:
   Gender:
   Race/ethnicity:
   Geographic location (country, state, county, city):
   List all degrees held and majors:
   First language:
   Please list any other languages:

Q2   As you already know, our survey is specifically interested in understanding various medical professionals and those who work with medical professionals, and how they are trained in media writing and editing. With this in mind, which of the below categories best represents your current position?

   Medical faculty
   Medical student
   Medical resident
   Medical writing support staff (examples in this category include journal editor, writing center tutor who works with medical students in a medical school writing center or regular writing center, medical copyeditor; PMW, etc.)

Q3   In the space below, please explain in two or three sentences what your primary medical writing and editing experience is.

Q4   How many articles or abstracts have you published (or assisted with that were published) in the last 5 years?

   0
   1
   2
   3
   4+

Q5   Regarding the manuscripts you coauthored, how many authors, on average, were involved?

   1
   2–4
   5–7
   8+

   Thanks for those answers. Now, we'd like to start with some rather broad questions, just to get you thinking more about medical writing and editing. Based on your experience, could you tell us in your own words…

Q6   What are the main writing and editing challenges facing people in your position?

Q7   In your work, what types of documents are you expected to produce/help with producing? Please check all that apply.

   Abstracts
   Journal articles
   Blog posts and/or commenting on blogs
   Patient communications
   Popular articles/editorials

Research proposals
IRB/QI protocols
Grant proposals
Pamphlets
Booklets
Editorials
Reviews
Proceedings papers
Catalogues
Encyclopedia articles
Other

Q8   What format does the majority of your work take on?
Print
Online
Both

Q9   Of these types of documents, how would you rate the importance of each type for your own personal career advancement? Please rate each one on a scale of "1" for "not at all important" to "10" for "extremely important."
Abstracts
Journal articles
Blog posts and/or commenting on blogs
Patient communications
Popular articles/editorials
Research proposals
IRB/QI protocols
Grant proposals
Pamphlets
Booklets
Editorials
Reviews
Proceedings paper
Catalogues
Encyclopedia articles

Q10 For academic publishing, how familiar are you with the following publication indices? Please indicate on a scale of "1" for "not at all familiar" to "10" for "extremely familiar."
Altmetrics
Eigen factor
Hirsh index
Google Scholar metric
SC Imago journal rank indicator
Immediacy index
Scientometrics
Journal impact factor

We are particularly interested in how medical writing and editing have changed with newer technologies. Our next questions will focus on the influence of technology on media writing and editing.

Q11   First, please review the different ways that medical writing is published today—many of these represent new genres of medical writing made possible by communication technologies and novel communication platforms. Of those below, please check each of the response options that apply with respect to your personal experience.

Possible response options:

    1. I was trained formally on how to use this platform for medical writing.

    2. I was socialized informally on how to use this platform for medical writing.

    3. I have read medical writing using this platform.

    4. I have shared medical writing using this platform with others.

    5. I have published medical writing on this platform.

    6. I generally respect the medical writing that I have seen on this platform.

Facebook

Twitter

Reddit

Podcasts

Online journal clubs

Wikis

E-books

Infographics

Video abstracts

Newsrooms

YouTube

Blogs

Personal websites

Webinars

Other

Q12   Which communication platform(s) do you personally use for medical writing and editing (check all that apply)?

Reddit

Facebook

Twitter

Skype

Zoom

EasyChair

Email

Dropbox

Others (specify)

Q13   Thinking about the technologies listed above, how would you say that new communication platforms have impacted the medical writing and editing process?

1 = Strongly disagree 2 = Disagree 3 = Slightly disagree 4 = Neither disagree nor agree 5 = Slightly agree 6 = Agree 7 = Strongly agree

Facebook

Twitter

Reddit

Podcasts

Online journal clubs

Wikis

E-books
Infographics
Video abstracts
Newsrooms
YouTube
Blogs
Personal websites
Webinars
Other

Q14 Per the choices below, how would you say that new communication platforms have impacted the medical writing and editing process?
1. These technologies have improved medical writing.
2. These technologies have made medical writing worse.
3. These technologies made medical writing unnecessary.
4. These technologies have allowed medical writing to be produced much more quickly.
5. These technologies have allowed for a diverse set of voices in medical writing.
6. These technologies created new genres.
7. These technologies are difficult to use for the purpose of medical writing.
   Reddit
   Facebook
   Twitter
   Skype
   Zoom
   EasyChair
   Email
   Dropbox
   Others (please specify)

Q15 How familiar you are with following collaborative writing platforms?
1. Never heard about it
2. Read about it
3. Read articles, produced by these platforms
4. Have used once or twice
5. Using it all the time
   Google Drive/Docs
   LaTex
   Overleaf
   Fidus Writer
   Authorea
   ShareLaTeX
   Git/Manubot
   Other

We're almost finished! Here, we would like to ask you a bit more about the types of support that medical writers need, especially as a way to cope with newer forms of medical publishing (such as through those technologies mentioned above).

Q16 What kinds of writing support do medical writers need (please choose all that apply)?
   One-on-one tutorial
   Editing services

     Statistical services

     Writing retreats and boot camps

     Ghostwriting

     Grants

     Computer spelling and grammar checkers

     Bibliographic assistance (Library)

     Training on the new collaborative publishing platforms.

     Other

Q17 If you had the opportunity to have technology-specific training for medical writing (e.g., AI, crowdsourcing, etc.) what would it be?

Q18 Thank you for your participation in this important survey! If you would like to be entered in a drawing for a Starbucks gift card, please provide your phone number and email address below.

References

1. Lee M, Yoon Y, Ryu GH, et al. Innovative distribution priorities for the medical devices industry in the fourth industrial revolution. *Int Neurourol J* 2018;22(Suppl 2):S83–S90.
2. Morgan J. *What is the fourth industrial revolution?* Forbes website. https://www.forbes.com/sites/jacobmorgan/2016/02/19/what-is-the-4th-industrial-revolution/?sh=3a41b6b2f392. February 19, 2016. Accessed January 31, 2021.
3. Kaku M. *The Future of Humanity.* New York, NY: Doubleday; 2018.
4. Schimanski LA, Alperin JP. The evaluation of scholarship in academic promotion and tenure processes: past, present and future. *F1000Research.* 2018;7:1605.
5. Niles MT, Schimanski LA, McKiernan EC, Alperin JP. Why we publish where we do: faculty publishing values and their relationship to review, promotion and tenure expectations. *PloS one.* 2020;15(3):e0228914.
6. Keen A. Writing for publication: pressures, barriers and support strategies. *Nurse Educ Today.* 2007;27(5):382–388.
7. Fleming LW, Malinowski SS, Fleming JW, Brown MA, Davis CS, Hogan S. The impact of participation in a research/writing group on scholarly pursuits by non-tenure track clinical faculty. *Curr Pharm Teach Learn.* 2017;9(3):486–490.
8. Brandon C, Jamadar D, Girish G, Dong Q, Morag Y, Mullan P. Peer support of a faculty "writers' circle" increases confidence and productivity in generating scholarship. *Acad Radiol.* 2015;22(4):534–538.
9. Jackson D. Mentored residential writing retreats: a leadership strategy to develop skills and generate outcomes in writing for publication. *Nurse Educ Today.* 2009;29(1):9–15.
10. Andresen K, Laursen J, Rosenberg J. Outlining and dictating scientific manuscripts is a useful method for health researchers: a focus group interview. *SAGE Open Med.* 2018;6:2050312118778728.
11. Franks AM. Design and evaluation of a longitudinal faculty development program to advance scholarly writing among pharmacy practice faculty. *Am J Pharm Educ.* 2018;82(6):6556–6556.
12. Rickard CM, McGrail MR, Jones R, et al. Supporting academic publication: evaluation of a writing course combined with writers' support group. *Nurse Educ Today.* 2009;29(5):516–521.
13. Barroga E, Mitoma H. Critical thinking and scientific writing skills of non-anglophone medical students: a model of training course. *J Korean Med Sci.* 2019;34(3):e18–e18.
14. Kramer B, Libhaber E. Writing for publication: institutional support provides an enabling environment. *BMC Med Educ.* 2016;16:115–115.
15. Kulage KM, Larson EL. Implementation and outcomes of a faculty-based, peer review manuscript writing workshop. *J Prof Nurs.* 2016;32(4):262–270.
16. Hosseini MJ, Bazargani R, Latiff L, Hanachi P, Hassan STS, Othman M. Medical researchers in non-English countries and concerns about unintentional plagiarism. *J Med Ethics Hist Med.* 2009;2:14–14.

17. Salamonson Y, Koch J, Weaver R, Everett B, Jackson D. Embedded academic writing support for nursing students with English as a second language. *J Adv Nurs.* 2010;66(2):413–421.

18. Pololi L, Knight S, Dunn K. Facilitating scholarly writing in academic medicine. *J Gen Intern Med.* 2004;19(1):64–68.

19. Barroga E, Mitoma H. Improving scientific writing skills and publishing capacity by developing university-based editing system and writing programs. *J Korean Med Sci.* 2018;34(1):e9–e9.

20. Barroga E, Vardaman, M. Essential components of educational programs on biomedical writing, editing, and publishing. *J Korean Med Sci.* 2015;30:1381–1387.

21. Marchington JM, Burd GP. Author attitudes to professional medical writing support. *Cur Med Res Opin.* 2014;30(10):2103–2108.

22. Cowles EL, Nelson, E. *An Introduction to Survey Research.* New York, NY: Business Expert Press; 2015.

23. Fowler FJ. *Survey Research Methods.* London, UK: SAGE; 2014.

24. Kothari CR, Gaurav G. *Research Methodology: Methods and Techniques.* New Delhi, India: New Age International (P) Limited Publishers; 2019.

25. Kostenko VG, Solohor IM. How to incorporate academic writing pedagogy in undergraduate and postgraduate medical education. *Wiad Lek.* 2018;71(2 pt 2):261–265.

26. Libraries at Texas Tech University Health Sciences Center. *Systematic Reviews and Meta-Analysis: Tips for Getting started.* Libraries at Texas Tech University Health Sciences Center. https://ttuhsc.libguides.com/systematic-reviews January 14, 2020. Accessed January 31, 2021.

PART II
Writing in Nursing

4

DEVELOPING STUDENTS' PROFESSIONAL IDENTITY THROUGH WRITING AND PEER REVIEW

Barbara J. D'Angelo and Barry M. Maid

Writing and communication are key components of the health professions. Nurses, in particular, work in interdisciplinary teams of varying expertise and training, whether the setting be clinical (such as hospitals, hospices, urgent care) or other types of organizations (home health, pharmacy, insurance, research lab, etc.). Recognition of the interdisciplinary nature of health-care practice, and the importance of "writing in the health professions," led to the collaborative development of two required writing courses for multiple health-care degree programs at Arizona State University (ASU). One, TWC361 Writing for Healthcare Management, was developed specifically for the RN-BSN online degree and on which we focus specifically for this chapter; the other was developed for undergraduate majors in a variety of other health science degree programs. Collaboration to develop and redesign the nursing course included faculty from the Technical Communication (TC) Program in the College of Integrative Sciences and Arts (CISA) and faculty from the RN-BSN degree program in the Edson College of Nursing and Health Innovation.

TWC361 is an online 7.5-week course taught in several sections per semester by multiple writing instructors; it is the required first course taken by newly admitted students in the RN-BSN Program. It emphasizes process pedagogy, critical thinking, and metacognition (reflection to promote teaching for transfer [TFT]) to engage students in writing experiences that develop an awareness of their professional identity as health-care professionals. One component of the course is the integration of a comprehensive and structured peer review process that emphasizes the development of skills related to giving, receiving, and using constructive feedback. The goals are multifaceted. In addition to helping students improve their writing, the peer-review process helps students to develop their ability to effectively collaborate and communicate within diverse groups and to develop critical thinking and metacognitive skills. As such, we are able to incorporate pedagogy that effectively addresses writing outcomes within a professional context, outcomes that align with accreditation criteria for nursing, and outcomes for intraprofessional practice.

Previously in Stevens et al.[1] and D'Angelo and Maid,[2] we described the original development of TWC361. In addition, we shared the results of the assessment of the course. In this chapter, we focus more specifically on the dynamics and challenges of redesigning the course within institutional constraints. The redesign was conducted within the paradigm of contextually driven institutional change within the two programs.

Commonly, narratives about curriculum change describe the exigence, the concept, and the process to develop the new curriculum. Then they often conclude with a presentation of assessment

DOI: 10.4324/9781003162940-7

data to evaluate the change. However, this chapter does not do that, as it is a report on a very different problem that fits more appropriately into the framework of institutional ethnography. While the report chronicled here is about curriculum change, the revision occurred primarily as a function of institutional/administrative changes that required the course to be redone. The idea of institutional/administrative contexts driving curriculum reform is a common theme in writing program administration scholarship. In these situations, the changes create a problem to be solved, ideally by still using the best disciplinary and pedagogical theories and practice. In the best of worlds, those changes would then still be assessed in a way that would produce data to be reported. However, in many cases, and this is one of them, the very institutional/administrative changes that initiated the revision work against the creation of an appropriate assessment system that produces quantitative data. Therefore, what we present here is our best solution to the problem within the realities of the new institutional constraints and within the theoretical framework of institutional ethnography, a qualitative methodology that attempts to uncover and make explicit the work of individuals in negotiating the everyday contexts of their workplace environment.

Literature Review

The redesign of TWC361 was informed by multiple branches of literature that converge to frame the theoretical underpinnings for the course. In this section, we will define institutional ethnography; we will also contextualize the literature related to writing within the discipline of nursing, the use of peer review in writing courses, and the concepts of transfer and threshold concepts.

Institutional Ethnography

Institutional ethnography (IE) as originally defined by the Canadian sociologist Dorothy Smith,[3] challenged the role of empirical models of social science research and developed a theoretical framework that focuses on peoples' work—work that is situated within an organizational context. IE allows individuals to understand how things come to happen as "people participate in social relations, often unknowingly; as they act competently and knowledgeably to concert and coordinate their own actions with professional standards."[4(p31)] Michelle LaFrance[5] has conceptualized IE for the field of writing studies, a field that is highly contextualized within and mediated by the organizational structures within which they exist. According to LaFrance, IE offers writing studies professionals the means to identify and understand the types of negotiation and coordination they do with others within their specific context to better comprehend how writing, writing instruction, and writers are shaped by their institutional context and culture. As such, IE is an ideal methodology for inquiry and understanding the relationships between locations and practices of writing. When articulating the work of different disciplines to negotiate curriculum design for a subject-based writing course (such as TWC361), IE is perhaps even more relevant as it facilitates understanding not only of the work done within the institution but also lays bare the professional identities, policies, and best practices to find common ground and achieve the desired outcome.

Writing in Nursing

Clear and effective written, verbal, and nonverbal communication using current and emerging technologies is an essential competency for nurses for the delivery of high-quality and safe patient care.[6] The American Association of Colleges of Nursing[7] identifies writing as a requisite skill for nursing practice. Written communication is important to academic and scholarly discourse to disseminate knowledge within the nursing community. In addition, to meet the growing need for patient care, nurses became increasingly responsible for providing care following the implementation of the

Affordable Care Act (ACA). This resulted in a need to increasingly work collaboratively on inter-disciplinary teams in which nurses communicate with other care providers (physicians, therapists, etc.) for improved health-care outcomes. As a result, employers began expecting a higher level of education; a BSN has become the standard entry into nursing practice, replacing the more tradi-tional route of an RN with an associate's degree.

BSN degree programs have used several strategies to facilitate student writing competence. These strategies include writing (or writing-research intensive) courses, writing tutorials as part of professional development (extracurricular), and collaborations with writing centers.[8-14] Further, metacognition and process pedagogy, common strategies in writing studies, have also been utilized in nursing courses in the context of writing. For example, Sasa[9] reported on a structured writ-ing assignment in which students composed low-stakes weekly reflections and a high-stakes case report using process pedagogy (scaffolded assignments based on the nursing process framework). Further, Rohan and Fullerton[10] instituted a Writing Tutor Round Table program as part of a writ-ing quality improvement project in which writing center tutors worked with groups of three to four doctor of nursing practice students who would go on to serve as clinical leaders and educators. (Collaborations with writing centers are featured in Chapters 6, 9, and 10.)

The nursing literature often refers to the concept of writing self-efficacy, which is deemed to contribute to a student's sense of agency as a writer and, theoretically, leads to improvement in learning outcomes related to it. This identification of self-efficacy aligns conceptually with the concept of *writing to learn* within the field of writing studies, which is a frequently used strategy in courses focused on "writing in the disciplines." As Fulwieler and Young[11(px)] explain, "Language pro-vides us with a unique way of knowing and becomes a tool for discovering, for shaping meaning, and for reaching understanding." It makes sense, then, that self-efficacy is increased when writing is used as a tool to enhance learning in the classroom: the more students use writing to learn, the more confident they become not only in their subject expertise but also in their writing (and in their agency as writers). In several studies, Miller et al.[12-14] explored writing self-efficacy in short-term contexts. Mitchell [15] also explored and assessed writing self-efficacy longitudinally across the nursing curriculum at their institution by examining one assignment from each year in the program and found that writing self-efficacy increased across the curriculum.

Process Pedagogy

Process pedagogy is widely accepted within the field of writing studies as the most effective ped-agogical approach for helping individuals improve their writing. Process pedagogy structures a course with small tasks, drafts, reviews, and revisions leading to a final product. The cycle of drafts-reviews-revisions is essential for writers of all experience levels. Indeed, one of the primary differ-ences between novice and experienced writers, as Flower and Hayes[16] note, is the amount and level of attention to process, both *whether* they revise and *how* they revise. In addition, no one intuitively knows how to give feedback; writers must learn the strategies that lead to giving it rhetorically—that is, to understand the context within which it is being given and to whom. In the classroom, that context is the assignment and grading criteria in addition to assignment and course outcomes. As Wiggins 2012[17] articulates, there are seven keys to effective feedback: it is goal-oriented, tangible and transparent, actionable, user-friendly (or understandable), timely, ongoing, and consistent. In addition, for revision to be effective, individuals must engage in deep revision; that is, they engage in metacognition—or reflection—to understand the feedback that they receive by reading it thor-oughly and making decisions about its usefulness. Just as giving feedback is rhetorical, so too is revi-sion. Revision takes place within a context: the goals, audience, and environment for the writing; it is not simply about proofreading to fix mechanical issues or typos.

Novice writers, however, do not approach this process intuitively nor with the language or experience needed to provide effective and constructive feedback to others. Nor do they intuitively know what to do with feedback received in order to improve their own work. One task for instructors, then, is to help students to learn the language needed to effectively provide feedback and, in turn, use it. Indeed, as Hattie and Timperley[18] explain, feedback on tasks and how to improve have more impact on student learning than do praise, rewards, or punishment. A curriculum that facilitates student engagement in process pedagogy through multiple small tasks in which students are asked to give guided and structured feedback and then develop revision plans facilitates learning on multiple levels: improvement in writing, engagement with their learning, engagement with one another, and learning the language, strategies, and moves needed to make learning transferrable to other contexts.

Process pedagogy can be integrated into a learning management system; both Canvas and Blackboard, for example, have "peer-review" functionality (depending on institutional settings). Further, a discussion board can serve as a means of conducting peer reviews. However, the structure and intended functions within these systems limit their capacity to do so effectively, as they are rarely (if ever) grounded in writing studies research or theory. In their collection, *Foundational Practices of Online Writing Instruction*, Hewett and dePew[19] present a solid introduction to teaching in online environments, including learning management systems. In addition, peer-review software such as Eli Review (www.elireview.com) was created by writing studies experts based on the fields' research, theory, and best practice to support peer learning environments using evidence-based teaching practices. Eli bolsters peer review and revision planning by providing a framework in which students engage with one another (anonymously) to first provide feedback and to then develop revision plans based upon it.

Importantly, the framework for reviews is created by the course instructor based on the assignment criteria and purpose so that students work through a structured rhetorical process. As such, they may be asked to make decisions on specific traits, rate aspects of a draft (and potentially comment on the reasoning for the rating), provide contextual comments, and final comments. A key to feedback is the emphasis on a heuristic for providing the contextual and overall comments: describe-evaluate-suggest. This heuristic teaches individuals how to provide feedback constructively by paraphrasing what was written (*describe*), assess it based on criteria (*evaluate*), and then making targeted specific suggestions for improvement (*suggest*). Similarly, after receiving feedback, revision plans are guided by a heuristic of select-prioritize-reflect, so students need to read and reflect on the feedback they received before implementing it. Eli, then, meets the seven characteristics that Wiggins identifies as effective feedback. Using this strategy, individuals are stepped through the metacognitive process of choosing which feedback to use (*select*) based on whether it effectively helps them to meet the goals of the assignment, place it in ranked order (*prioritize*, a sort of triage), and then *reflect* on what they will do to revise, how, and why.

TFT and Threshold Concepts

One of the recurring themes in writing studies' literature is the topic of transfer, which is also discussed in Chapter 5. Simply put, the question arises whether students can not only learn something in one class, typically First-Year Writing, but also carry those skills and knowledge with them and be proficient in another course. It is common, and has been so historically, for students to do well in First-Year Writing and then have problems with writing in other courses—especially advanced discipline-based courses. It has also been historically common for students who have taken a disciplinary-based, upper-level writing course, such as business or technical communication, and then demonstrate difficulty in transferring those skills in other discipline-based courses.

There are multiple reasons for the problems associated with transfer. However, over the last decade, two different but related areas of research in writing studies speak to the specific problem of teaching and curriculum design to facilitate student transfer of learning to other venues (courses or workplace). Yancey et al. in *Writing across Contexts*[20] report on their study to create what they call a TFT curriculum for First-Year Writing. Drawing on Yancey's previous work on "reflective transfer" in *Reflection in the Writing Classroom*,[21] the three researchers incorporate a strong emphasis on reflection/metacognition. They then demonstrate that their TFT curriculum does indeed support transfer in students.

Related to transfer, but looking at it from a different perspective, is the idea of threshold concepts (more fully reviewed in Chapter 7). In the edited collection *Naming What We Know*,[22] writing studies scholars defined for the first time possible threshold concepts for writing studies. This text has become foundational to the discipline as it relates to the concept of transfer of learning. Similarly, the identification of threshold concepts is being applied pedagogically and in research on disciplinary teaching, learning, and practice in nursing. For example, McAllister et al.[23] identified threshold concepts for nursing using a review of the nursing literature. However, the rigor of their and others' approaches has been questioned, as they did not clearly link or articulate their research or process to identify them, as Crookes et al.[24] note. Martindale's[25] dissertation (which was supervised by Ray Land) utilizes the threshold concept theoretical framework for her study on nursing student education in the United Kingdom within the context of learning evidence-based practice and research. While she does not identify threshold concepts specifically, she does identify five themes utilizing the threshold concepts framework. Threshold concepts, then, are familiar to nursing as a field and as a pedagogical underpinning, as they are in writing studies.

Institutional Context and Initial Course Development

Since IE situates the work individuals do within the context of the individual workplace, it is important to articulate the context in which the redesign of TWC361 took place. ASU is a Research I university with four physical campuses in the metropolitan Phoenix area, several satellite locations around the globe, and a large online presence through an entity known as ASU Online. The initiative discussed in this chapter was developed through the collaboration of two of the ASU Online degree programs: the TC Program in CISA and the RN-BSN Program in Edson College of Nursing and Healthcare Innovation (CONHI).

In 2010, RN-BSN faculty approached the TC Program about creating a required writing course for their degree program, which they were moving from hybrid delivery to become fully online. We have described the collaboration that led to the design and development of the course elsewhere,[1] as well as how the course met outcomes and objectives.[2] The highly collaborative development resulted in an online professional writing course, TWC361 Writing for Healthcare Management, blended outcomes from both disciplines (writing and nursing), addressed writing contexts that nursing students would potentially encounter in health-care workplaces, and placed significant emphasis on process and reflection. RN-BSN students take the writing course as the first in the degree program; therefore, we were cognizant of the need to facilitate students' sense of disciplinary identity as professional nurses and the role of writing in that process. Students may take First-Year Writing prior to other disciplinary courses; however, it is structured within curricula as a general education course. It is rare for disciplines to structure a degree program with a required course taught through and by another degree program. If we contextualize our work through the lens of IE, the placement of the course as the first and required in the degree is an indicator of success, as we negotiated disciplinary similarities and differences in terms of reaching a mutual understanding of the definition of writing and goals for the course in the context of disciplinary standards and practices for both nursing and writing studies.

One of the more successful aspects of the initial design of the course was a writing assignment during the first week. The assignment asked students to analyze and reflect on the role of writing as a "hallmark of professionalism" for nurses, building on the week's readings and videos. The intent was to help students to immediately engage with the course, to facilitate an understanding of how writing and communication develops professional ethos, and to show how discourse is part of disciplinary practice and varies based on audience. In an end-of-term final assignment, students were then asked to return to their first-week reflection to analyze their own learning and to reflect upon how their understanding of writing had changed over the course of the term. The use of these bookended reflective assignments is indicative of the pedagogy of TFT[21] in which students are asked to look back and to look forward as a way to encourage reflection on what has been learned and how it will apply to future contexts. In between these two assignments, students stepped through a scaffolded set of tasks to develop a final product geared toward a specific audience (patients).

In addition to anecdotal evidence, assessment data showed that TWC361 was successful in meeting goals and that students met course outcomes. In our chapter in *Metaliteracy in Practice* (D'Angelo and Maid[2]), we report on a case study in which metacognitive statements from multiple sections of the course were assessed by two faculty (one from nursing, one from TC) who were not involved with teaching it. In addition, portfolios were coded to uncover how students met outcomes. Results indicated that students met outcomes in finding, using, and presenting information to communicate to different audiences using different genres of writing. We had intended to continue to assess the course and to use that assessment data to continually improve it, as is best practice in writing studies. However, as both the RN-BSN Program and the TC Program underwent organizational change, the course was placed on the back burner until fall 2018 when ASU's change of learning management system from Blackboard to Canvas served as an impetus to revisit the course, which was now in its seventh year. In the spring of 2019, one of the authors, Barbara, took on the redesign of TWC361.

Course Redesign

A scaled-down version of the previous design process was used partly due to organizational and personnel changes. Within the IE framework, this is known as "ruling relations"—that is, institutional patterns, hierarchies, allocation of resources, and work processes within which individuals negotiate their activities and work. The shifts in the ruling relations of our own environment were a topic of conversation for us as we formed to begin working on the redesign. At the institutional level, changes in provost and dean led to a reorganization of units and programs within CONHI. CISA also underwent similar organizational changes as programs were shifted and/or merged with other units. In addition, changes in program leadership occurred due to retirement or program heads stepping down. At the same time, other faculty in the RN-BSN Program either retired or left the university. In addition, by the time of the redesign, the RN-BSN and TC faculty members from the original course development who remained had established a fairly solid working relationship. The relationship was established during the original creation of the course via multiple meetings, discussions, and sharing of information related to disciplinary standards and practice. This initial work led to a degree of disciplinary ethos that carried over to the redesign. That relationship was maintained as communication was ongoing between the head of the RN-BSN Program and Barbara (as course coordinator). As a result, we did not need to engage with a full-blown and time-consuming process for the revision; instead, the head of the RN-BSN Program selected one faculty member to represent their group, and Barbara took the lead for the TC Program. The faculty member from the RN-BSN Program and Barbara met several times to discuss course goals in the context of changes in RN-BSN Program needs and student populations.

The shift in the population of those who take the course had become a factor in course redesign. Initially, the RN-BSN Program served a student population of working RNs who were returning to school to complete their BSN to meet the expectations of the ACA's impact on health care. Over time, however, the population of students enrolling in the degree expanded to include concurrent students (traditional-age students completing their RN at a community college while simultaneously beginning coursework for the BSN at ASU), as well as new RNs. This meant that there were fewer experienced working nurses in the course and more inexperienced or new to the workforce students. In addition, ASU Online continued to ramp up efforts to recruit students from outside of Arizona.

Further, subtle shifts had taken place in curricular priorities within CONHI. Clearly, the need for new practicing nurses in health-care settings continued. But the need to recruit students for graduate school to feed the pipeline of nursing faculty also became a concern for the nursing faculty as current academics were retiring. This manifested itself in a couple of ways. TWC361 had originally been developed with the intent of being a professional writing course within the specific context of nursing. As time progressed, the RN-BSN faculty began to express that a shift in the desired emphasis to be more focused on academic writing was needed. This desire was a double-edged sword, however, as the desire to facilitate students' learning of and engagement with professional workplace writing remained. A common question from the RN-BSN faculty was "can't they learn both in one course?" Within the IE framework, this was manifested in our ability to negotiate "standpoint"—the acknowledgment of situated experience and knowledge; in this case, how to define writing and the teaching of it. For those in writing studies, standpoint allows the writing researcher to situate herself or himself as a professional experienced in managing and teaching writing. As such, she or he can negotiate requests, such as those we faced in which disciplinary faculty seemingly want students to "learn it all" in one course.

Of course, from a writing studies perspective, that was not possible (or at least problematic) since the rhetorical exigence for workplace versus academic writing is distinct. Yet, despite the tension evident in the desire for students to learn academic/scholarly writing and workplace writing, the overriding concerns related to the writing course did not differ significantly from our original collaboration. Nor did the commitment on the part of the RN-BSN faculty to the writing course as the first (and required) course in the degree program to emphasize the importance of writing and communication in the work—professional and scholarly—that nurses do. As a result, we found ourselves on the same page in terms of using process pedagogy and developing students' ability to understand rhetorical contexts for writing; to adapt style, tone, and content to those contexts; to learn good organization; to write concisely but clearly; and to understand and use appropriate genre conventions. Clearly, one of our collaborative approaches to addressing the tensions that arose was through the use of a clear definition of writing so that we could define goals and approaches to meet them. Just as students cannot conduct peer reviews or create revision plans without knowing the language to do so, course developers need to articulate the language used to develop a clear, mutually acceptable definition of writing, as well as the goals for the course. All of these are necessary in order to have agreement on strategies and techniques.

The importance of academic style and how much it should be incorporated into the course remained part of the conversation, though, throughout the redesign. From an IE framework perspective, we clearly had an issue that was "problematic." American Psychological Association (APA) style, in particular, continued to be a thorny issue due to the increased emphasis on recruiting students to enter graduate programs where scholarly writing would be of greater importance than it would be to students who would become or would remain practitioners. That is not surprising given the emphasis on APA in the nursing discipline, in particular, the elements of style that are used. On the other hand, writing studies places emphasis on the rhetorical aspects of an academic style as well, as on the conventions. What we needed to arrive at together (nursing and TC representatives) was a socially recognized breakdown of a complex practice.

One advantage that we had in our discussions about redesigning the course was that they took place within the overall context of the entire RN-BSN curriculum and how the course would feed into the introductory foundations nursing course that followed it. As a result, we decided that we would continue to emphasize primarily professional writing in the course but that we would also ask students to use APA style for citation practices only. In this way, we could address the rhetorical context of citation style; that is, how disciplinary discourse and practice adopts a particular style and that being a member of that discipline requires one to use it appropriately. This "introduction" to APA prepped students for the more stringent emphasis in their next course, which focused more on the mechanics of conventions and formatting. This approach, we hoped, would help students learn that using a citation style was not simply about avoiding plagiarism. Instead, citation and writing styles are part of being a member of a profession and its associated discourse community; using the style correctly is a part of being a professional in the field.

One aspect of the course that we did not alter was the final week's metacognitive statement in order to facilitate student reflection about what they were learning and how they might transfer it both to other courses in the BSN program and their workplaces. This assignment, in addition to the reflection required during the process revision planning, allowed us to maintain the emphasis on metacognition in the TFT spirit but also emphasized how writing is connected to identity formation within one's profession.

We had built the course originally using the structure of a term-long scenario in which students role-play as working nurses. We continued the use of a term-long scenario in the redesign; however, we adopted a new context in which students would work together more collaboratively through brainstorming and researching. We hoped that this additional collaboration would emphasize that process and peer review can take place at any stage of the writing process, not just when doing the actual composition. Each week during the course, as students worked through a task associated with the scenario, they submitted a draft, conducted peer review, developed a revision plan, and ultimately submitted the final product, as illustrated in Table 4.1.

TABLE 4.1 Overview of the redesigned course

Module 1	Video: Introduction	Discussion 1: Building a culture of peer feedback		
Module 2	Memo draft: Critical thinking and reflection	Memo peer review	Memo revision plan	Final revised memo
Module 3	Topic selection brainstorming	Topic selection peer reviews	Research log draft	Research log peer reviews	Research log revision plan
Module 4	Poster draft	Poster peer reviews	Poster revision plan	
Module 5	Handout draft	Handout peer reviews	Handout revision plan	
Module 6	Poster and handout final revision	Metacognitive memo		

The intent of the increase in the use of process was multifold. While TWC361 had always incorporated process via the use of a scenario, the 7.5-week online course format made managing the draft and peer review process challenging, in particular for instructors teaching four to five courses per semester. We adopted the use of Eli Review in the redesign to facilitate a more structured review process, which also allowed us to ground it in disciplinary theory, research, and best practice. In addition, we increased the number of peer reviews required in the course from one to four to emphasize that engaging in process—drafting, reviewing, revising—and the collaborative role in it, is important for all writing at all stages, not just for proofreading and editing the final draft. In the previous iteration of the course, students engaged in discussion forums, a standard strategy in online courses.

However, discussions seemed to engender limited engagement as students worried more about the number of posts, number of words, and number of replies to peers needed to get a grade rather than on substance or engaging with one another. Reframing engagement around peer reviews meant that we eliminated all but one (out of seven) of the discussions; we hoped that in peer reviews, students would more actively engage with their writing and, equally, with each other in a more meaningful and effective way. Next, we intended that the increase in emphasis on peer reviews would help students to learn how to effectively give and receive feedback and collaborate with one another as professionals. While important for all professionals, nursing students work in teams; learning how to constructively give meaningful feedback to others and how to use received feedback are important skills. An enhanced benefit was that the use of peer review crossed disciplinary boundaries and was reflected in course outcomes related to writing, as well as in interprofessional outcomes for nursing students. Finally, the adoption of the more robust peer review through Eli Review was intended to enhance opportunities for students to engage in metacognition beyond the first and last weeks' assignments.

To help both instructors and RN–BSN faculty colleagues learn about Eli Review and the pedagogical principles associated with it, we along with the director of professional development at Eli Review, conducted a workshop at the end of the spring 2019 semester. Although one component for this workshop was to help course instructors to use Eli in their sections, the primary goal was to introduce writing process pedagogy more fully and specifically to both writing instructors teaching the course and nursing faculty members so that they would understand the goals and purpose. While we did not formally assess the workshop, we did receive feedback from participants from the RN–BSN faculty. In a personal communication, the program head, H. Sanborn, commented that the workshop had provided inspiration for working toward greater use of the pedagogy in other BSN courses. In addition, K. Vana, the senior director of all the undergraduate nursing programs, indicated that she would schedule additional workshops for faculty in their other programs.

Discussion

Although the previous version of the course had incorporated process pedagogy through a scenario scaffolded into multiple tasks leading to a large final project, only one of the assignments incorporated peer review and revision. In recognition of the need to enhance student engagement and learning related to process, as well as to have the students engage more with one another, incorporating more peer review and revision planning became a major goal of the course revision.

First, in the former version of the course, the students seemed to take the use of the draft-peer review-revision as a "one-off" rather than learn the importance of engaging in the process for all of their writing. Based on our experience using Eli Review in other courses, we knew that we could use it to meet multiple challenges in TWC361. Increasing the number of assignments that were peer-reviewed allowed us to emphasize that peer review and revision aren't just "one-offs"; instead, they are a part of the process of writing that can and should be used in all contexts whether in school or at work. Indeed, we intended this to showcase how process is an important foundational concept for writers at all levels—indeed, perhaps a threshold concept—including professional nurses, whether they were working in clinical-level positions delivering patient care or in an administrative capacity doing more managerial-level writing. Harkening back to the first assignment in the course, in which we had asked students to reflect on how writing is a hallmark of nursing, we hoped that students would make the connection between writing and their identity as professional nurses who write in multiple genres to various audiences.

Second, although the previous version of the course used peer review, the use of technology such as Eli Review allowed us to enhance the structure of reviews by requiring multiple forms of feedback (trait yes/no responses, ratings, and comments) in a way that could be aligned to assignment grading criteria. Doing so made the review process not only more structured but also more closely aligned with what students would ultimately be graded on. It also provided students who felt insecure or uncertain about how to conduct reviews with the structure they needed to give them the confidence to give effective feedback. As is evident from the TFT pedagogy, an important factor in learning is the need to learn the language needed to accomplish tasks. The heuristic model of describe-evaluate-suggest for review comments provided students with guidance about *what* to say in their reviews. As such, we intended that students would feel more confident, increasing their self-efficacy as they began to take control of and agency over their own process of writing, review, and revision to identify writing as part of their professional nursing identity.

Third, the revision planning heuristic aided the learning of metacognition since students were placed in the cognitively challenging task of evaluating the feedback they received in order to make decisions about how to put them into immediate action to revise and improve. Metacognition has been identified as a key to learning by Bransford et al.[26] and is commonly used as a pedagogical strategy to facilitate transfer. As Yancey et al.[21] point out, TFT curricula helps to foster metacognition.

Fourth, the increase in the use of draft-peer review-revision enhanced student opportunities for engagement in a meaningful way (achieving goals) by allowing them to work together to develop as writers through constant reading, writing, and revision. While we reduced the number of discussions in the course to accommodate the increase in the process cycle, we believed it was worth the trade-off. By providing students with an opportunity to engage with one another in peer review and revision planning, we gave them a meaningful, transparent, and actionable way to collaborate for improvement in an environment that was relatively risk-free (minimal potential impact on grades). It also provided students with the opportunity to both learn and use the discourse of process writing and the discourse of nursing since the creation of review comments and revision plans necessitated that students read closely both drafts and the feedback they received.

Fifth, the use of APA is taught as a way to develop an identity within a discipline; understanding it as more than a template to be followed religiously but rather a set of disciplinary conventions that have emerged out of the needs of a particular disciplinary discourse community. Understanding discipline-based threshold concepts helps with understanding the need for the conventions in an academic style such as APA.

Where Are We Now? IE

As we've worked with the creation, development, and revision of the two courses, it has become increasingly clear to us that traditional university courses that emphasize one disciplinary discourse community are naturally insufficient when disciplinary discourse communities overlap. Curriculum development becomes even more complicated when, as we've seen through the evolution of TWC361, the nursing faculty members do not have a clear consensus on what kinds of writing needs to be taught (mainly because writing in multiple genres for multiple audiences are all necessary and appropriate). We're also very aware that students in nursing programs only have room for so many writing courses.

Using IE, we wonder if it may not be best to visualize the courses as the area where the Venn diagrams of the universes of the discourse communities of writing studies and nursing professions intersect. How does that impact what the two courses look like now? We have discovered over the past 10 years that not only do the courses evolve but the relationship between the two disciplinary faculties is also one of constant evolution, just as institutions themselves evolve. Where might we go next? Certainly, assessment is needed to ensure the redesign is working—both to achieve outcomes and to identify if the goals of increasing self-efficacy and professional identity were achieved. Perhaps working with health-care faculty members to make more content courses Writing In the Disciplines-like? That's only one possibility. Most likely the answer will be determined by the interests, both pedagogical and programmatic, of the faculty involved in the discussions, as well as the changing institutional vision for these pedagogical collaborations. That realization alone helps us to understand that IE is a crucial framework to apply to ongoing research and development in curriculum.

References

1. Stevens CJ, D'Angelo B, Rennell, N, Muzyka D, Pannabecker V, Maid B. Implementing a writing course in an online RN-BSN program. *Nurse Educ.* 2014;39(1):17–21.
2. D'Angelo BJ, Maid. Metaliteracy learning of RN to BSN students. In: Jacobson TE, Mackey TP, ed. *Metaliteracy in Practice.* Chicago, IL: Neal-Schuman; 2016:47–71.
3. Smith, D. *Institutional Ethnology: A Sociology for People.* Walnut Creek, CA: Altamira, 2005.
4. Campbell M, Gregor, F. *Mapping Social Relations: A Primer in Doing Sociology and Social Welfare.* Walnut Creek, CA: Altamira, 2002.
5. LaFrance M. *Institutional Ethnography. A Theory and Practice for Writing Studies Researchers.* Louisville, CO: University of Colorado Press, 2019.
6. American Association of Colleges of Nursing. *Essentials of Baccalaureate Education for Professional Nursing Practice. American Association of Colleges of Nursing* website. https://www.aacnnursing.org/Portals/42/Publications/BaccEssentials08.pdf. Updated October 20, 2008. Accessed January 25, 2021.
7. American Association of Colleges of Nursing. *The Essentials of Baccalaureate Education for Professional Nursing Practice.* American Association of Colleges of Nursing; October 20, 2008. https://www.aacnnursing.org/Portals/42/Publications/BaccEssentials08.pdf. Accessed April 15, 2021.
8. Luthy KE, Peterson NE, Lassetter JH, Callister LC. Successfully incorporating writing across the curriculum with advanced writing in nursing. *J Nurse Educ.* 2009;48(1):54–59.
9. Sasa RI. Nursing care paper as a writing intensive requirement in clinical nursing courses. *Teach Learn Nurs.* 2020;15:137–144.
10. Rohan A, Fullerton J. Interdisciplinary peer mentorship: an innovative strategy to enhance writing competency. *J Nurs Educ.* 2020;59(3):173–175.
11. Fulwieler T and Young A eds. *Language Connections: Writing and Reading across the Curriculum.* Urbana, IL: NCYE; 1982.
12. Miller LC, Russell CL, Cheng, AL, Skarbek AJ. Evaluating undergraduate nursing students' self-efficacy and competence in writing: effects of a writing intensive intervention. *Nurs Educ Pract.* 2015;15(3):174–180.
13. Mitchell KM, Harrigan T, McMillan DE. Writing self-efficacy in nursing students: the influence of a discipline-specific writing environment. *Nurs Open.* 2017;4:240–250.
14. Mitchell KM, Harrigan T, Stefansson T, Setlack H. Exploring self-efficacy and anxiety in first-year nursing students enrolled in a discipline-specific scholarly writing course. *Qual Adv Nurs Educ.* 2017;3(1):4

15. Mitchell KM. A curriculum-wide assessment of writing self-efficacy in a baccalaureate nursing program. *Nurse Educ Today* 2018;70:20–27.
16. Flower L, Hayes J. A cognitive process theory of composing. *CCC*. 1981;34(4):365–387.
17. Wiggin SG. Seven keys to effective feedback. *Educl Leadersh*. 2012;70(1):10–16.
18. Hattie J, Timperley H. The power of feedback. *RevEdu Res*. 2007;77:81–112.
19. Hewett BL, dePew KE, eds. *Foundational Practices of Online Writing Instruction*. Ft. Collins, CO: WAC Clearing House; 2015. doi:10.37514/PER-B.2015.0650.
20. Yancey KB, Robertson L, Taczak K. *Writing across Contexts: Transfer Composition, and Sites of Writing*. Logan, UT: Utah State UP; 2014.
21. Yancey KB. *Reflection in the Writing Classroom*. Logan, UT: Utah State UP; 1999.
22. Adler-Kassner L, Wardle E, eds. *Naming What We Know: Threshold Concepts of Writing Studies*. Logan, UT: Utah State UP; 2015.
23. McAllister M, Lasater K, Stone TE, Levett-Jones T. The reading room: exploring the use of literature as a strategy for integrating threshold concepts into nursing curricula. *Nurse Educ Pract*. 2015;15(2015), pp. 549–555.
24. Crookes PA, Lewis PA, Else FC, Crookes K. Current issues with the identification of threshold concepts in nursing. *Nurse Educ Pract*. 2020;42:article 102682. doi:10.1016/j.nepr.2019.102682.
25. Martindale L *Threshold Concepts in Research and Evidence-Based Practice: Investigating Troublesome Learning for Undergraduate Nursing Students*. Durham, UK: Durham University Theses; 2015. http://etheses.dur.ac.uk/10998/1/Threshold_concepts_in_research_and_evidence-based_practice.pdf?DDD29+. Accessed January 25, 2021.
26. Branford JD, Ann L Brown AL, Cocking RR, eds. *How People Learn: Brain, Mind, Experience, and School*. Washington, DC: National Academy Press; 2000.

5

NURSING SIMULATIONS AND INTERMEDIARY GENRES

Bridging Students' Classroom and Clinical Writing

Lillian Campbell

Like many health-care professionals, nurses do not necessarily see writing as central to their clinical role. And yet, they rely on and contribute to a wide range of genres—nurse's notes, patient charts, insurance forms, etc.[1,2] This raises an important question for writing in the health professions—what kinds of writing assignments should nursing students learn in the classroom?

This chapter investigates how junior-year nursing students draw connections between their writing experiences in three different contexts: classrooms, clinical simulations, and hospital placements. I argue that if leveraged appropriately, writing in clinical simulations—where students provide care for a robotic patient in a structured scenario—can help students to conceptually bridge their classroom and clinical writing experiences. As a result, they come to value their classroom writing more highly. My analysis draws on a yearlong qualitative study of junior-year nursing students, including a collection of student writing, document-based interviews, and observations and video recordings of 30 clinical simulations totaling 90 hours.

The writing students do in simulations is an example of what Tachino[3] has called an "intermediary genre," which "can be used to connect and mobilize two otherwise unconnected genres to make uptake possible."[p456] Through their positioning in an experiential learning context between classroom and clinic, simulation texts mediate between these spaces. They provide opportunities to practice negotiating importance and communicating importance, two of the tasks that challenge students most in their classroom writing. At the same time, they anticipate the audience and stakes of future professional contexts, helping students to see the value of their classroom writing.

The chapter begins with an overview of the challenges of teaching writing in nursing and discussions of transfer of learning. I introduce Tachino's theory of intermediary genres and apply it to the simulated patient health record, showing how its features mediate between classroom and professional writing tasks. Next, drawing on 4 sets of interviews with my 5 focal students, I report on how students articulated connections between class assignments, writing in simulations, and hospital writing and discuss how the intermediary nature of simulation writing helped support this connection-making. Finally, I conclude by considering the implications of these findings for instructors who teach writing in the health professions.

DOI: 10.4324/9781003162940-8

Field Context

Nursing education has a rich history of incorporating simulations into training in order to provide students with an opportunity to practice hands-on care. My research focuses specifically on simulations that are "sequential decision-making classroom events" and utilize high-tech robotic manikins that respond to care both physically and verbally.[4(p15)] These computerized manikins are programmed to have physical features like breath sounds and pulses that respond to student intervention. For example, a manikin's temperature might rise to indicate that an infection is worsening or its pulse might quicken in response to a medication. Meanwhile, during simulations, a facilitator speaks from a microphone in a control room connected to the manikin's mouth, so students can converse with the manikin and hear its reactions.

This chapter is based on a yearlong investigation of clinical nursing simulations at a mid-sized private university in the Pacific Northwest. I observed and video recorded three simulation sequences by ten groups of junior-year baccalaureate nursing students (30 simulations total) over the course of the 2014–2015 academic year. These nursing students were beginning their clinical placements at local hospitals simultaneously and, thus, were able to compare classroom, simulation, and clinical experiences during interviews. Data collection included observations and field notes of clinical simulations and debriefs and interviews with instructors and 5 focal students who indicated an interest in study participation during recruitment. I also collected focal student classroom writing—a care plan based on their clinical experiences—and documents that circulated during the simulation like student charting on whiteboards. This study was exempted by the human subjects board at my institution and the institution where it took place. I use pseudonyms for my participants throughout to preserve their anonymity.

During simulations, students in my study were immersed in a patient narrative set up by the coordinator, Maura. For example, their first simulation of the year featured an elderly patient, Eliana, who was diabetic and had recently had surgery on her leg. On her way to the hospital she tripped and twisted her ankle. Over the course of 20 minutes, a group of 2 to 3 students cared for the patient while the patient's condition worsened. Eliana had low blood sugar and would become increasingly disoriented until students provided food. Care included both verbal conversations with each other, the patient, and other providers, as well as physical care such as wound dressing and catheter insertion. Students documented care on several large whiteboards in the classroom, which acted as the patient's health record.[5] While one group provided care, the other two groups sat in a nearby classroom watching a live video stream of the simulation. After each group's turn, the students, clinical instructor, and simulation coordinator reconvened in the classroom for a debrief conversation before the next group began care.

Challenges of Teaching Writing in Nursing

Throughout this chapter, I will use the word "genre" to refer to groups of texts that share common purposes and textual features. Rhetorical scholars who work in genre studies emphasize the importance of attending to social context when analyzing genres. That is, rather than just categorizing texts by shared organization patterns or formatting, one should consider the role they play in a social group, the values they imbue, and the relationship between structure and social practice.[6]

Writing scholars argue that genres function quite differently in classrooms than in the "real world." In professional and public contexts, genres participate in complex systems that include other genres, people, and practices.[7] In contrast, instructors are the primary audience for classroom writing and an individual's grade is the main goal. Even when instructors ask students to write for an imagined audience in some workplace or public context, their writing is still ultimately evaluated by the instructor.[8] Wardle[9] describes these as "mutt genres," texts that look like public genres, but within the classroom "their purposes and audiences are vague or even contradictory."[(p774)]

Nursing students are expected to produce a lot of writing in their undergraduate courses and that writing takes a wide variety of different forms. The students I interviewed catalogued a range of assignments—summaries of their nursing philosophy, reflections on communication practices, article summaries, and clinical care plans, to name a few. Meanwhile, classroom nursing genres come with their own unique challenges tied to the community's values and practices.

First, since technical correctness is so critical to the nursing profession, lower-order concerns like formatting, citation, and grammar tend to be overemphasized, making it hard for students to see inter-textual connections to professional genres. Ariail and Smith[10(p258)] show the parallels between nursing instructor's worldview and their approach to writing instruction using the metaphor of a Foley catheter insertion:

> Nursing faculty outline structure and criteria for grading. In standardizing the genres their students produce, these health care professionals treat writing as they treat insertion of a Foley catheter. Sure, it may have a certain unpleasantness associated with it, but there is a procedure that can be followed. [(p259)]

In my interviews, students discussed how instructors had them use sections to organize their care plans that sometimes did not feel closely tied to their experiences in clinicals. Savannah noted that the distinctions between subjective and objective information in a subjective, objective, assessment, and plan (SOAP) notes assignment felt arbitrary, while Kira said of her care plan: "I'll typically just like go down the list and fill it out [...] the order kind of makes sense but kind of not."

Another challenge is finding a balance between teaching students to present information objectively while also supporting their future role as patient advocates. Focal student Liz discussed how writing had been a means for her to engage with topics like social justice in high school. Thus, Liz struggled with the neutral stance of her nursing writing: "You have to be very succinct and straight to the point [...] and that's pretty difficult for me especially if it's something that I care about." Ariail and Smith[10] found that faculty shared in this sense of loss regarding more creative or open-ended writing. In trying to help students learn the genres of the field with explicit assignments and guidelines that focus on form or structure, instructors "wonder if they are sacrificing the more humanistic, creative attributes for which the profession is valorized."[(p245)]

Of course, this is a larger tension for nursing as a field given its positioning within a community that includes medical professionals from a range of different backgrounds and with a wide variety of priorities. Heifferon[11] advises health students, "Emotion in charts is unadvisable; if you have particular difficulties with patients, it's best to air those in your team meetings."[(p294)] Her comment demonstrates how the fact-based, list-oriented genres of nursing exist to facilitate interdisciplinary communication. However, this means "the texts that grow out of nurse-patient interactions might not be accurate depictions of the core helping relationship."[10(p262)] Ultimately, the tension between teaching students how to communicate effectively with other health-care professionals and how to interact compassionately with patients and family undergirds the range of assignments that under-graduate nursing students encounter.

It may also be the case, however, that both nursing instructors and students are not recognizing and valuing the opportunities for fostering rhetorical awareness and a nursing identity that exist even in less creative or open-ended assignments. Focal student Kira expressed frustration with an article summary assignment, saying, "I'm like, why does this matter? Like spitting out this article?" Most writing instructors would quickly respond with skepticism to Kira's view of the summary as straightforward or neutral. Summaries ask students to make strategic choices about which information to foreground based on their assessment of what is valued within a community. Thus, they are deeply situated and rhetorical, relying on students' burgeoning understanding of disciplinary relevance. Teaching summaries as flexible and situated counters students' entrenched orientation to this genre as proof that they have done the reading. As a field, nursing has tended to prioritize technical and content-based correctness,[10] but there are certainly ways to approach even summary assignments to emphasize the development of disciplinary identity and possibilities for rhetorical flexibility. Ultimately, this chapter demonstrates how a focus on intermediary genres might help both students and instructors to recognize connections between classroom writing and professional writing and, thus, to value classroom writing more.

Simulation Genres as Intermediary Genres

Recognizing the immense complexity of classroom-based genre teaching, some scholars like Dias and Pare[7] have argued that professional writing cannot be taught outside of its original context. Others, like Bawarshi,[12] have discussed ways to assign genres that have social functions to play within the classroom context. In contrast, this chapter calls for scholars to consider how the writing that happens in in-between spaces, like experiential learning contexts, could help mediate between classroom-based and professional writing, creating stronger connections between the two and helping students to recognize the value of their classroom work.

In her review of scholarship on the transfer of learning, Moore[13(p2)] calls for more attention to collateral transitions: "multi-directional movements between concurrent activities, such as the daily transition from school to a part-time job." Since students participate in simulations at the same time as coursework and their clinical placements, their writing experiences in these contexts occur simultaneously. At a single moment in the semester, for example, they might be working on a nursing philosophy statement for a class, practicing taking nursing notes during a clinical simulation, and using the patient health record at their hospital placement to input patient documentation.

Tachino's[3] theory of intermediary genres focuses on genres that exist in the in-between. As Tachino[3(p456)] explains, a "genre can be used to connect and mobilize two otherwise unconnected genres to make uptake possible." For example, a press release facilitates the uptake of an organization's information by the press. His example of an intermediary genre is focused on an investigation into a wrongful conviction that led to judicial reforms in Canada. Accordingly, he tracks citations in the commission report to show how it mediated between scholarly research in psychology and public policy. While Tachino's work has been applied to other public writing contexts to understand the relationships between scientific and public texts,[13,14] its applicability to academic writing contexts has been undertheorized. Tachino's theory can help instructors to recognize and value the ambiguous nature of in-between texts that occur in experiential learning spaces that are neither fully classroom nor fully workplace.

According to Tachino,[3] when performing an analysis of intermediary genres, it is necessary to identify the source genre and the target of uptake, as well as the text that bridges the two. For this analysis, the source text is classroom nursing assignments, specifically the care plan. The target of uptake is hospital writing and more precisely, patient charting, frequently done in an electronic health record (EHR). And the intermediary genre is the simulated patient health record documented on a large whiteboard during the course of a simulation. Next, I provide brief context on all three texts before moving into my analysis of their relationship.

1. Care Plan

   Care plans, also called clinical write-ups, are genres used by nursing instructors to teach students to think about patients through the framework of the nursing process. Nurses share a similar decision-making structure, the nursing process, which is guided by the acronym ADPIE: assessment, diagnosis, planning, implementation, evaluation. While instructor expectations vary, the clinical write-up typically involves focusing on one patient who is under a student's care at their clinical placement. Students choose several conditions to unpack and then describe the pathophysiology of those conditions, a plan of care, interventions, and assessment of those interventions. Essentially then, the care plan asks students to track the nursing process across one or two conditions for a single patient.

2. Patient Health Record

The patient health record (or EHR) is a flexible genre that varies significantly even within a single hospital, floor by floor and patient by patient. Most hospitals use some variation of an electronic system with similar sections: "progress notes, I/O (Input/Output) records, checklists for admissions and transfers, blocks or pages for narratives, nurse worksheets, and daily and patient assignment sheets."[11(p104)] Thus, the health record is a cross-disciplinary text that transfers information between different health care providers to guide their collaboration around patient care. Health record systems are also strategically designed to guide providers through the process of clinical decision-making. Schryer[15] describes the "Problem Oriented Medical Record" system, which "offers new physicians a heuristic that reflects the actual problem-solving structures" of health care.[(p117)] Thus, the patient health record moves providers through a recursive process documenting patient information, formulating interventions, and evaluating those interventions, similar to the nursing process.

3. Simulated Patient Health Record

Most simulation labs use makeshift strategies to support patient charting, from preformatted Excel sheets to large whiteboards. At my field site, students relied primarily on one large whiteboard (approximately 4′ by 6′) and occasionally a smaller board (2′ × 3′) to document patient vital signs, changes in status, and interventions. Interestingly, students were given free rein over how to organize the board and document information about their patients. After their orientation to the simulation room, Maura would instruct the full group to work together to design a charting template. Students would converse about the design, choosing a layout that made sense for this patient and the simulation space.[5] Templates varied widely, with some groups laying out their boards to emphasize the three groups moving through the simulation and others clustering information around categories like vitals and interventions. As I will discuss next, instructors highlighted the nursing process as a guiding heuristic for chart design and organization.

Analysis

This section draws on four sets of interviews—an opening interview and one after each of the three simulations during the academic year—with my five focal students, as well as observations of their simulations. I rely heavily on data from my final interview in spring 2015 when I had students bring a care plan from their class and conducted a document-based interview[16] in addition to discussing their experiences with the third simulation. Overall, I show how the intermediary simulated patient health record enabled students to practice negotiating importance and communicating importance, two of the most challenging aspects of their classroom care plan.

Negotiating Importance

First, in composing their care plans, students struggled with making strategic choices about which conditions to track. As I mentioned earlier, the assignment typically asked students to choose several conditions from a patient at their clinical site and to track those conditions through the nursing process from assessment to interventions. As newcomers to the discipline, students struggle to identify which conditions are most relevant. For example, Kira described the challenge of interpreting one patient's EHR to determine what the real problem was:

> I looked it up and I was like, "Oh, backache like that's why you're here? Main problem—backache?" And it wasn't until I looked up a Physical Therapy note that they were like, "Oh yeah, he has spastic tetraplegic cerebral palsy" and I was like, "Really? Of course his back hurts! He just had a reconstructive surgery for cerebral palsy!"

Kira's lack of familiarity with the EHR at her hospital made it extremely difficult for her to know where to find relevant information. As she describes, the most important problem appeared buried in a note, rather than spotlighted in the main sections of the record. This created a struggle in identifying which condition to prioritize in her care plan. Ultimately, her care plan tracked three conditions—cerebral palsy, dorsal rhizotomy (the reconstructive surgery and recovery), and "backache."

Meanwhile, Savannah explained how it was difficult for her to recognize which diagnoses go together when working on her care plans. She would pick one condition to track and then receive feedback from instructors that she needed to include others that co-occurred with that condition. She commented, "The [instructor] is always like 'Well, these three things go together so if you mention this thing you have to mention these other two things' and I was like, 'Well I never knew that!'"

Both Kira's and Savannah's struggles will resonate with those familiar with learning theory. Indeed, one of the key epistemological challenges for newcomers to the nursing field is how to take in large amounts of patient information and quickly determine what to prioritize for intervention.[17] In Benner's[18(p23)] description of the advanced beginner nurse, she notes their tendency to "integrate as many attributes and aspects as possible, but […] ignore their differential importance."

In contrast, important patient information in the simulated patient health record was usually clearly identified by previous groups. Students would often use situated and immersive means to highlight key information on the whiteboards like stars, different colored markers, etc. As Ryan explained, it was much easier to look at the simulated patient health record and identify the most important notes:

> Everything [the previous group] thought was pertinent was already on the board […] I would step over and then look at the board and I saw what the other people wrote down and what they thought was important for me and I can kind of see the highlights.

Comparing Ryan's comments to Kira's struggle to find her patient's main diagnosis, one can see how the format of the simulated patient health record is more accessible, and important patient information is unlikely to be buried in unexpected sections.

At the same time, students still had to make decisions in simulations about which information from their shift to highlight for the incoming group. Thus, the simulated patient health record provided them with an opportunity to collaboratively negotiate importance, deciding together what patient information should be documented and highlighted in their charting. Typically, toward the end of their turn with patient care, a group would stand together at the whiteboard, collaboratively taking stock of patient information and talking through next steps.

For example, in the following conversation, four students check in and document their care for the next group at the end of their simulation. The conversation begins as one student finishes assessments of the elderly, diabetic patient and ends with their collaborative negotiation of what they should include in their patient health record.

S1 [*Writing on board. Turns to the student who is still assessing*] Is there anything you want to add about physical findings?

S2 Okay, so she has PERLA [pupils are dilating appropriately]

S1 Anything abnormal?

S2 Abnormal? She has a weird-sounding heart. It's a slow heart rate.

S1 [*Looks at telemetry machine and confirms normal heart rate*] No it's fine.

S2 It just sounds weird. I don't know how you would describe that…. Okay well, her cap[illary] refill in her finger is four sec and her feet is five. [*Walks over to the whiteboard and begins watching other students document on the board.*] There's no cyanosis [skin discoloration]. Her skin feels warm. She says her leg is nontender.

S1 What was it? Four sec.?

S2 It's four in her fingers and five in the toes.

S1 Okay.

S3 [*Skimming columns on the board*] Okay so last change of dressing…last PRN…

S4 Can say we were going to change her dressing, but we didn't have time?

S3 And her insulin time she said was this morning before breakfast.

S1 That's not something we found though. That's in the chart.

S3 That's true.

S1 So I don't think we need to put that.

Here, the student who is documenting for the group acts as the primary decision-maker about what they should include, overriding other group members' suggestions based on their lack of urgency. She prioritizes abnormalities and numerical data (number of seconds for capillary refill, for example) and reminds groups members that some information will be available elsewhere. Group 1's final documentation is visible in the first column of Figure 5.1. Their negotiation is visible in the decision to include capillary refill numbers but not specifics about the patient's eye dilation, lung sounds, or the insulin that she took at home.

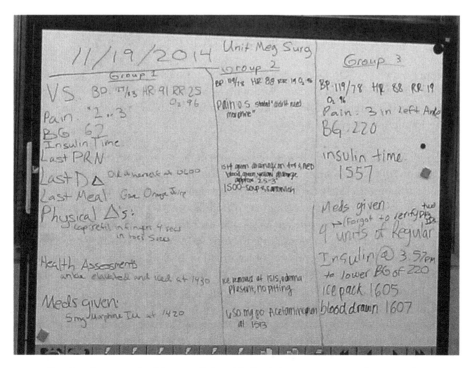

FIGURE 5.1 Simulated patient health record for elderly diabetic patient at the end of the simulation
Photo by Author.

Whether this group made the "right" decisions about what should be documented is less relevant than the fact that students were given the opportunity to work together to negotiate the importance of information, practicing one of the most difficult cognitive moves for disciplinary newcomers.[19] The conversation they had during this simulation is an example of the internal dialogue many students will have to perform when working on their care plans for classes and when navigating the patient health record in hospital contexts. By providing students with an opportunity to enact this negotiation, then, the simulated patient health record bridges their experiences with classroom care plans and their future hospital documentation, making the process external and collaborative rather than internal and individual.

Communicating Importance

After they had established which conditions to focus on in their care plan, the next step for students was to diagnose that condition and decide on an intervention (the D through I in ADPIE). Acquiring the language of diagnosis was difficult since oftentimes students did not know how the condition would be described in their field. Savannah explained the challenge of using their nursing diagnosis book:

> It's just hard to learn the nursing diagnosis that goes with it because you can be like, "Oh well they have decreased sensation in their fingertips because they have poor circulation" but then the nursing diagnosis is something completely differently worded and you have to find it in this big book.

Thus, another key tenet of disciplinary participation—knowing the jargon—was a significant barrier for students working on their care plans.[18]

Along similar lines, students were expected to explain their choice of conditions and their interventions in the care plans. According to Liz, instructors insisted that their interventions be accompanied by a "rationale" that closely tied them back to the patient's situation:

> So before I would say, "Oh kidney failure [...] monitor intake and output" and that would be it and [my instructor] would be like, "Well why would you do that?" And so you have to really go down into the Patho[physiology] and then how your patient's presenting and explain why that's an important intervention.

Sometimes this rationale had its own designated column in their care plans. In the care plan Michelle brought to discuss, there were separate columns for "Interventions" and "Rationale." Paired with the intervention "monitor closely for hemorrhage and signs of bleeding," then, Michelle included the explanation, "clients at risk for bleeding may include those >60 years of age, previous bleeding episode, HTN, low platelets, active malignancy, renal/liver failure, and NSAIDs" and cited Ackley, 2014. Other versions had a single column titled "Nursing Interventions with Rationale(s)" where students were expected to include both sets of information. In both cases, moving from the book's abstract description of a diagnosis and intervention to the particulars of the patient's situation and an argument for the intervention was challenging for new nurses.

However, in their experiences during simulations, students practiced this very kind of rationalization – elaborating upon the information they had documented in their patient health record. During their handoff to the incoming group, the patient health record often became a primary object of reference as both groups gathered near the board. In the following conversation, the first group featured in the previous section uses their board to help the next group prioritize care (emphasis added):

s1 This is Eliana Ruiz who is in initially for a dressing change but on her way here she tripped and hurt her other ankle. We checked her blood glucose, and it was pretty low, so we gave her some orange juice. *You might want to keep an eye on that.* We also gave her some morphine for her pain. Um, how much did you guys give?

s2 Five milligrams. Intramuscular.

s3 And then we put ice on her ankle that she hurt. It's pretty bruised and swollen *so take that off in fifteen minutes or so.* And then…

s1 *Did not get time for a dressing change. There's also an order in there for a foley catheter if you have time.*

Here, we see the group both rationalizing their interventions and prioritizing interventions for the next group based on their experience with the patient. For example, they explain that their decision to give the patient juice was based on their assessment of low blood sugar. They also encourage the incoming group to continue monitoring Eliana's blood sugar, with the implication that they may need to give insulin or more food depending on her levels. Notably, during their conversation, the information that was not documented (i.e., pupil dilation, lung sounds, skin tone) did not show up. Even some specifics they did document—like capillary refill—were not prioritized because they were not tied to a specific action item for the next group. In this way, as students communicate during a handoff, they continue making decisions about importance but this time with the goal of convincing a new audience of incoming students about its relevance as well.

Thus, the simulated patient health record also provided scaffolding in communicating importance, a skill that students practiced with varying degrees of success in their classroom care plans but which will be extremely important in hospital contexts. Students will need to communicate importance in both the patient health record and in handing off care to other providers. During an interview, Kira was able to make a direct connection between the rationalization work that is happening in care plans and the kinds of explanations that nurses need to offer when doing a handoff to one another:

> If you say, "Hey, keep an eye on room twenty, they're super fidgety" then obviously the [other nurse would] be like, "Okay, why do you think they're fidgety? What do I have to look out for? What are you sending me into?"

However, other nurses are not the only audience for communicating importance. As I previously discussed, the genres of nursing exist in a network of interdisciplinary providers with different roles and responsibilities. Savannah noted that because of the nurse's close proximity to the patient, she was often much more in tune with their immediate needs, and thus other providers trusted her to be a patient advocate:

> I actually saw it on Tuesday that doctors have so many patients and they write the orders, which are very important, but a lot of times the orders need to be updated. So my nurse was actually really on top of that and when she saw the doctor she was like "Oh can you please change this order?" […] And the doctors really trust them and they're like "Oh okay I'll definitely change that order."

Part of the value of students experiencing classroom, simulation, and clinical experiences concurrently was their ability to make these genre connections in real time. They were not just imagining future conversations they might have with a doctor but seeing them happen during their clinical placements. Meanwhile, I attribute both Kira's and Savannah's abilities to see a connection between the care plan and the hospital context to their experiences communicating importance with the simulated patient health record. Its bridging role between classroom and workplace supported students in recognizing its relevance and the skills they could transfer.

Discussion

Returning to Tachino's[3] definition of intermediary genres, he argues that these texts facilitate the uptake of other genres in either "form or content."[(p459)] Based on my analysis in the two previous sections, I would argue that simulated patient health records support the uptake of content more than form. Communicating importance looks different in the classroom, simulation, and workplace given the different media at play (an academic paper, a whiteboard, an EHR). However, simulations bridge the content in care plans and patient health records, providing practice in negotiating and communicating importance. I would also argue that because Tachino's[3] focus was primarily on expert communication, he has not adequately accounted for the advantageous role that intermediary genres might play in relation to classroom writing. The simulated patient health record helped novices to value their classroom writing more and helped instructors begin to imagine revisions to their assignments that would better support student transfer.

As previously discussed, there are a number of reasons why it is often difficult for nursing students to recognize the value of their classroom writing. These include instructor emphases on technical correctness and struggles to incorporate assignments that reflect the unique nurse-patient relationship. That said, many of my focal students were able to articulate clearly how care plans contributed to helping them "think like a nurse," indicating that the goals of the assignment and its relationship to future work were exceptionally clear to them. Scholarship on the transfer of writing knowledge suggests that this kind of connection-making is both unusual and especially difficult.[8,18,20] The fact that so many focal students were able to explicitly identify the logic behind the care plan as transferable, then, is truly exceptional!

Overall, students' experiences with the simulated patient health record as intermediary genre reinforced this valuing of the care plan assignment by providing opportunities to see how the nursing process guided their care and supported their patient documentation and handoffs. Simulation coordinator Maura frequently used the nursing process to guide the group's debrief conversations, sometimes even writing ADPIE on the board and asking the group to describe what they had assessed, diagnosed, etc. During the third and final set of simulations for the year, Maura observed two groups who used ADPIE to organize their whiteboard—putting vital signs and systems down the left side of the board and assessment, plan, and interventions across the top. After that, she began recommending this layout to students. While I argue elsewhere that providing a template for charting limited student genre learning in certain ways,[21] this shift also highlighted the relationship between the simulated patient health record and the nursing process. In doing so, the template bridged students' experiences using the nursing process to write about patient conditions in the care plan and their communication in their future workplace. (For a comparable perspective from undergraduate medical education, see Chapter 1.)

Not only that, but my research also demonstrated that simulated genres could actually provide instructors who may be far removed from professional contexts with reminders about the way that texts support action in their fields of practice. After watching two groups of students move through the geriatric simulation, one instructor, Cleo, began to consider the SOAP note writing assignment she had been giving students to reflect on their clinical experience. She said that she was beginning to feel that SOAP notes, which require the separation of subjective and objective information about the patient followed by an assessment and a plan, seemed detached from the communication students were doing on the job.

Specifically, Cleo was interested in how students struggled with using the situation, background, assessment, and recommendation (SBAR) format to have conversations with the physician in simulations. SBAR is a shared heuristic for communicating patient information across interdisciplinary lines and requires that the speaker begin with the most important and relevant patient information and then provide general background. As with the care plans, one of the biggest challenges for novice nurses was leading with relevant information and not overwhelming the physician with background on the patient. Watching these struggles, Cleo wondered if "they should move towards more SBAR writing for clinical and focus on a resident with a changing condition." Thus, another simulation genre prompted her to think more strategically about the kinds of assignments that might support the transfer of learning between classroom and clinic.

Recommendations for Instructors

Cleo's revelation is one that I hope can inform readers of this chapter from both nursing and other health professions, especially those teaching courses that are linked to other experiential contexts like labs, work placements, or service learning. My analysis demonstrates that intermediary genres in experiential learning contexts can help bridge students' learning in the classroom and the workplace, encouraging them to recognize and value classroom learning. In order to support this connection-making across contexts, I recommend three directions for instructors of writing in the health professions.

Consider Opportunities for Concurrent Transfer in Experiential and Extracurricular Contexts

As Moore[20] argues, those researching the transfer of writing knowledge have had a tendency to overlook student's concurrent writing experiences, prioritizing backward-reaching and forward-reaching transfer. Instructors may make a similar mistake when we focus primarily on student's future workplace writing without considering their current extracurricular and workplace experiences.[22] Indeed, health science students are often participating in a myriad of experiential and extracurricular activities, from practicing palpation during a hands-on lab, to volunteering in a traveling urban clinic, to tutoring in the campus writing center. These experiences come with the advantage of transmitting embodied knowledge that makes their audiences and the stakes of their communication physically tangible. We might even think of extracurricular contexts as transmitting what Rice[23] calls "para-expertise," "experiential and embodied knowledge [that] allows individuals to articulate exigencies by validating real needs, problems, and experiences."[(p131)] Opening space in the classroom to discuss these concurrent embodied experiences and building connections to writing assignments has the potential to help students value their new communication skills in immediately relevant ways. (Chapter 4 throws additional light on the challenges of transfer.)

Design Writing Tasks That Authentically Coordinate Classroom Activities

In addition to facilitating connection-making to other experiential learning contexts, instructors can also consider how they might use simulated writing tasks within their own courses to bridge more traditional classroom writing and future workplace communication. While Wardle[9] warns about introducing inauthentic "mutt" genres into our writing courses, simulated writing assignments are unique because they actively support classroom practices. As I have argued[5] in previous analyses of writing in nursing simulations, "a true simulation genre would not just mimic outside texts; it would be purposeful within the simulated framework and play a role in coordinating activities."[(p260)] The simulated patient health record's active role in facilitating student charting and handoffs is a perfect example of this authentic coordination.

Another example comes from a colleague who had students in their writing course linked to a biology course collaboratively design study guides for an upcoming test with attention to a range of visual and spatial elements. The class even voted on the best guide, providing immediate critical peer feedback to support learning. Overall, instructors should consider how to empower students to design genres that are responsive to the rhetorical situation of their classrooms, rather than asking them to mimic professional genres.

Identify and Articulate Shared Heuristics in Writing Assignments

The nursing process was an ever-present heuristic that informed students' care plans, their simulated patient health records, and even the design of electronic patient health records in the workplace. And instructors were explicit about this heuristic, reminding students to use it to shape their documentation and writing. Therefore, when asked about the value of their care plans, students were able to talk clearly about how it was shaping their thinking for future work. Undoubtedly, instructors in the health sciences are working with similar heuristics that inform their curriculum and assignments. However, it is also probably less common that we: (1) Clearly articulate these heuristics to our students, explaining the logic that informs an assignment's structure, and (2) show them how that heuristic will carry through to workplace contexts. Indeed, researchers have found that a key barrier to the transfer of writing knowledge is inconsistencies in how we describe assignments— i.e., a research paper might mean one thing in a sociology course and something entirely different in political science.[8,18,20] This research points to the value of devoting time as a department to not only deciding what to call different kinds of writing but also articulating the thinking processes that we hope students will engage in while completing them. The more we can clearly describe these processes to ourselves and one another, the better we will be able to explain them to students and help them to see the transferability of this thinking, even when writing tasks might take different forms across contexts.

References

1 Gimenez J. Beyond the academic essay: discipline-specific writing in nursing and midwifery. *J Engl Acad Purp*. 2008;7(3):151–164.

2 Opel DS, Hart-Davidson W. The primary care clinic as writing space. *Writ Commun*. 2019;36(3):348–378.

3 Tachino T. Theorizing uptake and knowledge mobilization: a case for intermediary genre. *Writ Commun*. 2012;29(4):455–476.

4 Hertel JP, Millis BJ. *Using Simulations to Promote Learning in Higher Education: An Introduction*. Herndon, VA: Stylus Publishing, LLC; 2002.

5 Campbell L. Simulation genres and student uptake: the patient health record in clinical nursing simulations. *Writ Commun*. 2017;34(3):255–279.

6 Bawarshi AS, Reiff MJ. *Genre: An Introduction to History, Theory, Research, and Pedagogy*. West Lafayette, IN: Parlor Press; 2010.

7 Dias P, Paré A. eds. *Transitions: Writing in Academic and Workplace Settings*. Cresskill, NJ: Hampton Press; 2000.

8 Russell DR. Rethinking genre in school and society: an activity theory analysis. *Writ Commun*. 1997;14(4):504–554.

9 Wardle E "Mutt genres" and the goal of FYC: can we help students write the genres of the university? *CCC*. 2009;60(4):765–789.

10 Ariail J, Smith TG Concept analysis: using an academic nursing genre for writing instruction in nursing. In: *Rhetoric of Healthcare: Essays Toward a New Disciplinary Inquiry*. New York, NY: Hampton Press; 2008:243–263.

11 Heifferon B. *Writing in the Health Professions*. Harlow, UK: Longman Publishing Group; 2005.

12 Bawarshi A. *Genre and the Invention of the Writer: Reconsidering the Place of Invention in Composition*. Boulder, CO: University Press of Colorado; 2003.

13 Bray N. How do online news genres take up knowledge claims from a scientific research article on climate change? *Writ Commun* 2019;36(1):155–189.

14 Rachul C. Digesting data: tracing the chromosomal imprint of scientific evidence through the development and use of Canadian dietary guidelines. *J Bus Tech Commun*. 2019;33(1):26–59.

15 Schryer CF The lab vs. the clinic: Sites of competing genres. In: Freedman A, Medway P eds. *Genre and the New Rhetoric*. London, UK: Routledge; 1994:105–124.

16 Prior P Tracing process: How texts come into being. In: *What Writing Does and How It Does It: An Introduction to Analyzing Texts and Textual Processes*. London, UK: Routledge; 2009

17 Dowding D. Examining the effects that manipulating information given in the change of shift report has on nurses' care planning ability. *J Adv Nurs*. 2001;33(6):836–846.

18 Nelms G, Dively RL. Perceived roadblocks to transferring knowledge from first-year composition to writing-intensive major courses: a pilot study. *WPA: Writ Prog Adm*. 2007;31(1-2):214–240.

19 Benner PE. *From Novice to Expert: Excellence and Power in Clinical Nursing Practice*. Boston, MA: Addison-Wesley Publishing Company; 1984.

20 Moore J. Mapping the questions: the state of writing-related transfer research. *Composition Forum*. 2012; 26.

21 Campbell L. Textual mediation in simulated nursing handoffs: examining how student writing coordinates action. *J Writ Res*. 2019;11(1):79–106.

22 Brittenham R. The interference narrative and the real value of student work. *CCC*. 2017;68(3):526–558.

23 Rice J. Para-expertise, tacit knowledge, and writing problems. *Coll Engl*. 2015;78(2):117–138.

6

"SEMI-EMBEDDING" WRITING CENTER SPECIALISTS IN A MASTER'S-LEVEL NURSING COURSE TO IMPROVE PERCEPTIONS OF WRITING SUPPORT

Sarah Kosel Agnihotri, Tracey Chan, Neal Haldane, Caleb Lalinsky, and Jennifer Weaver

In nursing, there is often a gap between students' current writing skills and what they need to excel academically and professionally.[1–3] Nursing programs do not consistently incorporate direct instruction on writing, which can create additional challenges due to nursing students' varied levels of experience with academic writing.[2,4–6]

It is not uncommon for nursing and composition faculty to collaborate, such as by implementing Writing Across the Curriculum (WAC) or Writing in the Disciplines (WID) approaches. WAC/WID approaches incorporate scaffolded writing instruction and assignments into discipline-specific classes, supporting students who are learning to write in their respective disciplines and faculty who teach in those disciplines.[7] While showing promising results, those collaborations can be labor-intensive in both design and implementation.[3,8] Perhaps as a result, although the number of WAC programs has increased over the last 30 years, a significant percentage of responding surveyed institutions still did not have one.[9]

Writing centers, as resources that already exist on many campuses, have the potential to assist with teaching "writing in the health professions" through partnerships with nursing programs. For example, writing center staff can provide one-on-one instruction, writing workshops, and other resources, as mentioned in Chapters 9 and 10. Writing centers may be particularly useful at institutions without a WAC/WID program.[10,11] However, the limited research on writing centers and nursing suggests that students must perceive the writing center as beneficial and relevant to their needs to be willing to use it.[12–17]

Our university is a small, liberal arts institution with an established writing center and a nursing program that offers bachelor of science in nursing (BSN), master of science in nursing (MSN), and doctor of nursing practice (DNP) degrees (including a BSN-to-DNP option). There is not an official WAC/WID program, and the writing center often becomes the default resource for any WAC/WID initiatives, as can happen with writing centers at small colleges.[11] Although our writing center employs both undergraduate peer tutors and professional tutors with advanced degrees (called writing center specialists in our context), it has been rare for graduate-level nursing students to make use of the available resources. During the two academic years prior to our study (2018–2019 and 2019–2020), only 1.9% of the tutoring sessions (62 out of 3,321) had been with graduate nursing students. Other researchers also found nursing students could be reluctant to use writing centers on their campuses.[8,9,18,19]

DOI: 10.4324/9781003162940-9

This led us to launch a pilot study examining the impact of an adapted model of embedded tutoring on the perceptions of the graduate MSN students, nursing faculty, and writing center specialists. By understanding the expectations and perceptions of each of the stakeholders, the hope was the nursing students would become more open to working with the writing center specialists, and the writing center specialists would feel more confident working with papers written for the nursing discipline. The nursing faculty also hoped they could better support the students whose writing skills needed more attention by partnering with the writing center specialists. Future research could investigate whether the partnership resulted in improved writing outcomes for the students, as well as how an adapted embedded tutor model could be optimized.

Literature Review

In preparation for the collaboration, we examined research on writing instruction in nursing and what partnerships had been documented between writing specialists (whether writing center tutors, composition faculty, or writing program administrators) and nursing programs. We knew nursing faculty at our institution and in the literature had expressed concern about their students' writing abilities[1-3] and that while writing centers were often part of those discussions, they were not always considered particularly helpful resources.[12,13,19] We were interested in finding out what options had been explored at institutions like ours where there existed a writing center but not a formal WAC/WID program. Therefore, the literature review primarily examined partnerships between writing specialists or writing centers working with BSN/MSN nursing programs, rather than full-scale WAC/WID program collaborations with nursing departments.

Writing Instruction in the Nursing Discipline

Research in the field of nursing consistently refers to the importance of teaching nursing students how to write—and specifically, how to write like nurses.[1-3] This is especially true at the graduate level; the American Association of Colleges of Nursing (AACN) lists writing as an essential component of master's level nursing education programs, emphasizing the importance of strong writing abilities for academic scholarship, professional communication, and advocacy work.[20] Long and Beck highlight the importance of learning to write within the nursing discipline, making the connection between writing like a nurse and thinking like a nurse in their argument for the importance of nursing students learning how to write well.[21]

While nurse educators recognize the need for their students to possess proficient writing skills, no single solution for how to provide such instruction has been implemented as standard practice across programs. Mitchell examined the typical approaches nursing faculty take to teaching and evaluating student writing, noting that many instructors focus on grammar and other surface-level mistakes, with writing considered a product rather than a process interconnected with learning. In such instances, nursing educators may overlook the fact that as experts in their field, they understand the expectations and conventions of writing in their discipline in a way that newcomers to the discipline will not.[2] (Narváez-Cardona and Chois-Lenis, in Chapter 2, further describe this process of enculturation.) Other researchers reviewed how writing was taught in individual courses involving writing development and where learning to write in the nursing discipline was integrated into courses throughout the program. They found WAC/WID interventions being used to emphasize writing in connection to learning and help students more fully develop skills for writing in their discipline.[22]

Recognizing the need for improved writing instruction, increasing numbers of nursing educators have turned to the WAC/WID movement for ideas about how best to teach writing. WAC philosophy states that writing instruction needs to be integrated into the entirety of a student's course of study and taught at various points and in multiple ways.[7] At institutions where WAC/WID practices have been incorporated into the nursing curricula, these approaches resulted in beneficial outcomes for students. One set of researchers conducted a study in which they provided nursing students with assignments that built upon one another, guiding the students to meet increasingly challenging writing requirements. The combination of sequenced assignments, feedback from instructors, and peer review led to better writing outcomes overall and noticeable gains related to voice and organization. However, it was noted that these interventions could be challenging to implement due to the amount of effort required.[3] Other researchers also observed that redesigning nursing courses to incorporate WAC/WID elements can be time-consuming.[8]

One acknowledged shortcoming in the literature is the lack of assessment to find out which method of writing instruction provides measurable improvements in nursing students' writing abilities. Two studies explored how nursing students are taught to write, and while a variety of methods were noted, only a small portion had been evaluated to determine how well they worked. The researchers emphasized the need for assessment so the uneven approach to teaching scholarly writing that occurs across nursing programs could be addressed.[1,23] Other researchers have confirmed this and have begun to fill the gaps in the literature with empirical studies so more evidence-based strategies can be identified and hopefully implemented on a large scale.[3,24]

Expectations and Abilities of MSN Student-Writers

Concerns around nursing students' writing abilities exist at all levels of nursing education, yet at the master's level, students are expected to already have a strong grasp of academic writing to build upon. Without that foundation, they will struggle with the increased writing demands as they become nursing scholars ready for advanced practice, further graduate studies, or research.[25] As suggested above, the AACN identifies writing development as a high priority for nurses obtaining a master's degree, charging nursing programs to ensure their graduates are prepared for scholarly and professional communication.[20] Yet students starting MSN programs have varied writing backgrounds and abilities, and they are commonly underprepared for graduate-level writing.

Similar to students entering doctoral programs (discussed in the next chapter), students entering master's programs may have had little writing instruction during their undergraduate courses, and they often are returning to school after a period of time spent working. This situation also causes a dilemma for the nursing faculty, who are often not prepared to support writing development for these students.[4–6,16] One set of researchers assessed MSN students' knowledge, skills, and attitudes (KSAs) related to scholarly writing in nursing and found that most students knew the KSAs but did not always apply them. Therefore, the authors recommended additional instruction and scaffolded opportunities to practice writing through a variety of assignments.[26] While effective, however, these interventions do require additional time and resources to implement.

A common approach has been the use of peer review, as it can support student-writers while reducing the load on faculty. The students' shared disciplinary expertise can make peer review helpful, as long as the students are provided guidance on how to effectively provide feedback on each other's work.[3] Peer review can also be aided by a manuscript checklist in order to provide disciplinary context to the students.[27] Another benefit of peer review is that it is often less stressful or intimidating than when an instructor responds to a paper since the students understand the content being discussed yet remain at an equal level of authority. (See Chapter 4 for additional discussion on feedback practices, including peer review.)

Despite its widespread use and recognized benefits, peer review does have some shortcomings. One team of researchers found not everyone in the nursing class they were observing received useful feedback because the students were not equally proficient in writing.[28] The question of students' perceptions of peer review has also been studied in contexts outside of the nursing field. One study discovered students did not always trust the ability of their peers to offer reliable feedback on papers; furthermore, the researchers found that without careful instruction on how to provide a peer review, the exercise tended to become one of proofreading and editing rather than a holistic discussion of the paper.[29]

Nursing Partnerships with Writing Specialists, Writing Programs, and Writing Centers

Collaborations between nursing and writing faculty can improve the methods used for teaching writing in the health professions. At two institutions in Canada, faculty from nursing and composition came together to examine the research on best practices for teaching writing in the nursing discipline.[30] They found many similarities between their core beliefs about writing instruction but discovered "that although the team was mostly speaking the same language, different members spoke different disciplinary dialects of it."[30(p204)] From this discovery, they developed a synergistic course that drew on the disciplinary expertise of both fields. The result was improved writing instruction for the nursing students that highlighted the connection between general academic writing and nursing-specific academic writing.[30]

At other institutions, English faculty have supported their colleagues in nursing through various partnerships. Writing specialists and nursing faculty at one institution formed a writing team and offered workshops for students and professional development for nursing faculty, eventually creating an online resource center for writing in nursing as well.[13] Another nursing program created a short writing course, taught by nursing faculty but developed in collaboration with the campus writing specialist, to help bridge new MSN students' writing abilities up to the appropriate level. It began as an optional in-person course, with eventual plans to convert it to a mandatory online course due to its success.[12] In each of these scenarios, writing specialists shared strategies for teaching writing, while nursing faculty layered on their expertise in scholarly writing for nursing; these partnerships led to better support for the struggling graduate students and less frustration for the nursing faculty.

Writing centers also have the potential to support nursing students, although the type of writing center and the perception of its value can impact the success of the collaboration. A qualitative systematic review of how nursing students perceived scholarly writing found nursing students often considered general campus writing centers to be limited in their helpfulness because of staff who were not experts in nursing.[18] Similar findings appeared elsewhere in the literature, often noting that while writing centers could assist with mechanics, formatting, and citations, they lacked the discipline-specific and/or graduate-level expertise the students wanted.[12,13] McMillan and Raines explored the benefits perceived by nursing instructors when their students utilized campus resources, including writing centers, but noted mismatched expectations around what the faculty hoped the writing centers would help with versus what they could provide.[19] Thonus investigated the conflicting perceptions tutors, instructors, and students can possess when it comes to writing center sessions, as well as the importance of reconciling those divergent views so everyone has a productive and beneficial experience.[31] Just as composition and nursing faculty need to understand each other's goals and the methods for reaching those goals in order for their collaborations to be successful,[30] discipline-specific faculty, writing specialists, and students need to understand what should be expected of a writing center tutorial for it to succeed.

When writing centers staff had some amount of disciplinary expertise, students had more positive impressions. One writing center at a medical university was designed specifically for students studying to become health-care professionals. Students considered the writing center a valuable resource because of the faculty members' expertise in the health professions and in graduate-level writing.[14,15] Another institution developed an academic-community writing center for students in the BSN and MSN programs. Although their writing center employed community members without a nursing background, the individuals did have expertise in writing and were given resources and training on the particulars of scholarly writing in nursing. Here, too, the writing center was perceived positively by the nursing students.[16] Writing centers do not have to be discipline-specific to have a positive reception though. A writing center, library, and nursing program collaboration involved a graduate-level writing specialist working in the writing center who received insight from the nursing faculty regarding the assignments and expectations for writing in nursing before the course began. This preparation and collaborative model led to the writing center support being positively received by the students.[17]

In WAC/WID literature, scholars have examined the effects of embedding tutors within discipline-specific courses to support both students and faculty in the course.[32] Gladstein examined the embedded tutoring program at her institution, looking specifically at the negotiations that happened when writing specialists worked with students in a writing-intensive science course. She found that the writing specialists were able to come up with creative approaches to help the students, and she also found that the faculty also benefited by learning how to more effectively design their writing assignments and teach discipline-specific writing based on their discussions with the writing specialists.[33] Although writing centers at institutions lacking a WAC/WID program might not have the resources to embed tutors across the curriculum, there is potential for those approaches to be adapted to fit the local context.

Our adapted model of "semi-embedding" writing specialists into a graduate nursing class was guided by the literature. Considering that partnerships between nursing faculty and writing specialists often lead to better outcomes for nursing students but that the resources necessary for those collaborations are not always available, a partnership with the writing center seemed logical. Writing centers already have resources and staff to support student-writers, yet nursing students may be reluctant to use them unless they see a direct link between the writing center and their discipline-specific writing. Writing centers could therefore use an adapted model of semi-embedding tutors in a nursing class to encourage the students to make better use of the resources already available.

Institutional Context and Methods

Our institution had for years used a writing assessment administered and scored through the writing center to evaluate writing in new graduate nursing students to ensure they all entered the program with comparable writing skills. The assessment was a 90-minute timed writing exercise, with students responding to a prompt and expected to demonstrate graduate-level writing skills and appropriate use of American Psychological Association (APA) formatting. It was scored by three composition faculty using the same rubric. This assessment was developed at the nursing department's request due to concerns over the entering students' writing abilities; if students scored below a certain threshold on the writing assessment, they were required to enroll in a supplemental writing class to develop their writing skills. Despite this procedure, however, nursing faculty found some students were still underperforming on master's-level writing tasks.

In response to this situation, the nursing faculty developed an online one-semester foundational course with one credit focused on writing in the nursing discipline. The first semester this course was taught, students had a weekly short, prompted writing assignment, and use of the writing center was recommended but not required. Formulating the course this way was burdensome, as well as ineffective in developing students' writing skills since the assignments were not adequately scaffolded and covered different topics weekly. In the next offering of the course, the number of writing assignments was decreased to every other week and again the writing center was recommended but not required. This offering was better, but faculty still did not perceive students developing the expected graduate-level writing skills.

At this point, the nursing faculty and the writing center decided to partner to semi-embed writing center specialists within the course. This idea developed from the writing center's desire to highlight the unique resource graduate students had access to in the writing center specialists and the nursing faculty's concern that the writing assessment had not been effective in ensuring all new graduate students could write at the appropriate level. Multiple meetings occurred starting in early 2020 between the course faculty and the writing center staff to determine how to best formulate the course, and as part of those discussions, the writing assessment requirement was eliminated in favor of semi-embedding writing center specialists in the course and requiring the students to use the writing center.

Our adapted version of embedded tutoring ("semi-embedded" tutoring) was different from the traditional approach of having tutors participate in weekly class sessions. Instead, the writing center specialists joined the initial class to introduce themselves and provide supplemental writing resources, while the students were expected to make appointments with the specialists in the writing center during their regular shifts. This approach allowed the writing center to use staff and resources it already had while still increasing the writing center specialists' interaction with the nursing students. The students were required to meet with a writing center specialist during the first 2 weeks of the course prior to submitting a writing assignment. The writing center specialists used those meetings to understand each student's level of writing experience and explain the role the writing center specialist would have within the course. It was also decided that three writing assignments of 3 to 5 pages each, which would be scaffolded into a longer paper, would be adequate for the course. The students would be required to meet with a writing center specialist at least once for each assignment.

The two nursing professors team-teaching the nursing course met with the writing center coordinator and the two designated writing center specialists throughout the spring and summer in order to plan for the fall 2020 class. As the course was traditionally offered online, the writing center specialists were added to the course's learning management system so they could introduce themselves, see the assignments, and join select class sessions where writing would be discussed. Since the students would be expected to schedule appointments with the writing center specialists at the writing center, the specialists' schedules were provided, along with instructions for using the writing center's online scheduling system.

Prior to the course starting, the nursing faculty and writing center specialists also devoted time to discussing the faculty's goals around the assignments, the structure and time line of the assignments, and what were reasonable expectations for the support that the writing center specialists could provide. The specialists discussed their emphasis on addressing topics like organization, focus, and development of the whole paper rather than providing line-by-line editing; the fact that students would need to plan in advance and potentially make multiple appointments to allow adequate time for feedback; and the importance of the papers remaining the students' responsibility. This alignment of expectations and goals before the semester started was intended to help the faculty and writing center specialists reach a shared understanding of how the writing center specialists could be of assistance to the students during the course.

This planning phase also allowed time to prepare additional resources. The nursing faculty mentioned that incoming graduate students often struggled with making the transition from undergraduate to graduate writing and that they frequently needed refreshers on using APA formatting. Subsequently, the writing center specialists created online modules on those topics that could be used in the nursing course but also were made available to all students using the writing center. An important consideration throughout this collaboration was how to use writing center resources that were already available or how to create resources such as handouts and online modules for the nursing course that could also be used more broadly by the writing center.

One unexpected complication was the COVID-19 pandemic. While initial discussions had started before the pandemic impacted our state, most of the planning occurred during months when the campus was shut down and the writing center was limited to virtual appointments. During the fall 2020 semester when the nursing class was offered, the writing center reopened in a hybrid format but the unusual circumstances left resources stretched thin. The writing center switched from offering drop-in sessions and appointments both in-person and online to requiring appointments and only offering limited in-person options, a change that also reduced the total number of tutoring sessions available for students on any given day. The nursing course had already been planned in an online format but had its own stressors, as many of the students were working on the front lines of the pandemic while simultaneously starting their graduate studies. The biggest impact was the significant reduction in the time that the writing center staff and nursing faculty had to plan the pilot collaboration during the summer and then check in with each other on progress during the fall.

To analyze how the collaboration impacted how students perceived the value of scholarly writing and the semi-embedded writing center specialists, we distributed a survey at the end of the semester. We reviewed the literature for potential surveys but none were found that fit exactly what we were looking to measure. Subsequently, we developed a survey around two main research questions:

- How did the structure of the writing assignments and instruction in this course influence the way students perceived scholarly writing in the nursing discipline?
- Did the students perceive the writing center and writing center specialists' support in this course as helpful?

On the survey, students were asked to indicate their level of agreement for 13 statements related to scholarly writing and writing center support in their nursing course. Each statement was followed by a visual analog scale that students could use to indicate their level of agreement, with 0 equal to "do not agree at all" and 100 equal to "completely agree." There were two open-ended questions at the end of the survey.

The survey was piloted with the nursing faculty and writing center coordinator prior to distribution to the students. The survey was administered online at the end of the course, and 9 students responded out of a total class size of 24.

Survey Results

The statements on the survey and the response mean, range, and standard deviation (SD) are as follows:

1. Work throughout this course allowed me to realize that learning to write is a process. (Mean 76.9, Range 55–100, SD 13.5)
2. Work throughout this course allowed me to realize the importance of prewriting activities, such as outlining, searching the literature, or thinking about the topic. (Mean 66.7, Range 37–100, SD 20.3)

3. I value the connection between scholarly writing and advancing nursing science. (Mean 64.4, Range 10–100, SD 31.2)
4. The structure of the writing assignments within this course helped to improve my scholarly writing. (Mean 73.2, Range 13–100, SD 28.9)
5. I feel this course increased my confidence in my writing ability. (Mean 73.3, Range 34–100, SD 25.6)
6. I valued the writing modules that were a part of the course. (Mean 64.2, Range 17–100, SD 23.8)
7. Having support from the writing center allowed me to write a paper without feeling fear or distress. (Mean 31.9, Range 8–65, SD 23.6)
8. I feel the writing specialist increased my confidence in my writing ability. (Mean 37.4, Range 5–100, SD 31.6)
9. I can accept feedback on my writing. (Mean 96.9, Range 81–100, SD 6.2)
10. I value having assistance from writing specialists who were embedded in the class during the writing process. (Mean 37.9, Range 10–74, SD 24)
11. I found the requirement to go to the writing center helpful. (Mean 27.8, Range 0–65, SD 24.9)
12. I had issues with being able to access the writing center. (Mean 71.1, Range 28–100, SD 27.3)
13. I felt there was a discrepancy between writing experts and course faculty feedback. (Mean 66, Range 0–100, SD 34.2)

The students then commented on the most and least valuable aspects of working with the writing center specialists. Students found that the specialists were able to assist with grammar (n = 2), proofreading (n = 3), writing process (n = 1), and APA style (n = 2). The aspects they found least helpful were related to nursing content (n = 1), finding time to schedule (n = 3), and inconsistencies between writing center specialists and nursing faculty feedback (n = 3). Some specific comments included the following: "Brought a process to writing that I did not consider (e.g. different ways to organize; set a goal to write 3 paragraphs/day; taking thoughts and streamlining them)," "Reviewing APA accuracy, writing flow," and "The times were a bit limited, I also got some conflicting information from the writing center vs feedback from professors at times." Students also experienced issues with being able to access the course-dedicated writing center specialists.

Students who responded (n = 9) felt that integrating writing assignments into an early graduate nursing course was helpful for improving their writing. Students also found value in writing three shorter papers that fed into a longer paper at the conclusion of the course. It should be noted that the mean scores on the three short papers that were reviewed with a writing center specialist improved throughout the course with the first assignment having a mean score of 86.6 (range 71.5–97.8), the second having a mean of 90.6 (range 57–100), and the third having a mean of 92.3 (range 72–100). Multiple factors could have contributed to the improved writing scores, including work with a writing specialist, nursing faculty feedback on previous assignments, or simply repetition of writing.

Reflections from the Writing Center Specialists and a Nursing Faculty Member

Only 9 participants responded to the survey out of a total class size of 24, which made it difficult to calculate measures of validity. To triangulate the data, one of the nursing faculty members and both of the semi-embedded writing center specialists provided written reflections on their experiences in this pilot study. The reflections are summarized next.

The writing center specialists felt that during the pilot program, nursing students' perceptions of the prewriting and draft process were largely positive, as were their perceptions of their own skills and improvements, which could be directly tied to their experiences working with the writing center. Nursing students internalized reviewing their work with a tutor as part of their course and writing expectations, eventually developing their own drafting processes around the relationship. Over time, working with the writing center became an intentional part of the nursing students' planning. The writing center specialists also observed that after initial contact was made and a familiarity with the staff and procedures of the writing center was established, nursing students were able to anticipate their appointments based on these shared expectations and areas of feedback. As the minimum length and rigor of the sequenced writing assignments increased, requiring more attention and effort from the nursing students, planning ahead for return writing center appointments become more frequent. Nursing students learned to approach their appointments with ownership, rather than a sense of requirement, learning when and how they needed the most help with each draft. The average number of pages and depth of discussion increased during these recurring tutoring sessions, as both nursing students and writing center specialists became better aware of the requirements for working together and possible outcomes.

The nursing faculty teaching the course valued the input of the writing center specialists, as they were able to offer students a different perspective on writing. She was able to focus more on content within the paper and help students refine that while the writing center specialists assisted with the mechanics of writing. Students did resist being required to meet with the writing center specialists, but the faculty continued requiring it and noted improvements in writing throughout the term. Students complained of issues with scheduling to meet with the writing center specialists; the faculty had known that could be an issue and had encouraged students to make appointments early in the term, suggesting they use those as deadlines for writing, but many students waited until the last minute to try and get an appointment. As a result, some of the students may not have been able to see one of the writing center specialists. Being graduate students, they needed to understand time management and not wait to do an assignment that had to be reviewed by a writing center specialist prior to submission. In the future, the nursing faculty will consider putting in required writing center visit dates a few days prior to the actual due date to assist with this. The nursing faculty felt that semi-embedding the writing center specialists into the course was beneficial for both students and faculty and indicated this model will continue with enhancements as necessary, including a more objective evaluation of students' writing.

The nursing faculty member also felt the structure of assignments was appropriate. Students were able to pick a topic they wished to write on and were provided writing prompts to address the topic, such as ethical concerns related to their topic. Since writing is a process, being able to spread three shorter papers over the first 10 weeks of the course allowed faculty time to review the assignment and provide adequate feedback, as well as for students to have time to spend on the writing process. This also allowed a few weeks for students to spend compiling material from the first papers, refining and expanding on it to have a final comprehensive paper on their chosen topic.

Discussion

Our findings align with literature indicating that nursing students are not likely to perceive writing centers as helpful if there is not an obvious connection to the nursing discipline. In our case, future collaborations could be optimized by making the institutional partnership more evident to the students, emphasizing the role of the writing specialists in the course.

A possible next step to refine the semi-embedded tutoring model at our institution would be to create a separate survey for the writing center specialists and nursing faculty. Such a survey could show us how their perceptions of the writing center and tutoring process were communicated to nursing students and how these perceptions changed throughout the program. That could also be important for reducing the students' perceptions of mismatched feedback from the nursing faculty and writing center specialists. Since the literature showed that writing centers do not necessarily need to be discipline-specific for nursing students to have a positive perception of them, a future refinement to our collaboration could be familiarizing the writing center specialists more with "writing in the health professions" and evangelizing our work to students more effectively.

Limitations of this study were the small sample size, not collecting data prior to the course, and using a survey that we developed ourselves instead of a standardized one. In the future, it could be beneficial to conduct a similar study using pre-post data, examining not just perception but also changes in writing ability as shown by a validated tool. Although we will need more robust assessments in the future, these survey results and reflections provide a starting point for considering ways to refine the writing center/nursing program partnership and continue to improve graduate nursing students' perception of the writing center.

Recommendations for Instructors and Administrators

Writing centers at small schools without a WAC/WID program could support teaching writing in the health professions by embedding or "semi-embedding" writing specialists in specific courses to improve students' perception of the writing center as a valuable resource. A trend that emerged in the literature and that was reinforced by the findings in our study was the importance of nursing faculty, writing specialists, and graduate nursing students having a shared understanding of the type of support the writing center can provide. If students do not consider the writing center relevant to them and view it as unable to help with their specific disciplinary writing needs, they are unlikely to use it. Although aspects of the writing specialists' involvement were recognized by students as good qualities of the course in our study, such as the emphasis on writing as a process through scaffolded assignments and the supplementary writing resources, the students did not seem to realize the connection to the writing center itself. If writing centers and nursing faculty are planning a collaboration, taking time to jointly decide their goals and expectations and determining the best way to communicate those aligned expectations to the students would be important.

Ensuring the writing center is accessible for graduate nursing students is also important, especially because they are often juggling full-time jobs and other commitments that leave them with little extra time. We were optimistic about this aspect initially because the writing center normally was open 50 hours per week, including weekend and evening hours, for in-person or online sessions. One concern was whether the course-designated writing specialists' schedules would match up with the students' schedules, as much about this first collaboration was guesswork, and we did not know whether two specialists would be enough support. The COVID-19 pandemic complicated everything, as did confusion caused by introducing a new online scheduling system in the writing center that semester. It is not surprising that the nursing students were frustrated by the inaccessibility of the writing center, and that would be an important factor to consider for future collaborations.

While this pilot collaboration had its share of unexpected complications from the pandemic, it provided an exciting opportunity to start building a strong partnership between the writing center and the graduate nursing program at our institution. It was understood from the beginning that there would be trial and error to figure out the best ways to support the MSN students' writing development, but what we learned about the importance of shared goals, clear communication with students about how the writing center can help, and the benefits of keeping an open line of communication between the writing specialists and the nursing faculty shows promise.

References

1. Oermann MH, Leonardelli AK, Turner KM, Hawks SJ, Derouin AL, Hueckel RM. Systematic review of educational programs and strategies for developing students' and nurses' writing skills. *J Nurs Educ Thorofare*. 2015;54(1):28–34. doi:10.3928/01484834-20141224-01

2. Mitchell KM. Constructing writing practices in nursing. *J Nurs Educ Thorofare*. 2018;57(7):399–407. doi:10.3928/01484834-20180618-04

3. Miller LC, Russell CL, An-Lin C, Zembles S. Testing the efficacy of a scaffolded writing intervention with online degree-completion nursing students: a quasi-experimental design. *Nurse Educ Pract Kidlington*. 2018;32:115–121. doi:10.1016/j.nepr.2018.06.011

4. Murrock CJ. Innovative short group writing assignments to enhance scholarly writing skills. *J Nurs Educ*. 2019;58(1):61. doi:10.3928/01484834-20190103-11

5. Walker M, Tschanz C. Stories are like water: an academic writing workshop for nurses. *Creat Nurs Minneap*. 2013;19(2):81–85.

6. Bastian H, Fauchald SK. Confronting the challenges of blended graduate education with a WEC project. *Across the Disciplines*. 2014;11(3):n3.

7. International Network of WAC Programs. *Statement of WAC Principles and Practices*; 2014. https://wac.colostate.edu/docs/principles/statement.pdf Accessed February 20, 2020.

8. Luthy KE, Peterson NE, Lassetter JH, Callister LC. Successfully incorporating writing across the curriculum with advanced writing in nursing. *J Nurs Educ*. 2009;48(1):54–59.

9. Thaiss C, Porter T, Zugnomi M International WAC/WID Mapping Project: 2015–2020 Survey. 2020. https://mappingproject.ucdavis.edu/content/2015-2020-survey Accessed January 18, 2021.

10. Harris M. The writing center and tutoring in WAC programs. In: McLeod SH, Soven M, eds. *Writing Across the Curriculum: A Guide to Developing Programs*. The WAC Clearinghouse; 2000. https://wac.colostate.edu/books/landmarks/mcleod_soven/. Accessed January 15, 2021.

11. Stay BL. Writing centers in the small college. In: Murphy C, Stay BL, eds. *The Writing Center Director's Resource Book*. Mahwah, NJ: Lawrence Erlbaum Associates; 2006.

12. Cone PH, Van Dover L. Shaping how graduate nursing students write. *Nurs Educ Perspect*. 2012;33(4):272–274.

13. White BJ, Lamson KS. The evolution of a writing program. *J Nurs Educ*. 2017;56(7):443–445. doi:10.3928/01484834-20170619-11

14. Ariail J, Thomas S, Smith T, Kerr L, Richards-Slaughter S, Shaw D. The value of a writing center at a medical university. *Teach Learn Med*. 2013;25(2):129–133. doi:10.1080/10401334.2013.770739

15. Smith TG, Ariail J, Richards-Slaughter S, Kerr L. Teaching professional writing in an academic health sciences center: the writing center model at the Medical University of South Carolina. *Teach Learn Med*. 2011;23(3):298–300. doi:10.1080/10401334.2011.586937

16. Latham CL, Ahern N. Professional writing in nursing education: creating an academic--community writing center. *J Nurs Educ*. 2013;52(11):615–620. doi:10.3928/01484834-20131014-02

17. Bernstein M, Roney L, Kazer M, Boquet EH. Librarians collaborate successfully with nursing faculty and a writing centre to support nursing students doing professional doctorates. *Health Inf Libr J*. 2020;37(3):240–244. doi:10.1111/hir.12327

18. Mitchell KM, Blanchard L, Roberts T. Seeking transformation: how students in nursing view their academic writing context—a qualitative systematic review. *Int J Nurs Educ Scholarsh*. 2020;17(1). doi:10.1515/ijnes-2020-0074.

19. McMillan LR, Raines K. Using the "write" resources: nursing student evaluation of an interdisciplinary collaboration using a professional writing assignment. *J Nurs Educ Thorofare*. 2011;50(12):697–702. doi:10.3928/01484834-20110930-01

20. American Association of Colleges of Nurses. *The Essentials of Master's Education in Nursing*; 2011. https://www.aacnnursing.org/portals/42/publications/mastersessentials11.pdf Accessed February 27, 2020.

21. Long TL, Beck CT. *Writing in Nursing: A Brief Guide*. New York, NY: Oxford University Press;2016.

22. Troxler H, Vann JCJ, Oermann MH. How baccalaureate nursing programs teach writing. *Nurs Forum*. 2011;46(4):280–288. doi:10.1111/j.1744-6198.2011.00242.x

23. Hawks SJ, Turner KM, Derouin AL, Hueckel RM, Leonardelli AK, Oermann MH. Writing across the curriculum: strategies to improve the writing skills of nursing students. *Nurs Forum*. 2016;51(4):261–267. doi:10.1111/nuf.12151

24. Mitchell KM, Harrigan T, McMillan DE. Writing self-efficacy in nursing students: the influence of a discipline-specific writing environment. *Nurs Open*. 2017;4(4):240–250. doi:10.1002/nop2.90.

25. Gazza EA, Hunker DF. Facilitating scholarly writer development: the writing scaffold. *Nurs Forum*. 2012;47(4):278–285. doi:10.1111/j.1744-6198.2012.00275.x

26. Gazza EA, Shellenbarger T, Hunker DF. MSN students' self-assessed use of the knowledge, skills, and attitudes of scholarly writing. *Nurs Educ Perspect*. 2018;39(6):350–354. doi:10.1097/01. NEP.0000000000000363.

27. Hirschey R, Rodgers C, Hockenberry M. A program to enhance writing skills for advanced practice nurses. *J Contin Educ Nurs*. 2019;50(3):109–114. doi:10.3928/00220124-20190218-05.

28. Schlisselberg G, Moscou S. Peer review as an educational strategy to improve academic work: an inter-disciplinary collaboration between communication disorders and nursing. *Work*. 2013;44(3):355–360. doi:10.3233/WOR-121512.

29. Brammer C, Rees M. Peer review from the students' perspective: invaluable or invalid? *Compos Stud Chic*. 2007;35(2):71–85, 142–143.

30. Feltham M, Krahn MA. Breathing life into the syllabus: the collaborative development of a first-year writing course for nursing students. *Collect Essays Learn Teach*. 2016;9:199. doi:10.22329/celt.v9i0.4444.

31. Thonus T. Triangulation in the writing center: tutor, tutee, and instructor perceptions of the tutor's role. *Writ Cent J*. 2001;22(1):59–82.

32. Hughes B, Hall EB. Guest editor introduction. *Across the Discip*. 2008;5. doi:10.37514/ATD-J.2008.5.2.01.

33. Gladstein J. Conducting research in the gray space: how writing associates negotiate between WAC and WID in an introductory biology course. *Across the Discip*. 2008;5. doi:10.37514/ATD-J.2008.5.2.02

7

WRITING-RELATED THRESHOLD CONCEPTS IN DOCTORAL NURSING EDUCATION

Deborah E. Tyndall

Teaching writing in the health professions can be challenging, especially in doctoral programs. Graduates of doctoral programs are expected to create and disseminate knowledge, secure grant funding, and engage in academic presentations to advance the science of nursing. Yet these expectations depend on strong competencies in scholarly writing,[1] and research indicates that, for many doctoral students, scholarly writing is a struggle.[2,3] While there are efforts to mentor faculty on their own skills,[4,5] they may receive less mentoring on how to effectively teach scholarly writing to students. Consequently, nursing faculty may feel underprepared to teach writing conventions required for the discipline, leading to trial-and-error types of instruction. To support writing development in nursing students, collaborations with writing experts are common,[6–9] as mentioned in previous chapters.

I often talk with my colleagues about doctoral students' challenges with scholarly writing, and I repeatedly hear, "They should already know how to write": so, why do students enter our programs so seemingly unready? For starters, undergraduate and graduate nursing curricula are often focused on preparing clinical practitioners, and writing competencies are not prioritized. Writing assignments are typically limited to review by the course instructor, and feedback may be inadequate to help the students meet the demands of a broader scholarly audience. Additionally, nurses may take time off from their studies before returning for their doctorate.[10] All of these factors may make it more difficult to develop and refine scholarly writing skills.

Understanding the writing-related challenges that doctoral students face can provide insight into best pedagogical practices for entry-level students. Building students' scholarly writing competencies as they embark on their PhD journey is critical to support a successful transition into the genres of doctoral writing. Early identification of writing strengths and weaknesses can position both students and faculty to address gaps before arriving at the dissertation stage when students conduct independent research. At this stage, students often feel isolated and insecure[11,12] and are at more risk of falling behind, especially if their writing competencies have not been strengthened over the prior years.

Entry PhD courses have been beneficial in introducing nursing students to the writing conventions for doctoral study.[13,14] The introductory course I describe in this chapter was created to assist PhD nursing students with development of writing competencies they need as novice nurse scientists. This course has been crucial in our program, as 80% of PhD students enter with no experience with peer-reviewed, scholarly writing (i.e., manuscript and grant writing). In this chapter, I report

DOI: 10.4324/9781003162940-10

research findings based on 5 years of instruction with entry-level PhD students and strategies that have been successful in their writing development.

Threshold Concepts

Since beginning my academic career, I have had opportunities to teach undergraduate, master's, and doctoral writing. Teaching across the curriculum has given me a unique perspective on the role of faculty in supporting student transfer of writing knowledge between education levels. The study described in this chapter examines how threshold concepts might relate to the discipline of nursing, especially for the research-doctorate. I argue that a "threshold concepts in writing" framework provides a conceptual understanding of troublesome concepts doctoral students encounter as they begin to think and write like nurse scientists. This research is a collaborative effort with colleagues from the university's writing program and my research mentor who co-taught the introductory course before her retirement. This research has increased our understanding of writing-related threshold concepts and their impact on teaching and learning in entry-level PhD students. (As Chapter 4 shows, threshold concepts can be applied at other levels as well.)

Threshold concepts were first introduced by engineers Meyer and Land,[15] who based this framework upon the premise that certain disciplines have "conceptual gateways" or "portals": challenging but important concepts that learners must master.[16(p373)] These portals result in some students having a transformational learning experience, while others get "stuck." Threshold concepts can be *integrative*, *bounded* to context, and *irreversible*[15]; however, the characteristics of *troublesome* and *liminal*[15] may be of particular interest in doctoral education.

The characteristic of *troublesome* means that new knowledge may be conceptually difficult and emotionally charged, perhaps requiring learners to make an identity shift to fully embrace learning. The characteristic of *liminal* describes an "in-between state" in the learning process, which is understood as nonlinear. The idea is that, first, learners encounter a threshold concept that may be troublesome and unfamiliar. This is a *preliminal* state. Then, as learners engage with it, such as through additional study or practice, they enter a *liminal* state. Here, they oscillate between prior knowledge and new knowledge, finding ways to integrate them—or getting stuck. In time, learners can "cross the threshold": they can enter a *postliminal state*, where a threshold concept is mastered, and the learning is transformational.[17]

The framework of threshold concepts has been used predominately in undergraduate education within a variety of disciplines. Scholars began applying the framework to doctoral education in 2009[18] by examining faculty experiences with student learning challenges related to research. As such, some scholars have used *liminality* to describe doctoral writing practices.[19] This scholarly dialogue continues as more research unfolds related to threshold concepts in doctoral education.[20,21] In a recent integrative review in this area, student writing development was a significant factor in facilitating conceptual threshold crossing.[22]

Experts in the discipline of writing studies have noted writing-related threshold concepts. These threshold concepts are applicable to writing across the disciplines and include (1) writing is a social and rhetorical activity, (2) writing speaks to situations through recognizable forms, (3) writing enacts and creates identities and ideologies, (4) all writers have more to learn, and (5) writing is a cognitive activity.[23] In a previous publication, my colleagues and I examined these threshold concepts specific to writing and their applicability to doctoral nursing education.[24] We took the perspective that doctoral students experience liminal states while writing new genres, and if students stay too long in these liminal states, it can hinder their writing development. Examining writing through the lens of these five writing-related threshold concepts also offered insight into challenges doctoral students experience and what factors may contribute to "crossing the threshold."

Writing Is a Social and Rhetorical Activity: At the doctoral level, students must consider both social and rhetorical contexts. That is, they must respond to the needs of an audience and *write for the reader*. Understanding this writing-related threshold concept can better equip doctoral students to position themselves as members of the research community and make meaningful contributions to science.

How can we help students learn this threshold concept? One way is peer learning, as learning from peers has been associated with scholarly writing development in doctoral students.[12,25] Indeed, doctoral students have been successful in the mastery of threshold concepts when they learn from experienced peers who are already in the "zone" of becoming a scholarly writer[26] and when they receive feedback from multiple readers.[27]

Writing Speaks to Situations through Recognizable Forms: The genres that nurse scientists must learn to write are grounded in the broader community of nursing. Mastery of this writing-related threshold concept is essential for doctoral students to transition from being consumers of knowledge (novices/students) to become both consumers and producers of knowledge (scholars/scientists). Scaffolded instruction has been effective in facilitating learning in master's and doctoral students,[28–31] including the development of nursing students' scholarly writing abilities.[32,33] Scaffolding is the sequencing of steps to support a student throughout the learning process, emphasized in Chapter 6, among others. Scaffolded instruction to support scholarly writers involves the decreasing of support over time as writing competencies are developed.[32]

Writing Enacts and Creates Identities and Ideologies: Doctoral students develop identities and ideologies through the process of writing within their discipline. Creating spaces where students can practice writing fosters the development of their researcher voices and positioning. Writing and learning communities, such as writing groups[34] and peer-review groups,[35] can offer spaces for writing-oriented practices to support doctoral students in the liminal states of learning. Communities where doctoral students write and learn together also foster reflective practice[36] and have been effective in shaping their identities as scholars.[37]

All Writers Have More to Learn: At the doctoral level, challenges with writing may result from a lack of exposure to complex genres, such as empirical research reports and literature reviews. Most doctoral students are shifting from readers to composers of these genres in order to disseminate new knowledge. To cultivate this shift to composers, doctoral students need opportunities to learn about themselves as writers. Feedback is an essential component to support awareness of voice and construction of writer identity.[38] Faculty should consider the type of feedback provided to doctoral students, as students report negative emotions and vulnerability when submitting early examples of writing.[39]

Writing Is a Cognitive Activity: Doctoral nursing education promotes the development of the intellectual habits necessary for students to become research scholars. Metacognitive activities, such as reflective writing, can help students to "think about thinking," better regulate their thinking, and work through troublesome knowledge and liminal spaces.[40,41]

The Doctoral Introductory Course

To foster the scholarly writing competencies of entry-level PhD students, a 3-semester-hour introductory course was developed at my university, a midsized public research institution in the eastern United States. This introductory course, Nursing Scholarship and Discovery I, is intended to assist students with building novice research and writing competencies to promote a successful transition into doctoral studies. PhD students, who enter the program in cohorts of 6 to 10, enroll in this course during the summer before beginning their core classes in the fall semester. This writing-intensive, 11-week hybrid course consists of weekly engagement via face-to-face class meetings, individual virtual meetings with faculty, and asynchronous online assignments. The course includes various assignments focused on the process of writing, peer review and critique, and developing the practice of revision through a final scholarly paper. To build novice researcher and writing competencies during the course, strategies including scaffolded assignments, metacognitive activities, and peer review are used.

Scaffolded Assignments

A series of scaffolded writing assignments were created to support PhD students in producing a final scholarly paper. These writing assignments break down the steps of writing a literature review: constructing a research question, creating a literature matrix, outlining the synthesis, drafting, peer-reviewing, revising, and presenting findings. In the first few weeks of the course, students work on constructing a research question to guide their literature review. PhD nursing students generally have research interests based on their clinical practice or other scholarly experiences. Many students build upon these early ideas cultivated during the course to develop a more focused area for dissertation research.

Next, students create a literature matrix that provides a structure for synthesizing the literature and identifying gaps in nursing research. Students learn to look for "gaps" in the literature, practice writing what is known about a research topic, and demonstrate the ability to sort and organize content into a cogent and relevant structure for a literature review. Finally, students practice the process of writing through drafting and revising. While the course includes a high-stakes final writing assignment (i.e., review of literature), low-stakes writing activities, such as peer review and scholarly presentation, are scaffolded throughout the course to engage students in learning the process of writing. These low-stakes writing activities provide an earlier view of how students are learning the course material and give faculty an opportunity to intervene when students are struggling.

Metacognitive Activities

Metacognitive activities prompt students to become aware of their thinking. In this course, students keep a reflective learning journal to encourage a habit of reflection. Students are encouraged to document their thoughts as they read, respond to class discussions, and explore their scholarship interests. To guide their reflection, students are given weekly prompts, which are designed to foster students' awareness of how they think. Students are encouraged to journal a minimum of twice weekly during the course. (For another kind of reflective journaling, see Chapter 13.)

Along with the reflective journal, other course activities are assigned to promote metacognitive thinking. Students examine a quantitative and qualitative PhD dissertation in an area of research in which they have an interest. After reviewing a dissertation, students respond to reflective prompts to capture their reactions (e.g., excitement, anxiety). This activity helps students begin to get a sense of the expectations for scholarly writing required for a research-doctorate. Students also complete weekly readings and exercises guided by Goodson's *Becoming an Academic Writer*[42] to develop productive habits of writing and awareness of writer identity. At the end of the course, students complete a writer's memo to reflect upon their processes for writing the literature review. This memo invokes metacognitive thinking about the writing choices students engage in, providing insight about themselves as writers.

Peer Review and Critique

During the course, we introduce "Critical Friends" to the PhD students, facilitating the processes of giving and receiving critique. Critical Friends is a six-step peer review protocol that allows time for feedback, reflection, and active revision processes.[35] To familiarize the students with the process, readings are assigned and guest speakers who use the protocol are invited to class. Then students are ready to try it for themselves. Among their peer group, students provide a draft of their literature review assignment, and critique is based on "tuning questions" that are provided before the review session. Tuning questions, which are crafted by the students, are queries and/or commentary provided to peer reviewers to solicit the desired feedback.

Students engage in the peer-review process with 3 to 4 peer learners who are paired with a faculty facilitator. Each individual review is allotted 35–40 minutes. Students are limited to two peer reviews to be mindful of their course workload. Faculty serve as facilitators, allowing students to lead the discussion while faculty supplement feedback by role modeling scholarly critique. At the end of the course, students' work is assessed through their review of the literature. The faculty assesses whether students applied feedback appropriately, identified a potential gap in knowledge, and discussed implications for student research.

Little research currently exists on how doctoral nursing students, who often do not receive direct instruction on scholarly writing, develop as writers or how they interact with crucial threshold concepts while doing so. The purpose of this chapter is to report findings from empirical data on troublesome knowledge identified by five cohorts of entry-level PhD nursing students. Specifically, troublesome knowledge students experience while constructing their researcher and writer identity will be explored.

Research Design and Data Collection

This chapter builds on earlier work that examined threshold concepts identified by entry-level PhD nursing students as they began to think and write like nurse scientists.[43] This mixed-methods case study uses writing-related threshold concepts as critical instruments for teaching and learning. The research was approved by the university's Institutional Review Board, and students signed informed consent forms to give permission for their reflective journals to be included in this research. These informed consent forms were collected from a member of the research team not affiliated with the course. Findings were generated from content analysis of multiple data sources collected from 5 cohorts of PhD students (n = 40). Data sources include 432 pages from student reflective learning journals, course evaluations, and faculty formative assessments of student writing.

Student Liminal Spaces during the Course

In earlier work, research exploring troublesome knowledge for entry-level PhD nursing students identified three threshold concepts for the research-doctorate: *developing new ways of knowing, constructing researcher and writer identity*, and *positioning within the nursing research community*.[43] While these concepts were interrelated and interdependent, the analysis indicated that entry-level students find the threshold concept of *constructing researcher and writer identity* most troublesome during the course. The juxtaposition of identities associated with expert practitioners and novice scientists created states of liminality for students. Here, I delve deeper into the data to unpack the liminal spaces students experienced within this threshold concept. To illustrate how the experience of constructing a researcher and writer identity created states of liminality, I provide reflective notes from PhD student journals kept during the course.

Writing the Literature Review

Students began to construct their research and writer identities in the course by undertaking the literature review, a liminal space where students often got stuck during the course. These findings are consistent with research conducted in other disciplines, citing the writing of a literature review as a threshold concept for doctoral students.[20,44,45] When the course first originated, scaffolded assignments were designed to support students with the process of a literature review. However, course faculty learned that our expertise was somewhat hindering our understanding of what was challenging for the students. As disciplinary experts, we had mastered the threshold concept of writing the literature review and did not fully understand the level of scaffolding needed to support students' thinking and writing (see also Chapter 2). As a result, we had not included enough instruction and guidance. This was evident upon end-of-course assessments when we found that students' literature review findings lacked a logical synthesis and discussions were not insightful. Understanding that students were encountering new knowledge (*preliminal state*) required faculty to think about more effective strategies to support students with the challenges they were experiencing (*liminal state*).

> It was a little uncomfortable. I wasn't sure how to set up the matrix or write [a literature] review. I find myself stressing out over being worried about submitting something that is way off the mark and looking stupid [...]. Are professors going to question whether they should have chosen me to be in their program? [...] This assignment certainly showed me some areas that I will need to get better at and strengthen.
>
> (PhD Student Journal)

Students struggled with creating a feasible research question to guide the literature review and most found themselves "in the ocean" with their ideas. We found students needed more guidance on constructing a research question before they were immersed in the literature.

> Hindsight and pride! I wish I had reached out to faculty and refined my question a bit more before presenting—I think it would have helped me not be in the ocean and be closer to the research question I really want. It also would have helped with my anxiety.
>
> (PhD Student Journal)

Meyer and Land's notion of threshold concepts helped the course faculty reconnect with what it meant to be a novice scientist and scholarly writer. This reconnection led to insights on teaching writing conventions more effectively. Course activities were revised to include additional scaffolding to create smaller steps. Individual sessions were added to create a space where students could brainstorm with faculty, receive immediate feedback, and seek clarification. This type of scaffolding also fostered collaboration, helping students link connections with the value of community-based learning early on.

> After meeting with [faculty] yesterday, I had mixed emotions but a better sense of direction for my literature review. I could not help but laugh a little bit when [faculty was not able to] "road map" what I wanted to tell my reader. I could see [her] struggling to link everything together [...]. To a novice like myself, it sounded great at the time [...]. I have felt some growing pains over the last week and realize [...]. I still have to learn to think from the perspective of defining terms that are taken for granted, and asking myself questions to anticipate reader concern.
>
> (PhD Student Journal)

While most students completed a literature review in their graduate studies, writing this genre at the doctoral level is more complex, as students are expected to generate research to address a gap in knowledge. Until this course, students had mostly regurgitated literature findings that were produced in a course assignment. The stakes are higher in doctoral education, as students must make a cogent argument to support dissertation research.

> I feel like I'm running in quicksand today. Everything seemed to take SOOO long to complete. The learning curve is steep, and I have a lot to accomplish. I know it will take practice […]. So far, I feel like I've never done a real literature review […]. I totally didn't expect to get this literature review right the first time and appreciate the revision process.
>
> (PhD Student Journal)

Another strategy to support student learning was the use of example literature reviews in class. In the first couple of years teaching the course, students were provided various types of literature reviews as examples to guide their processes. We found that students still struggled to understand the concept of synthesizing and identifying a gap. In year 3, we used an integrative review the course faculty had coauthored and published.[46] This strategy seemed to help students make connections between the processes in writing a literature review. Dissecting each component of the review gave students insight into the processes of how faculty had identified a problem and systematically reviewed the literature. Discussion included our analysis strategies, which led to identifying gaps in knowledge and how those gaps led to our recommendations for future research.

These scaffolded activities resulted in better-quality literature reviews (products) and improved writing processes. Summative evaluations indicated final papers had a more logical synthesis of nursing research, knowledge gaps were better articulated, and discussions were more insightful. These findings indicated the scaffolding of assignments supported students during the procedural bottlenecks of writing a literature review.

Transitioning to a New Researcher and Writer Identity

As students began transitioning to new researcher and writer identities required of novice nurse scientists, they experienced liminality. For many, the process of developing new identities was perplexing, as the transition required the surrendering of expert identities. Vulnerability occurred as students left the comfort of their known practice community and began positioning themselves into the research community. The reflective learning journal offered a space for metacognitive thinking and for students to uncover thoughts and feelings associated with the transition. Reflective writing also stimulated students' thinking about their ethos as writers and how their new researcher identities could make a meaningful contribution to the community.

Many students struggled with reflective writing, so the journal assignment was submitted at three different time intervals during the course. This gave course faculty an opportunity to keep a finger on the pulse of student frustration and identify areas of "stuckness" during the course. To assist students with becoming reflective scholars, faculty provided prompts to guide students beyond superficial responses and toward in-depth critical reflections.

> I've come to appreciate the process of reflection […]. When I start writing and reflecting, I want to read more. I enjoy the reciprocal process of reading and writing and how both inspire profound thought and a thirst for lifelong learning. Of course, what I like about writing may also be what I dislike. It is not always a fluid process for me. Sometimes the questions that are provoked through writing are not easily answered. This can be frustrating.
>
> (PhD Student Journal)

Examining both qualitative and quantitative dissertation studies assisted students with envisioning their new identities as researchers and scholars. This early exposure of what a "PhD" means facilitated the understanding of what it means to become a researcher and belong to a community of scholars. Through writing, students began to develop their own voices and viewpoints. Journaling gave them a safe space to tease out these new perspectives as they grappled with the tension between the forces of becoming and belonging. Toward the end of the course, students were better positioned as new members of the research community. Student reflections demonstrated a decrease in anxiety as they gained the writing skills needed for novice scholars.

> I am looking through a new lens. Perhaps, it is the amount of reading and writing I have done in the past month....Whatever the reason, I noticed it and I am excited that I have seen this change in myself […]. I am SO glad that we got to take this course. I feel much more prepared and grounded in expectations […]. I have learned a lot about writing.
>
> (PhD Student Journal)

The course assisted students with collecting a toolbox for their PhD journeys. Writing can be viewed as one of the most important academic tools for a scholar. During the course, students were confronted with the stark reality of writing expectations for the life of a scholar. This reality triggered feelings of anxiety, inadequacy, and vulnerability when they found themselves stuck when exposed to new writer expectations. Course activities were geared toward minimizing these emotional bottlenecks triggered by liminality so students could more effectively assess writing as an academic tool.

> I have dedicated an enormous amount of time to improving my time writing and eliminating my self-critique of every word I write. Unfortunately, I have likely left my writing tool kit in the shed. The tool bag is covered in dust and spiderwebs. Matter of fact, I believe a spider has made it her home for babies, an undisturbed area in the dark recesses of the shed. There is a small hole in the roof leaking in the resent rain fall on already rusting tools. The tips are dull from prior use and put away without cleaning or care. There are tools missing. Maybe I never had them, or maybe they have been misplaced along the way.
>
> (PhD Student Journal)

Reflective writing served as a mechanism for students to negotiate the construction of their researcher and writer identities. Many found journaling as a way of working through stuck places and bringing clarity to their ideas. Students were encouraged to "wallow" in their thinking and enjoy the PhD journey. Journaling offered a safe space to promote the process of writing and learning, thus creating a transformative approach to writing practices. Students found that journaling helped to clear their thinking by eliminating the "mental clutter," which often contributes to the dreaded writer's block.

Contributing to Research Community as a Peer Reviewer

Data analysis revealed doctoral students got stuck while engaging in the practice of giving and receiving constructive feedback on writing. To make meaningful contributions to the research community, doctoral students require peer review competencies. In the introductory course, the Critical Friends peer-review protocol is used to introduce students to common disciplinary practice in a supportive space. Writing and learning together are promoted by situating student-peer relationships alongside faculty.

> The one really nice thing about peer review is the feeling of support. The feedback I received this week was needed and not totally unexpected […]. Reviewing the work of other students

was helpful in that I was able to use their well-thought-out structured paragraph [as a guide] to structure my own work in certain places. I also learned that there are so many different styles of writing and many audiences. I never realized how important it is to know your audience and to always keep this in mind as you write.

(PhD Student Journal)

Faculty served as facilitators of the protocol and provided role modeling of PhD-level critique for scholarly writing. The protocol encouraged presenters to remain silent while listening and taking notes as their peers discussed their draft papers. Although students expressed receiving feedback using this method was challenging, this step in the protocol facilitated a supportive, respectful learning environment.

The presenter having to keep quiet was the most difficult part. Not that I am much of a talker, but one tends to feel a little defensive when being critiqued. I think the silence requirement is helpful in making the presenter actually take in what is said, process it, and consider it before replying to or gaining clarification on the person's point.

(PhD Student Journal)

Fostering student development as a peer reviewer was supported through a culture of peer learning. A culture of peer learning moved beyond a vertical approach to learning toward a horizontal, community-based learning approach. The course supported the valuing of peers, along with faculty, to assist students with research community positioning. For example, PhD students at different stages in the program were invited to class meetings to present strategies for organizing a literature matrix and share lessons learned from publishing a literature review.

One "Ah Ha" moment was understanding rewrites are not about pursuing perfection. They are about incorporating different points of views that make it easier for people in your audience to understand your topic. I see a peer group as an essential part of my toolbox. The best part is I don't feel alone in my writing anymore. I feel like I have a team of people to help me succeed.

(PhD Student Journal)

Nurse scientists are expected to share their scholarship through scholarly presentations. At the end of the course, students presented their findings from their literature review assignment and proposed potential ideas for student research. A peer-review panel composed of faculty and third-year PhD students provided constructive critiques to student presenters regarding how to cultivate their ideas moving forward. The activity of presenting their literature reviews gave students an authentic experience of early positioning within the research community. Translating their written work into the verbal expression of ideas supported the students' sense of agency, as they began to develop their voices as nurse scientists.

The [peer review] process is a gift to a young academic writer [like] myself for several reasons. First of all, as an immature scientific writer, I am not well versed in the social contracts of the research world […]. I welcome the constructive commentary. Growth will come from this recursive process.

(PhD Student Journal)

The use of the Critical Friends protocol received high remarks on course evaluations. Most students felt their experience with peer review was helpful in their scholarly writing development.

Reflective notes also indicated student insight into the benefits of peer review as a scholar. Analysis of faculty assessments indicated students' ability to consider and apply peer feedback.

Conclusion and Recommendations for Instructors

This chapter shared findings from data collected from PhD students who were enrolled in an introductory course designed to build novice research and writing competencies. Analysis of data indicated entry-level PhD students found the threshold concept of constructing researcher and writer identities most troublesome during the course. This chapter unpacked the liminal spaces students experienced within this threshold concept. States of liminality occurred while students were writing the literature review, transitioning to new research and writer identities, and contributing to the research community as a peer reviewer.

Faculty who teach writing in the health professions must work to advance pedagogies that support scholarly writing development. However, disciplinary experts may have trouble understanding the type of support doctoral students need to facilitate their learning. As such, faculty must be willing to endure student challenges with writing and be open to exploring strategies to support writing development. Scaffolded instruction has been a useful strategy to assist entry-level PhD students with the procedural bottlenecks that occur when exposed to complex genres of writing. It is recommended to layer assignments, along with creating opportunities for feedback and revision, to support students' evolution of thinking and foster scholarly writing development.

Students experienced vulnerability as they left the comfort of their expert identities within the practice community and began positioning into the research community. Reflective writing served as a safe space for students to negotiate the construction of their research and writer identities while experiencing the emotional disciplining that occurred. Faculty should consider incorporating metacognitive activities, such as reflective learning journals, to offer students a space to work through liminality. While some students may be hesitant to the idea of keeping a learning journal, introducing this activity early in their studies can cultivate the intellectual habits necessary for the rest of their PhD journeys.

Peer-review opportunities should also be introduced to PhD students early in their studies. Protocols, such as Critical Friends, can provide structure for students to learn how to give and receive constructive critique. Peer review supports peer learning and offers unique opportunities to develop scholarly writing in doctoral students while fostering awareness of writer identity and voice. The strategies discussed in this chapter have the potential to support writing development for research-doctorates who will be expected to advance the science of nursing. A first step in preparing these students for success during their doctoral studies is the consideration of writing-related threshold concepts and liminal states of learning.

References

1. American Association of Colleges of Nursing. *The Research-Focused Doctoral Program in Nursing: Pathways to Excellence.* Washington, DC: Author; 2010.
2. Graves JM, Postma J, Katz JR, Kehoe L, Swalling E, Barbosa-Leiker C. A national survey examining manuscript dissertation formats among nursing PhD programs in the united states: manuscript option format for nursing dissertations. *J Nurs Scholarsh.* 2018;50(3):314–323.
3. Taylor LA, Terhaar MF. Mitigating barriers to doctoral education for nurses. *Nurs Educ Perspect.* 2018;39(5):285–290.
4. Smith L, Hande K, Kennedy BB. Mentoring nursing faculty: an inclusive scholarship support group. *Nurse Educ.* 2020;45(4):185–186.

5. Webber E, Vaughn-Deneen T, Anthony M. Three-generation academic mentoring teams: a new approach to faculty mentoring in nursing. *Nurse Educ.* 2020;45(4):210–213.

6. Bernstein M, Roney L, Kazer M, Boquet EH. Librarians collaborate successfully with nursing faculty and a writing centre to support nursing students doing professional doctorates. *Health Inf Libr J.* 2020;37(3):240–244.

7. Cowles KV, Strickland D, Rodgers BL. Collaboration for teaching innovation: writing across the curriculum in a school of nursing. *J Nurs Educ.* 2001;40(8):363–367.

8. Feltham M, Krahn MA. Breathing life into the syllabus: the collaborative development of a first-year writing course for nursing students. *CELT.* 2016;9:199.

9. Singleterry L, Kalkman B, Chrenka L, Courtright-Nash D. Nursing faculty development: building a common grading rubric to evaluate writing. *Nurse Educ.* 2016;41(5):222–224.

10. Robert Wood Johnson and the American Association of Colleges of Nursing for the Robert Wood Johnson Foundation New Careers in Nursing Scholarship Program. *Doctoral Advancement in Nursing: A Roadmap for Facilitating Entry into Doctoral Education.* Washington, DC: Robert Wood Johnson; 2013.

11. Starke-Meyerring D. Writing groups as critical spaces for engaging normalized institutional cultures of writing in doctoral education. In: Aitchison C, Guerin C, eds. *Writing Groups for Doctoral Education and Beyond: Innovations in Practice and Theory.* Florence: Routledge Ltd; 2014:137–165.

12. Wegener C, Meier N, Ingerslev K. Borrowing brainpower—sharing insecurities. Lessons learned from a doctoral peer writing group. *Stud High Educ.* 2016;41(6):1092–1105.

13. Armstrong DK, McCurry M, Dluhy NM. Facilitating the transition of nurse clinician to nurse scientist: significance of entry PhD courses. *J Prof Nurs.* 2017;33(1):74–80.

14. Salani D, Albuja LD, Azaiza K. The keys to success in doctoral studies: a preimmersion course. *J Prof Nurs.* 2016;32(5):358–363.

15. Meyer JHF, Land R. Threshold concepts and troublesome knowledge: linkages to ways of thinking and practising within the disciplines. In: Rust, C ed. *Improving Student Learning - Theory and Practice Ten Years On.* Oxford: Oxford Centre for Staff and Learning Development (OCSLD); 2003:412–424.

16. Meyer JHF, Land R. Threshold concepts and troublesome knowledge (2): epistemological considerations and a conceptual framework for teaching and learning. *High Educ.* 2005;49(3):373–388.

17. Land R, Meyer JHF, Baillie C *Editors' Preface: Threshold Concepts and Transformational Learning.* Rotterdam, The Netherlands: Sense Publishers; 2010.

18. Kiley M, Wisker G. Threshold concepts in research education and evidence of threshold crossing. *High Educ Res Dev.* 2009;28(4):431–441.

19. Wisker G, Savin-Baden M. Priceless conceptual thresholds: beyond the "stuck place" in writing. *Lond Rev Educ.* 2009;7(3):235.

20. Chatterjee-Padmanabhan M, Nielsen W, Sanders S. Joining the research conversation: threshold concepts embedded in the literature review. *High Educ Res Dev.* 2019;38(3):494–507.

21. McKenna S. Crossing conceptual thresholds in doctoral communities. *Innov Educ Teach Int.* 2017;54(5):458–466.

22. Tyndall DE, Firnhaber GC, Kistler KB. An integrative review of threshold concepts in doctoral education: implications for PhD nursing programs. *Nurse Educ Today.* 2021;99:104786–104786.

23. Adler-Kassner L, Wardle EA. *Naming What We Know: Threshold Concepts of Writing Studies.* Logan, UT: Utah State University Press; 2015.

24. Tyndall DE, Flinchbaugh KB, Caswell NI, Scott ES. Threshold concepts in doctoral education: a framework for writing development in novice nurse scientists. *Nurse Educ.* 2019;44(1):38–42.

25. Adamek ME. Building scholarly writers: student perspectives on peer review in a doctoral writing seminar. *J Teach Soc Work.* 2015;35(1-2):213–225.

26. Kiley M. Identifying threshold concepts and proposing strategies to support doctoral candidates. *Innov Educ Teach Int.* 2009;46(3):293–304.

27. Carter S, Kumar V. 'Ignoring me is part of learning': supervisory feedback on doctoral writing. *Innov Educ Teach Int.* 2017;54(1):68–75.

28. Huang K. Design and investigation of cooperative, scaffolded wiki learning activities in an online graduate-level course. *Int J Educ Technol High Educ.* 2019;16(1):1–18.

29. Negretti R, McGrath L. Scaffolding genre knowledge and metacognition: insights from an L2 doctoral research writing course. *J Second Lang Writ.* 2018;40(June 2018):12–31.

30. Salisbury JD, Irby DJ. Leveraging active learning pedagogy in a scaffolded approach: reconceptualizing instructional leadership learning. *J Res Leadersh Educ*. 2020;15(3):210–226.

31. Yu S, Jiang L. Doctoral students' engagement with journal reviewers' feedback on academic writing. *Stud Contin Educ*. 2020:1–18, https://doi.org/10.1080/0158037X.2020.1781610.

32. Gazza EA, Hunker DF. Facilitating scholarly writer development: the writing scaffold. *Nurs Forum*. 2012;47(4):278–285.

33. Sakraida TJ. Writing-in-the-discipline with instructional scaffolding in an RN-to-BSN nursing research course. *J Nurs Educ*. 2020;59(3):179–180.

34. Tyndall DE, Forbes III TH, Avery JJ, Powell SB. Fostering scholarship in doctoral education: using a social capital framework to support PhD student writing groups. *J Prof Nurs*. 2019;35(4):300–304.

35. Costantino T. The critical friends group: a strategy for developing intellectual community in doctoral education. *Ie(Wheeling, Ill)*. 2010;1(2):5.

36. Cahusac de Caux BKCD, Lam CKC, Lau R, Hoang CH, Pretorius L. Reflection for learning in doctoral training: writing groups, academic writing proficiency and reflective practice. *Reflec Pract*. 2017;18(4):463–473.

37. Murphy S, McGlynn-Stewart M, Ghafouri F. Constructing our identities through a writing support group: bridging from doctoral students to teacher educator researchers. *Stud Teach Educ*. 2014;10(3):239–254.

38. Inouye K, McAlpine L. Developing academic identity: a review of the literature on doctoral writing and feedback. *Int J Doct Stud*. 2019;14:1–31.

39. Wei J, Carter S, Laurs D. Handling the loss of innocence: first-time exchange of writing and feedback in doctoral supervision. *High Educ Res Dev*. 2019;38(1):157–169.

40. Cantwell RH, Bourke SF, Scevak JJ, Holbrook AP, Budd J. Doctoral candidates as learners: a study of individual differences in responses to learning and its management. *Stud High Educ*. 2017;42(1):47–64.

41. Medina MS, Castleberry AN, Persky AM. Strategies for improving learner metacognition in health professional education. *Am J Pharm Educ*. 2017;81(4):78A.

42. Goodson P. *Becoming an Academic Writer: 50 Exercises for Paced, Productive and Powerful Writing*. 2nd ed. Thousand Oaks, CA: Sage Publications; 2016.

43. Tyndall DE, Flinchbaugh KB, Caswell NI, Scott ES. Troublesome knowledge for entry-level PhD nursing students: threshold concepts essential for the research-focused doctorate. *J Prof Nurs*. 2021;37(3):572–577.

44. Chatterjee-Padmanabhan M, Nielsen W. Preparing to cross the research proposal threshold: a case study of two international doctoral students. *Innov Educ Teach Int*. 2018;55(4):417–424.

45. Feldon DF, Rates C, Sun C. Doctoral conceptual thresholds in cellular and molecular biology. *Int J Sci Educ*. 2017;39(18):2574–2593.

46. Tyndall DE, Firnhaber GC, Scott ES. The impact of new graduate nurse transition programs on competency development and patient safety: an integrative review. *Adv Nurs Sci*. 2018;41(4):E26–E52.

PART III

Writing in Allied Health and Pharmacy

8

WHEN THE CLASSROOM IS THE WORKPLACE

Developing Writing Curricula for EMS and Fire Service Training Programs

Elizabeth L. Angeli

Effective writing drives the patient care continuum because health-care providers at all levels write—from veterinarians, to transplant surgeons, to pharmacists, to prehospital providers. The patient health-care record informs medical decision-making and communication across health-care contexts and over time makes the written record a timeliness artifact.[1,2] To prepare providers for this distributed work, most writing initiatives in the health professions and corresponding writing research studies are designed for providers who earn 2-year and 4-year degrees, such as nurses and physicians.[3–7] Providers who earn these degrees are exposed to writing at multiple levels, including first-year writing courses; upper-division, writing-intensive courses; and writing-in-the-major courses. This focus misses other health professionals who complete certification or licensure programs, do not need to earn a degree, and are at the forefront of patient care, such as certified nursing assistants, medical assistants, surgical lab technicians, veterinary assistants, and emergency medical services (EMS) providers. As such, these populations have limited exposure to workplace writing instruction, and this chapter focuses on EMS providers to address this gap in "writing in the health professions" scholarship. (For an additional example of workplace research, see Chapter 12.)

Writing Initiatives on the University-Workplace-Community Continuum

To date, most scholarship in the field of writing studies *writ large* focuses on writing practice, pedagogy, and research that occurs within academic classrooms, in the workplace, or in community organizations. Inside the academic classroom context, theories of writing across the curriculum and writing in the disciplines (writing across the curriculum [WAC]/ writing in the disciplines [WID]), technical communication, and composition studies inform pedagogy and research. Outside the classroom, these theories inform writing practice and initiatives in community workshops and a myriad of workplaces from coal mines,[8] to public meetings,[9] to various health-care settings.[10]

However, writing practice and pedagogy happen in spaces that fall along the university-workplace-community continuum, such as spaces that are housed within a workplace and offer employees workplace-based education. This space is given little attention in writing studies scholarship and is tended to more fully in adult workplace education research, which is grounded in human resources, organizational management, situated learning, and education theories. Adult workplace education research focuses either on employees who are already on the job and have experience[11–14]

DOI: 10.4324/9781003162940-12

or on newly hired employees who have at least a 2-year college degree.[15,16] To date, though, two perspectives are under-addressed in adult workplace education research: a focus on writing training and a focus on recent high school graduates who are entering the workforce full time. Additionally, adult workplace education research is not yet in conversation with writing studies scholarship, and, as this chapter shows, this overlap shows great promise for both disciplines.

Despite these gaps, these fields overlap in important ways, especially as they relate to writing in the health professions. WAC, WID, and community-engaged researchers share commitments to sustainable and mutually beneficial partnerships and structures, and they are rooted in evidence-based scholarship.[3,17–24] Likewise, writing studies tends to the importance of situated learning and the material, social, emotional, and physical impact on the learning process.[25–30] Looking at the health professions specifically, rhetoric of health and medicine (RHM) scholarship highlights how WAC/WID, technical communication, and community engagement informs health-care writing practice, teaching, and curriculum building.[1,3,5–7,31–35]

These fields share a deep commitment to the transformative power of writing education—an education that builds habits of mind, skills, and knowledge that allow people to compose texts, respond to exigencies, effect change, and promote action. However, the frameworks used by these fields do not easily adapt to the hybrid workplace-classroom contexts of workplace training. As I outline in the following section, these frameworks are fully embedded in workplace or classroom contexts and rely on shared structures, such as a semester or course sequence. As such, they do not easily inform the building of a writing curriculum for a hybrid workplace-classroom space.

Turning to the Seven Tenets of Lean Technical Communication

To bring together writing scholarship and adult workplace education, I turn to Johnson, Simmons, and Sullivan's lean technical communication framework, specifically the seven tenets that support technical communication program success.[36] Informed by technical communication program administration, writing, and community engagement theories, lean technical communication "refers to a set of techniques and technologies that comprise an efficient, flexible, and visible model of technical communication program administration that is rooted in social responsibility."[36(p4)] The model upholds seven tenets that answer the question, "[W]hat sort of practices must happen to keep [a] program going"[36(p17)]?:

1. Starts with "value not deficit"
2. "Innovates and disrupts" procedures and practices in place
3. Are "rooted in local needs and aim at social responsibility"
4. "Regulates cost"
5. "Engages sustainability"
6. "Promotes efficiency"
7. "Enhances visibility"[36 (pp.18–29)]

Although these tenets are designed for academic classrooms and programs, they adapt to the exigencies and unique situations of the health professions workplace classroom that prepares technical communicators, like EMS providers.[31] Ultimately, the curriculum I outline is a technical communication curriculum that has "gone public"[37]: it is being taught outside the university classroom and inside the workplace classroom. In essence, the lean technical communication tenets are nimble and capacious enough to inform curricular design in this space, which is part workplace, part classroom.

The Research Site: The EMS-Fire Service Workplace and Classroom Training and Writing Practice in the EMS-Fire Service Workplace

In most areas of the health professions, providers develop many essential, lifesaving skills, such as intubating patients, suturing, and performing a physical assessment. As first responders, EMS providers learn these skills and earn their training and licensure through accredited programs offered through fire departments, private EMS agencies, community and technical colleges, or 4-year colleges and universities. Depending on the program structure and licensure level offered, the programs last between 3 months to 4 years. Basic EMS training covers foundational elements of prehospital medical care, such as anatomy and physiology, patient and scene assessments, and trauma and medical care. Advanced EMS training at the paramedic level covers more complex medical skills and decision-making, such as pharmacology and advanced airway management. Regardless of training level, all EMS providers are required to take state exams to earn their licensure. Some providers complete national-level exams to earn national licensure, allowing them to practice EMS outside their home state.

For every 911 response they complete, providers submit a patient care report (PCR). A well-written, effective PCR captures EMS providers' decision-making, interventions they performed (transferring a patient from a wheelchair to a stretcher, administering oxygen, taking vitals), results of those interventions, and rationales for the interventions that were performed. In an attempt to capture all of these decisions and actions, PCR interfaces are typically separated into two parts: drop-down menus and short text entry boxes, and a narrative section, which is a large text entry box. The checkboxes and shorter text entry boxes capture basic decisions, patient information, and intervention choices, and in the narrative portion, providers synthesize, justify, and contextualize the information inputted in the drop-down menus and short text entry boxes.

The PCR carries a heavy burden in the EMS workplace because multiple stakeholders use this document to inform writing tasks, actions, and decisions that impact patients and EMS agencies. The PCR allows health professionals to continue patient care, lawyers to represent patients or EMS agencies in lawsuits, billing experts to determine financial reimbursement for EMS agencies, insurance agencies to calculate medical coverage for patients, medical examiners to write death certificates, and organ procurement teams to determine if a patient is a viable donor. Ultimately, the PCR is a critical component used to coordinate patient care, and the document persuades stakeholders that the provider's actions were appropriate and effective. Implications of a poorly written PCR can lead to increased medical bills for patients, lower reimbursement for EMS agencies, and even patient death.[38] (In some ways, then, the PCR is comparable to the clinical notes taught in Chapter 1.)

Despite these implications, EMS training lacks effective, evidence-driven writing education. In the United States, training programs typically follow what writing specialists refer to as the inoculation model of writing instruction.[39–41] In this method, students are introduced to writing in a "one-dose" intervention, either in a few hours through an EMS-specific training course or a college-level English course if they complete training through a college. Regardless of where providers train, the inoculation method expects writers to be "vaccinated against" and prepared to "take on" writing challenges, including organizing thoughts clearly, synthesizing evidence persuasively, and avoiding grammar errors completely. In turn, this model reduces writing to a product to be perfected and shortchanges the rich, complex writing process in which disciplinary writers engage.[1,3,5–7,31–35,42–44] I work to counter this model in this research project, and I partnered with a local fire department's training academy to carry it out.

Creating a Partnership with MFD's Training Academy

My partnership with MFD and their training academy grew out of shared commitments to EMS education, and it was initiated through serendipitous events. A year before the partnership started, I had a campus visit at my current university, Marquette University, which is located blocks away from MFD's headquarters. During my research presentation, I discussed my now-published, then-under-review book, and I drew from my book's final chapter, which outlines writing-based classroom activities for educators in the health professions. After my presentation, a department faculty member, who is now my colleague, approached me and said, "My cousin is an assistant chief for MFD. Should this job work out for you and us, I think he'd be interested in meeting you."

A few weeks later, I accepted the university's job offer, and 10 months later during my first semester working there, my colleague and I met with her cousin, the assistant chief, and two deputy chiefs, another assistant chief, and a captain who ran MFD's training academy. To prepare for this meeting, I brainstormed a rather large research idea. Knowing that EMS training lacked formal, evidence-based writing curricula, I wanted to turn my book's last chapter into a full-fledged writing curriculum for their fire-EMS training program.

During the initial meeting with MFD, we discussed my research, and MFD officials shared their "pain points" about documentation training. They stressed that, although they are a fire service, MFD's primary role in the city is to provide emergency medical care to citizens (2017 annual report). Like other US agencies, MFD providers are required to write a PCR for patient interactions, but despite this prominence of report writing, their academy, like many US programs, lacked an evidence-based mechanism to teach PCR writing. The officials explained their academy's training structure, a model with which I was unfamiliar. MFD recruits students directly from high school and starting two months after their high school graduation, the students become MFD employees and are "cadets" in the academy. The academy is a 3-year training program in which cadets earn their paramedic and fire science licenses, two top-level licenses in these fields. Described as part boot camp, part medical school, the program includes classroom-based lectures, rigorous workout schedules, skills labs for EMS medical care and fire suppression and response, and field rotations at fire stations and various hospital departments, including rotations in the emergency department and surgery.

Given the relatively novel structure of this program and my unfamiliarity with the fire service, I proposed a 6-year longitudinal project organized into two 3-year phases that would start the following academic year. The first phase was dedicated to better understanding the academy's structure, culture, and the writing that cadets completed during training. Then, using those findings, I would develop and implement the writing curriculum in Phase 2. Within the following months, the project was Institutional Review Board approved (HR-3332), and I met with the 2017 cadet class to introduce the project and recruit participants for Phase 1.

Using Longitudinal Research to Gain Curricular Insights

A longitudinal approach made sense for this project for a few reasons.[45] First, longitudinal methods align with best practices of community-based writing, WAC/WID, and lean technical communication, which suggest researchers and program administrators build relationships with stakeholders. A longer research time line allowed me to do that. Second, because little scholarship exists about writing curricula in workplace training programs, I wanted to better understand the cadets' writing practices and their written assignments, such as class notes, study guides, and field notebooks. I did not want to impose writing curriculum structures that are informed by university teaching or community-based initiatives onto this space.

Following these reasons, I ultimately wanted to build a relationship with the academy so that they knew who I was, what I studied, and how I could add value to the training program. I knew the idea of a writing curriculum was new in EMS and fire science, and I would be asking a lot of the academy—to integrate a writing curriculum into an already-full, rigorous training schedule that had to meet national accreditation standards. Plus, I proposed this 6-year research project during my first meeting with MFD, a big, risky ask. Put another way, I basically proposed that they commit to a long-term relationship with me on our first date. Because they said "yes" so quickly, I knew they were as eager as I was to develop something that could change the way EMS education is taught nationwide, and they trusted me to do it. I wanted to take my time to do it well.

Informed by these rationales, Phase 1 involved spending time in person with the cadets, full-time instructors, and guest instructors, who often worked in the field and filled in at the academy when needed. When I met these instructors, I introduced myself, told them about the study, and they often would share their thoughts on EMS documentation practice and training. Some of them even showed me how they documented patient care on the department's field laptops.

During Phase 1, I conducted 26 hours of classroom observations, and 18 of the 26 cadets in the cohort completed a survey that asked them about their academic and workplace writing experiences and asked if they wanted to participate in the project as focal participants. Focal participants completed one 40-minute one-on-one interview with me and two 30-minute focus groups to discuss their writing process. Focal participants also submitted their class notes, clinical notes, and practice PCRs to me, and agreed to in-field observations during their paramedic field rotations. Of those 18 cadets, 6 cadets consented to be focal participants, and I conducted 48 hours of field observations where cadets practiced their paramedic skills and report writing under the supervision of MFD providers.

In addition to the practice reports participants completed for class, focal participants kept a separate paper notebook, the "study-assigned notebook," that was designed to support and facilitate their writing process. In this notebook, participants documented patient interactions using a model of report writing I am testing for another research study. Some focal participants also kept their own notebooks during field training, which I collected.

Identifying Structural Overlaps and Tensions

Phase 1 of the study illustrated key differences among academic, workplace, and training contexts and structures (Table 8.1).

The differences generated tensions, which ultimately informed Phase 2 of the study. Some of these tensions included the following:

- How can I build a curriculum that is not structured like a semester course but is more structured and sustained than a series of workshops?
- How can I offer feedback in a sustainable way that aligns with the academy's assessment structure?
- How can the curriculum support neurodiverse learners and address underlying writing anxiety or fears?
- How can I teach cadets rhetorical foundations of effective workplace writing without any shared introductory writing course?
- What data do I need to support the proposed curriculum, and what data will I need to measure its effectiveness?
- What structures will accommodate and adapt to the academy's changing schedules and leadership?
- What curricula can be built around the program itself and not on the interest of the current leadership?

TABLE 8.1 Structural differences between academic and workplace contexts

Structures*	Academic	EMS/Fire Service Workplace	Training Academy
Temporal structures	Semesters, trimesters, quarters	Shifts (i.e., 12 hours on, 12 hours off, 24 hours on, 48 hours off)	M-F 7 am-4 pm in class and cadets study on the weekend and at night; this schedule changes when cadets complete field rotations
Organizational hierarchy	President, board of trustees, provosts, vice provosts, deans, chairs, other university administration officials Programs, majors/minors, departments, colleges/schools	Chief, assistant chiefs, deputy chiefs, division chiefs, battalion chiefs, captains, lieutenants Divisions	Directed by MFD captains and lieutenants; instructors include firefighter/paramedics, lieutenants, captains The academy is under the purview of MFD
Assessment	Grades from quizzes, exams, projects, papers GPA	Performance reviews, raises, benefits, incentives	Grades on exams and quizzes, performance reviews on practical skills, paychecks, final ranking at the end of training, earning state and national licenses and certifications
Privacy regulations	Family Educational Rights and Privacy Act (FERPA)	Health Insurance Portability and Accountability Act (HIPAA)	HIPAA
Support mechanisms	Counseling and tutoring services, disability and academic success offices	Human resources	Human resources and the academy's instructors who are MFD providers and may not be trained/experienced educators
Technology	Email, learning management systems, telephone (calling, texting), smart classrooms, social media, video conference platforms	Email, telephone (calling, texting), PCR writing software	Email, smart classroom, learning management systems

* This list covers structures and examples relevant to this project and is not exhaustive.

To address these questions, I created targeted goals for informing curriculum development, and these goals started with the lean technical communication tenets of identifying a curricular space within the academy's structure and seeking stakeholder buy-in. To do that work, I needed data that was generated from the training academy itself.

Generating Locally Supported Data

To generate local data, I conducted surveys and focus groups that illustrated how the cadets' understanding of report writing aligned with departmental and professional expectations. To date, no formal research exists in this area of EMS and because my approach would "innovate and disrupt,"[36] in part by taking more time than the current writing training method and by focusing on process not product, I needed localized data to support the innovation.

MFD's approach to writing training is common in EMS: a lecture-based format that is between 1- and 2-hours long. The session introduces cadets to writing SOAP notes, which is a widely used writing mnemonic in health-care writing, and to other ubiquitous phrases in EMS report writing, like "paint a picture, tell a story," and "if you didn't write it down, you didn't do it." In an effort to follow tenets of lean technical communication, I first assessed how well the participants' retained and used this knowledge. These findings informed my conversations with the academy instructor team and the curriculum itself.

Assessing Participants' Knowledge from Training

About 10 months into the cadets' training, I conducted one-on-one interviews to assess what focal participants remembered about their report writing training, which was delivered a few months before interviews. Following report writing training, the cadets started their first set of field rotations on the ambulances and wrote practice PCRs. During interviews, I asked them, "How were you taught to write in EMS?" Despite all participants attending the same training a few months earlier, their responses were inconsistent. Some participants shared that they did not remember anything, a few remembered being shown example reports, one participant shared that they didn't feel like they learned anything at all, and others remembered brief tips and strategies, like writing in chronological order and how to use shorthand and abbreviations. Of note, though, no one remembered the mnemonic they were taught, SOAP.

Eight months later in focus groups, I asked a similar question. By that time, participants were completing their paramedic rotations, and they had completed an average of 197 hours on ambulance rotations and had an average of 75 patient interactions, all of which they documented in practice PCRs. They had not received additional report writing training between the interviews and focus groups. Despite their increased exposure to writing, most focal participants did not remember the SOAP mnemonic, suggesting that the one-time introduction to this mnemonic was not successful. In turn, this data point supported a rationale for multiple presentations and opportunities to practice writing in the new scaffolded writing curriculum.

Assessing Widely Used Health-Care Writing Mnemonics

In addition to the SOAP mnemonic, the phrase "paint a picture, tell a story" is a widely used writing tool in EMS. In turn, these devices become the frameworks in which report writers document patient care. In theory, both of these tools are meant to ease the cognitive workload of health-care providers and prompt them to detail pertinent information in the PCR. The challenge, though, is that these phrases have not been tested to see if they support EMS providers' writing process. In fact, the SOAP mnemonic has been replaced in some departments because it was not leading to satisfactory reports.[46]

To assess these two widely used tools, I developed a questionnaire for focal participants to complete during focus groups, and this questionnaire was developed based on preliminary data from another EMS writing study I am conducting. In that study, 16 EMS report readers were interviewed, including attorneys, medical examiners, medical directors, and billing specialists, to learn how and why they use PCRs and what they need from them. Those findings suggest that these audiences read narratives not only as a "painted picture" but also as a persuasive, data-driven argument that convinces them effective care was provided and appropriate decisions were made.

The questionnaire asked the six focal participants about how they, as writers, characterize their reports. When presented with the statement, "I think of my report as a persuasive argument," participants' average response was "disagree" (2.3 on a 5-point Likert scale). Alternatively, participants "agreed" with the statement, "I think of my report as a story" (4.3 on a 5-point Likert scale). These findings served as the biggest support for the shift in the curriculum because of the mismatch between writer and reader expectations. EMS report readers see the report as an argument: they need to be convinced that what is written in a report is true. However, participants, as the report writers, disagreed that their reports were an argument and, instead, agreed that their report was a story.

To further tease out these findings in focus groups, participants wrote words they associated with "picture, story" and "data, evidence, persuasive argument." In doing so, I aimed to learn what images, thoughts, or patterns came to their mind when they were prompted with familiar EMS writing words "picture" and "story" and the words EMS report readers used frequently in their interviews, "data," "evidence," and "persuade." Participants associated "data, evidence, persuasive, argument" with facts, numbers, vitals, time, place, trends, research, courts, lawyers, documentation, "trying to convince," and "if it's not written, it didn't happen." They associated "picture, story" with memories, events, details, general impression, chronological order, fiction, children, and laughter.

These findings suggest that participants associated appropriate elements of effective report writing with "data," "evidence," and "persuasive argument" more than "picture" and "story." For example, "data, evidence, persuasive argument" elicited more appropriate audiences ("courts, lawyers") than the audience that "picture, story" elicited ("children"). Additionally, the phrase, "If it's not written, it didn't happen" is a ubiquitous EMS writing phrase, which participants associated with "data" instead of "pictures." Finally, not all the words associated with "picture, story" were inappropriate, specifically "details," "events," "general impression," and "chronological order." These word associations suggest that these two frameworks may be more effective when used together, and the curriculum followed suit, building on widely held EMS writing traditions and integrating evidence-driven changes.

The EMS and Fire Service Writing Curriculum: Guiding Principles and Structure

The aforementioned data, my field notes, and writing studies research all informed the writing curriculum I am building for Phase 2. More specifically, tenets of lean technical communication helped me make sense of what I learned during Phase 1 in a context that is part workplace, part classroom. Table 8.2 outlines the seven lean technical communication tenets and details how I applied them in the EMS and fire service training workplace.

Guiding Principles

Informed by these tenets and the scholarship outlined in the previous section, the curriculum itself follows three core principles:

- Writing effectively is part of providing effective patient care
- Writing effectively relies on developing and cross-training habits of mind
- Scaffolding supports the first two principles, with a "low weights, high reps" approach built over 3 years

TABLE 8.2 Applying Johnson, Simmons, and Sullivan's lean technical communication tenets to the training classroom

Lean Technical Communication Tenets	Steps Taken in Curricular Development
Values not deficits	• Emphasize the transformative power of sustained writing engagement in initial meetings with administration; use locally generated data to further support that claim • Build on the strengths of the academy and the work EMS providers already do—e.g., showing how effective writing is part of effective patient care • Demonstrate how writing education can develop more than writing skills—e.g., writing education can cross-train other EMS and fire skills, such as collaboration and situational awareness
Innovates and disrupts	• Challenge the current "inoculation" model by creating a scaffolded curriculum • Bring in theories from writing fields that are not yet applied to EMS and fire science education • Integrate Eli Review into the curriculum, which has traditionally only been used in academic contexts (as in Chapter 4)
Rooted in local needs and aims at social responsibility	• Respond to the direct needs of the cadets as suggested by MFD's administration and educators and by Phase 1 data • Designed specifically for this program's 3-year structure, and could be adapted for other programs • Follow the academy's 3-year schedule • Use low-stakes assignments and assessments to encourage risk taking and failure without penalizing cadets' final course rankings • Integrate cadets' medical content knowledge and skills
Regulates cost	• Phase 1 was supported by an internal university grant • Currently working with Eli Review on a cost model for this unique setting • Most of the "cost" is my research time
Engages sustainability	• Find a balance between tailoring the curriculum for MFD and building in flexibility so other departments can adapt the curriculum • Consider how I can train EMS educators, university students or faculty, or others to teach the curriculum • Develop and embed assessment measures to routinely assess the curriculum's effectiveness and the cadets' engagement • Be flexible and account for necessary changes to the academy's structure and schedule
Promotes efficiency	• Integrate Eli Review to facilitate peer review • Embed activities into the academy's learning management system so I can engage with cadets remotely
Enhances visibility	• Incorporate writing curriculum activities and participation into the program's cadet ranking metric • Publish articles in peer-reviewed EMS and writing journals; present at EMS and writing conferences to raise visibility across disciplines • Spoke with my university's marketing and communications office about the partnership • Discuss the project with other fire departments with which I work

My previous research shows that patient care and writing in EMS involve several interrelated skills.[31] To treat patients effectively, document patient care, and thus continue the patient care continuum, providers must accomplish the following:

- Synthesize data and evidence gathered throughout a response, such as patient vitals, a patient's living environment, and bystander communication
- Remember and recall information
- Determine relevant information and pertinent negatives that support their decisions
- Hone their sensory and situational awareness
- Pay attention to detail
- Justify treatment and transport decisions
- Persuade multiple audiences that care was appropriate and effective

To support cadets as they learn these skills, the curriculum fosters growth in the following areas:

- Audience awareness
- Reflection
- Data collection
- Retention and recall
- Sensory awareness
- Situational awareness
- Empathy/emotional literacy
- Collaboration

These areas are habits of mind that providers need to develop, cultivate, and enact, and the curriculum aims at helping cadets see themselves as writers and EMS providers—that is, it helps them to see themselves as having disciplinary expertise that they showcase in their decision-making, patient care, and writing practice.

Structure and Assessment

As it is currently sketched out, the curriculum's structure includes a minimum of 12 hours of direct content delivery integrated over 3 years, and that number will most likely increase. Two years into Phase 1, I proposed a draft of the curriculum to the academy's lead instructors, and it included 12 hours of instruction because I did not want to ask for too much time of the already packed schedule. To my surprise, the instructors said I could have as much time as I needed. So, to learn how much time this curriculum really needs, I am conducting a soft launch of presentations and activities at the recommendation and support of the academy's instructors. At the end of each presentation, I ask the current cadets for feedback, and consistently, they say that they like hands-on activities, and they want more time to practice their writing skills.

In response to this feedback, the presentations, which I originally designed for 45-60 minutes, are now 60–120 minutes each, and regardless of the duration, the in-class instruction segments are organized into three parts:

- Lectures that include large-group activities
- Small-group activities where teams apply the concepts presented in lectures
- Time for reflection ("What did you learn? What will you do differently as a provider now?")

With the soft launch, I am delivering in-person presentations once every 6–8 weeks, depending on the academy's schedule and my schedule. Because so much time elapses between sessions, each session begins with a recap of "what we covered last time" as a way to bridge the sessions together, to help cadets recall what we covered, and to help them transition from the subject content covered that day to a focus on writing.

The assessment structure is still in progress. Unlike the traditional classroom, cadets do not earn traditional grades in the training program, even though they need to earn certain scores on exams, quizzes, and skills to pass the academy and to prepare for the state and national licensure exams. At the end of the training, cadets are ranked according to their exam scores and because they are paid employees, they receive a paycheck, which in itself is a form of assessment. If they are not meeting expectations, they are asked to leave the academy. I accounted for these assessment metrics because I did not want this curriculum to cause a cadet to risk their employment or ranking, especially because cadets are trying new skills and taking risks when learning how to write in EMS for the first time.

With that in mind, the current proposed assessment scheme does not convert to a grade. Instead, cadets' participation and completed assignments are worth 5% of the cadets' final rankings, thus making writing a visible part of their training but not worth enough to truly negatively impact their ranking if they are not the strongest writers. To encourage risk taking without penalty, assignments are assessed according to completion and address two criteria fundamental to EMS and the fire service: following all directions correctly and completing a task fully. So, cadets earn completion points for both these criteria, and this scheme is used for all assignments cadets complete.

This assessment scheme also directly responds to a captain's request. A previous cadet class was struggling to follow directions, and one day, the captain asked me, exasperated, "Can you teach them how to read, too?" In response, this assessment scheme encourages students to slow down, pay attention to details, and think about what they're being asked to do. My hope, too, is that this scheme will lessen writing anxiety and allow cadets to try out new forms of writing and learning.

In addition to assessing the cadets' writing, I will also assess the curriculum's effectiveness by asking cadets for their direct feedback, looking at changes in their writing, speaking with the academy's instructors, and following up with the cadets once they become MFD employees and begin to write in the field as licensed EMS providers.

Practical Takeaways

This research suggests that writing specialists are well suited to enter hybrid workplace/classroom spaces in the health professions. As ambassadors, we can build "writing in the health professions" training that prepares providers who are at the forefront of patient care, such as medical assistants and nursing assistants so that they engage in effective writing processes and practices.

Theories, research methods, and pedagogy from WAC, WID, technical communication, community engagement, and RHM can inform how we can develop responsive and sustainable writing initiatives along the university-workplace-community continuum. Likewise, the 7 tenets of technical communication[36] provide a flexible structure that can guide program development. Adding to these tenets, this research project suggests additional and related strategies for "writing in the health professions" training initiatives:

Build on common knowledge and experiences. In the EMS and fire service workplace, physical exercise analogies work well ("low weights, high reps").

If writing is seen as a burden or seems to be ignored/under-addressed, identify drives it.

- Do the instructors have teaching experience?
- Do they have experience teaching writing?

- Are the instructors teaching in the program by choice or is it by force, e.g., as an alternative duty?
- How comfortable and confident are the instructors with their own writing skills?
- Once you know those answers, consider ways to address them, perhaps by offering a workshop for instructors on why writing is challenging to learn, practice, and teach or on why writing is important in that specific health profession.

Know writing's value, purpose, and impact in the specific health-care workplace. The more you know about how writing works in that workplace, the stronger your ethos will be to the instructors and the students.

Revise, pivot, and adapt. Don't hold onto initial ideas too tightly so that you can allow your data and learnings to guide you.

Perhaps of most importance for implementing a "writing in the health professions" curriculum is understanding the local culture and knowing that writing studies *writ large* informs program development. These two points are symbiotic in that the local culture informs what theories and frameworks to use and vice versa. Ultimately, the foundations of effective, community-engaged "writing in the health professions" program building align with the core principles of writing studies: focus on process, build relationships with partners, train writers to develop effective habits of mind, and scaffold.

References

1. Opel DS, Hart-Davidson W. The primary care clinic as writing space. *Writ Commun.* 2019;36(3):348–378. doi:10.1177/0741088319839968
2. Schryer C. Records as genre. *Writ Commun.* 1993;10(2):200–234.
3. Berger M. Developing a writing across the curriculum program for a two-year nursing college. *TETYC.* 2015;42(4):400–409.
4. Campbell L. The rhetoric of health and medicine as a "teaching subject": lessons from the medical humanities and simulation pedagogy. *Tech Commun Q.* 2018;27(1):7–20.
5. Heifferon B. *Writing in the Health Professions.* New York, NY: Pearson; 2005.
6. Kenzie D, McCall M. Teaching writing for the health professions: disciplinary intersections and pedagogical practice. *Tech Commun Q.* 2018;27(1):64–79.
7. Long T, Beck C. *Writing in Nursing: A Brief Guide.* Oxford, Oxford University Press; 2016.
8. Sauer B. *The Rhetoric of Risk: Technical Documentation in Hazardous Environments.* New York, NY: Routledge; 2003.
9. Simmons WM. *Participation and Power: Civic Discourse in Environmental Policy Decisions.* Albany, NY: State University of New York Press; 2007.
10. Meloncon LK, Scott JB. *Methodologies for the Rhetoric of Health and Medicine.* New York, NY: Routledge/Taylor & Francis Group; 2018.
11. Billett S. *Learning in the Workplace: Strategies for Effective Practice.* Crows Nest, Australia: Allen & Unwin; 2001.
12. Billett S. Toward a workplace pedagogy: guidance, participation, and engagement. *Adult Educ Q.* 2002;53(1):27–43. doi:10.1177/074171302237202
13. Billett S. Workplace participatory practices: conceptualising workplaces as learning environments. *J Workplace Learn.* 2004;16(6):312–324. doi:10.1108/13665620410550295
14. Fenwick T. Workplace "learning" and adult education. Messy objects, blurry maps and making difference. *RELA.* 2010;1(1-2):79–95. doi:10.3384/rela.2000-7426.rela0006
15. Henderson A, Eaton E. Assisting nurses to facilitate student and new graduate learning in practice settings: what 'support' do nurses at the bedside need? *Nurs Educ Pract.* 2013;13(3):197–201. doi:10.1016/j.nepr.2012.09.005
16. Korte RF. How newcomers learn the social norms of an organization: a case study of the socialization of newly hired engineers. *Hum Resour Dev Q.* 2009;20(3):285–306. doi:10.1002/hrdq.20016

17. Bartlett LE, Tarabochia SL, Olinger AR, Marshall MJ, eds. *Diverse Approaches to Teaching, Learning, and Writing across the Curriculum: IWAC at 25.* Fort Collins, CO: WAC Clearinghouse; 2020.

18. Bean J. *Engaging Ideas: The Professor's Guide to Integrating Writing, Critical Thinking, and Active Learning in the Classroom.* 2nd ed. Hoboken: Wiley; 2011.

19. Brizee A, Wells JM. *Partners in Literacy: A Writing Center Model for Civic Engagement.* Lanham, MD: Rowman & Littlefield; 2016.

20. Flower L. *Community Literacy and the Rhetoric of Public Engagement.* Carbondale, IL: Southern Illinois University Press; 2008.

21. Goldblatt E. *Because We Live Here: Sponsoring Literacy Beyond the College Curriculum.* New York, NY: Hampton Press; 2007.

22. Grabill J. Infrastructure, outreach, and the engaged writing program. In: Rose SK, Weiser I, eds. *Going Public: What Writing Programs Learn from Engagement.* Boulder, CO: University Press of Colorado; 2010:15–28. doi:10.2307/j.ctt4cgpfh.4

23. McLeod S, Soven M, eds. *Writing across the Curriculum: A Guide to Developing Programs.* Fort Collins, CO: WAC Clearinghouse; 2000.

24. International Network of WAC Programs. Statement of WAC principles and practices. Published online 2014.

25. Angeli EL. Three types of memory in emergency medical services communication. *Writ Commun.* 2015;32(1):3–38. doi:10.1177/0741088314556598

26. Cooper MM. The ecology of writing. *College English.* 1986;48(4):364–375. doi:10.2307/377264

27. Rickert TJ. *Ambient Rhetoric: The Attunements of Rhetorical Being.* Pittsburgh, PA: University of Pittsburgh; 2013.

28. Rule HJ. *Situating Writing Process.* Fort Collins, CO: WAC Clearinghouse; 2019.

29. Prior P, Shipka J. Chronotopic lamination: tracing the contours of literate activity. In: Bazerman B, Russel D, eds. *Writing Selves/Writing Societies: Research from Activity Perspectives.* Fort Collins, CO: WAC Clearinghouse; 2003:180–238.

30. Seawright L. *Genre of Power: Police Report Writers and Readers in the Justice System.* Urbana, IL: NCTE; 2017.

31. Angeli EL. *Rhetorical Work in Emergency Medical Services: Communicating in the Unpredictable Workplace.* New York, NY: Routledge; 2019.

32. Campbell L. Simulation genres and student uptake: the patient health record in clinical nursing simulations. *Writ Commun.* 2017;34(3):255–279. doi:10.1177/0741088317716413

33. Forsa CQ. Writing about health: a health writing course that emphasizes rhetorical flexibility and teaches for transfer. *Double Helix.* 2018;6:1–21.

34. Gouge CC. Health humanities baccalaureate programs and the rhetoric of health and medicine. *Tech Commun Q.* 2018;27(1):21–32. doi:10.1080/10572252.2017.1402566

35. Sorrell J. Stories in the nursing classroom: writing and learning through stories. *Learn Lang Across Discip.* 2001;5(1):36–48.

36. Johnson MA, Simmons WM, Sullivan P. *Lean Technical Communication: Toward Sustainable Program Innovation.* New York, NY: Routledge; 2017.

37. Rose SK, Weise I, eds. *Going Public: What Writing Programs Learn from Engagement.* Boulder, CO: University Press of Colorado; 2010. doi:10.2307/j.ctt4cgpfh

38. Laudermilch DJ, Schiff MA, Nathens AB, Rosengart MR. Lack of emergency medical services documentation is associated with poor patient outcomes: a validation of audit filters for prehospital trauma care. *J Am Coll Surg.* 2010;210(2):220–227. doi:10.1016/j.jamcollsurg.2009.10.008

39. Paine C. *The Resistant Writer: Rhetoric as Immunity, 1850 to the Present.* Albany, NY: SUNY Press; 1999.

40. Rutz C, Lauer-Glebov J. Assessment and innovation: one darn thing leads to another. *Assess Writ.* 2005;10(2):80–99. doi:10.1016/j.asw.2005.03.001

41. Condon W, Rutz C. A taxonomy of writing across the curriculum programs: evolving to serve broader agendas. *Coll Compos Commun.* 2012;64(2):357–382.

42. Dayton D, Bernhardt SA. Results of a survey of ATTW members, 2003. *Tech Commun Q.* 2004;13(1):13–43. doi:10.1207/S15427625TCQ1301_5

43. Rainey KT, Turner RK, Dayton D. Core competencies for technical communicators. *Tech Commun.* 2005;52(3):323–352.

44. Henschel S, Meloncon L. Of horsemen and layered literacies: assessment instruments for aligning technical and professional communication undergraduate curricula with professional expectations. *Program Perspect.* 2014;6(1):3–26.

45. Rogers P. The contributions of North American longitudinal studies of writing in higher education to our understanding of writing development. In: Bazerman C, Krut R, Lunsford K, McLeod S, Rogers P, Stansell A, eds. *Traditions of Writing Research.* New York, NY: Routledge; 2009:365–377.

46. Randell D. New documentation mnemonic and rubric substantially improved documentation performance. *JEMS* Published May 12, 2020. Accessed May 28, 2020. https://www.jems.com/2020/05/12/new-documentation-mnemonic-and-rubric/

9

ONLINE INSTRUCTION ON SCHOLARLY WRITING AND LIBRARY RESEARCH IN A PHYSICIAN ASSISTANT PROGRAM

Laying the Foundation for Developing Academic Literacies and Examining Evidence-Based Research

Isabell C. May and Emilie M. Ludeman

From its inception, the physician assistant (PA) profession has focused on patient-centered care, a reaction to criticisms that the medical profession faced in the mid-twentieth century. Traditional medical practice was being accused of disregarding social and behavioral considerations when working with patients, in addition to ignoring preventive treatments and larger public health concerns. Similar to the roles of the nurse practitioner and the certified nurse-midwife, the separate role of the PA emphasized the ever-growing need to focus on the patients themselves, especially in rural areas and among populations of lower socioeconomic standing.[1]

Subsequently, PA programs developed in the United States during the 1960s.[2] The first PA cohort started in 1965 at Duke University, where graduates received a certificate in PA studies and a bachelor's degree in a different area.[2] This has remained common practice except for one change in recent years—namely, the introduction of master's degrees in conjunction with the PA certificate. In 1999, only three PA programs awarded master's degrees; by 2007, the majority did so.

This trend toward graduate-level education has introduced more research-oriented topics in the curriculum.[3] Traditionally, PA programs have not focused on educating their students in areas related to academic research.[4,5] The focus has predominantly, and often almost exclusively, been on preparing students for their professional lives as health-care providers. In addition, much has been published on developing the research skills of not just PA students but those of PA faculty.[4–6]

The demand for greater research skills has elevated the importance of information literacy and scholarly writing skills—significant areas in "writing in the health professions."[6] This importance is reflected in the standards of the Accreditation Manual of the Accreditation Review Commission on Education for the Physician Assistant, which accredited PA programs must meet. Standard B 2.10, for example, requires PA programs "to prepare students to search, interpret and evaluate the medical literature."[7] This standard emphasizes the need to cultivate students' skills in developing research questions, as well as in interpreting evidence-based research.

As a result, the current literature on PA education has started to interrogate how existing PA programs teach research skills, including information literacy and scholarly writing. Already in 2003, Cipher et al.[8] suggested that PA students should receive instruction on research skills early on in their education. Furthermore, some PA programs have developed models to include writing and research skills in the curriculum within already existing introductory courses.[9] However, much of the literature, and many PA programs, do not consider information literacy and scholarly writing as skill areas separate from research methodology. This realization prompted us to take a deeper look

DOI: 10.4324/9781003162940-13

into how we, as educators, can better meet the literacy needs of our PA students. We developed a model for course development based on the broader notion of academic literacies.

Literature Review

Academic Literacies

Overall, much of the curriculum in health-care education focuses on content and practice to prepare future health-care professionals. While we recognize these curricular necessities, we suggest that it does not necessarily take a lot of effort to develop courses or modules on "writing in the health professions" that integrate information literacy. Most students struggle with learning these skill areas via osmosis alone and would greatly benefit from targeted, well-developed, and research-based instruction in these areas.

The model of academic literacies, also discussed in Chapter 2, is one model to introduce health professionals such as PAs to research skills, information literacy, and scholarly writing. In this model, research skills and scholarly writing are built into the curriculum as part of a larger conversation around "meaning making, identity, power and authority."[10(p368)] Students are taught that writing is always situational and that it takes time and practice to be socialized into various academic and scientific genres—an essential concept when teaching writers highly specialized ways of writing.[10] Too often, writing instruction within health professions is reduced to grammar and sentence structure. For example, Kuntz et al.[12(p140)] discuss writing skills as an important area of evidence-based medicine but narrow writing skills down to "demonstrat[ing] appropriate grammar, sentence structure, word choice, and sequence of ideas in scientific writing," among other things. In addition, such a reduced approach to writing instruction ignores that "appropriate grammar" and "sentence structure" are culturally coded terms, which can perpetuate structures of inequality.[11,12]

With the academic literacies model at its center, we developed a framework for online course development that includes existing literature on information literacy curricula, graduate writing instruction, and online learning. This literature shaped our redesign of a required one-credit research and writing course in the PA program at the University of Maryland, Baltimore (UMB; Figure 9.1).

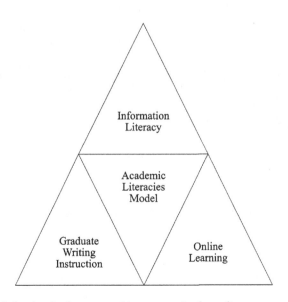

FIGURE 9.1 Framework for developing our writing course in the online program for PAs

Information Literacy Curricula

Instruction on information literacy plays a central role in the development of academic literacies among undergraduate and graduate-level students, especially in the context of writing in the health professions. Much of the research on assessing library instruction on undergraduate learning, offered frequently at the beginning of students' academic careers, shows a positive association between student learning outcomes and library use.[13-17] A recent body of research also offers guidance on how to structure information literacy instruction for graduate-level students.[18-21] Mostly, information literacy instruction takes place in one-shot instruction sessions with students.[22-24] However, such one-shot sessions often do not contribute to long-term retention[25] and are notoriously difficult to assess.[26] In addition, such one-shot sessions often focus on general library information outside of any specific course assignment contexts; however, information literacy instruction is most useful when it has a certain disciplinary specificity—e.g., locating information on evidence-based practice to create an integrative literature review for a nursing journal.[24]

Overall, the consensus in both undergraduate and graduate-level instruction on information literacy seems to be the same: frequent in-depth instruction with opportunities to practice and receive feedback seems to be most valuable for students, producing positive learning outcomes.[22] Well-designed library instruction sessions that are integrated into the curriculum present the ideal opportunity to make a lasting and meaningful impact in terms of students developing the necessary skills to work with evidence-based literature throughout their graduate careers.[27] As higher education has been witnessing an increase in online instruction, librarians are also delivering much of their content virtually, as the number of publications on various forms of online library instruction suggests.[28-31]

Since one of the main goals of information literacy instruction has to do with teaching students to select relevant and reliable sources to support their own writing and research, combining information literacy and writing instruction happens frequently. This often happens via collaborations between writing centers or writing programs and libraries. Such collaborations can consist of one-time workshops or workshop series that address the intersection of research and writing. For example, the Writing Center and Library at the University of South Alabama collaborated to develop an asynchronous online workshop to teach students about academic scholarship including appropriate citing of sources.[32] After viewing the workshop, students showed improved awareness of academic integrity; students also expressed increased awareness of the resources available through the library and writing center. In many cases, faculty solicit instruction on information literacy and writing skills to take place in their specific courses and can be quite impactful. For example, a program at Eastern Kentucky University involved a trilateral approach that involved librarians, writing center staff, and course faculty collaborating to effectively integrate sources into a first-year academic writing program.[33] Program evaluation showed improved scores in organization (cohesion) and information literacy; students engage more meaningfully with their sources

Teaching Writing Skills on the Graduate Level

Similar to the research on information literacy instruction, the literature on teaching basic writing skills is also very undergraduate heavy, although there is a growing body of literature on graduate professional programs beyond the baccalaureate, in which PA students fall.[34,35] The rich literature on writing across the curriculum and writing in the disciplines programs in undergraduate contexts in particular have informed much of the work on writing instructions for graduate students.[36-38]

Because of the lack of formalized graduate writing instruction, Rose and McClafferty[39] published "A Call for the Teaching of Writing in Graduate Education" in 2001. As the title suggests, writing instruction for graduate-level students was not a common part of the graduate curriculum in most academic disciplines. It seems that most graduate programs operated on the innate belief that students admitted to graduate programs would know "how to write." Since then, that assumption has been largely refuted, and three areas emerge from the literature on graduate-level writing, especially within the health professions, around effective curriculum design: genre theory, scaffolded writing assignments, and formative feedback.

Genre Theory

One of the most salient approaches in teaching writing to graduate students has been the use of genre theory.[40] Autry and Carter,[41] for example, used the theoretical concept of genre and genre systems to create thesis and dissertation support services for graduate students at North Carolina State University. In a broad sense, genres allow us to understand the socialization of writers into a specific discipline or community of practice. Genre-based teaching allows writing instructors to do a deep dive into often hidden assumptions and stylistic elements, often called "rhetorical moves," of widely used genres in a specific context.[10]

Such genre-based writing instruction is best understood as being part of the larger pedagogical goal of supporting students in developing academic or scholarly literacies.[42,43] The "academic literacies" model goes beyond understanding writing as just another study skill that students need to work on individually (often referred to as the study skills model) or as a process of acculturation into specific ways of writing (often referred to as the academic socialization model). It goes further by theorizing writing as a complex and diverse process of meaning-making in a wide variety of contexts, thereby emphasizing the dynamic and nuanced nature of writing, especially within highly stratified contexts such as academic disciplines and practices. Lea and Street[42] advocate for using the academic literacies approach when developing writing-based curricula; it foregrounds often underlying assumptions about what is expected in specific disciplinary contexts. A recent 3-year study, for example, on occupational therapy students in an embedded literacy program during their first year of graduate school showed improved writing skills and increased student satisfaction with their writing skills.[44]

Scaffolded Writing Assignments

A scaffolded approach to writing assignments goes hand in hand with a writing curriculum centered on genre theory and academic literacies that is based on transparency around expectations and conventions. As other authors in this collection have suggested, scaffolded assignments break down complex assignments into smaller, more manageable tasks by building on existing knowledge. The method of instructional scaffolding is based on the psychologist Lev Vygotsky's[45] theory of the "zone of proximal development," which, briefly put, is a theoretical concept that describes learners' current level of knowledge and what they can achieve with help. The use of scaffolded writing assignments has been widely discussed in the work of multilingual and second-language experts[46,47] as an effective method to teach academic writing and the cultural conventions around academic discourse in English to students for whom English is not one of their primary languages. Scaffolded journal writing assignments have also been used with students in medical and health care–related areas, with the explicit purpose of helping them explore connections between the course content, their own learning, and the further development of their writing skills.[48] (Chapter 7, for instance, shows how assignments like these can get students "unstuck" as they learn to write literature reviews.)

Formative Feedback

Lastly, much of the research on writing instruction suggests formative feedback when developing writing assignments. The concept of formative assessment is based on Bloom's Taxonomy for writing learning objectives, as well as on Vygotsky's theories, similar to the scaffolding of assignments.[49] (Bloom's Taxonomy also appears in Chapters 11 and 12.) Summative assessment, formative assessment's counterpart, tends to refer to assessment that determines whether students have achieved a certain outcome, most likely at the end of a curriculum or course. Formative assessment, on the other hand, tends to focus on the development of skills, often giving students the opportunity to revise and reorient their work. Research in K–12 education clearly demonstrates that formative assessment of writing leads to students improving their writing.[50] Some of the work focused on higher education also suggests that formative feedback leads to improved student writing but also emphasizes that formative feedback needs to be balanced in pointing out strengths and weaknesses so that students will not feel discouraged as they develop as writers.[51]

Despite this growing body of research around graduate-level writing, the focus within that research is predominantly on students pursuing a research-focused master's or doctoral degree. The articles, therefore, address the needs of graduate students to produce genres leading to future publications in their role as researchers and/or academics.[52–54] The discussion on graduate student writing in areas outside of these, such as graduate students in professional programs or health care–based/allied health training, has received virtually no attention.[44]

Online Instruction

To meet the growing need for writing instruction within the health professions, online writing courses offer some great opportunities. Even though some educators in higher education tend to perceive online teaching as academically less rigorous or even as being damaging to scholars' professional reputations, students, especially in graduate and professional schools, welcome, and at times even demand, online instruction for various reasons (e.g., convenience and flexibility).[55] As recent data show, the demand for online instruction is continually increasing, even though the last few years have seen a slower growth rate than previously recorded.[56] Online curricula in graduate-level education, for example, have enjoyed tremendous growth over the past decades.[57] Even Research 1 universities, whose offerings of online graduate programs used to be slim, have caught on to the trend.[58]

One area in online education has received a lot of attention and can be a great tool for online writing courses: online or video lectures. One of the most common genres used in online learning are video captures of narrated PowerPoint presentations or demonstrations of relevant applications (e.g., using a particular database for research), frequently referred to as video podcasts, which is the genre that we used in our course design. In recent years, more and more studies have emerged that investigate the effectiveness of video podcasts in online teaching. For example, recorded classroom lectures seem to have more positive than negative effects, both on instructors and learners.[59] Other research also suggests that video podcasts enhance student learning, especially in fostering independence, gaining technological or communicational skills, and increasing academic performance and self-reflection.[60] Additionally, research based on students' perceptions of learning content indicates that students see relevant multimedia content as enhancing their learning.[61,62]

Despite the positive impact of video and similar multimedia material in online classrooms, too many conflicting stimuli can lead to cognitive overload.[63] Cognitive overload in multimedia learning happens when "the learner's intended cognitive processing exceeds the learner's available cognitive capacity."[64(p43)] Fortunately, strategies exist that can prevent cognitive overload, such as presenting key definitions as narration with imagery instead of printed text or reducing the presenting material in shorter segments rather than in one long video.[64,65] In addition, producing videos interactive in nature (i.e., videos that are edited to include interactive elements such as quizzes, demonstrations of certain practices, and opportunities for application) seem to be particularly promising for students in health sciences programs.[66] Ultimately, educators' levels of technological literacies, as well as institutional support, both via instructional designers and the proper hardware and software, play a key role in delivering content successfully online.

Ultimately, the online environment represents great opportunities for information literacy and writing instruction.[67] Most graduate-level and professional schools require their students to master research-based writing effectively within their respective discourse communities. Many students must produce a thesis, dissertation, or similar capstone-type paper at the end of their program; however, most programs do not offer explicit instruction on writing, particularly for the thesis/ dissertation level.[68] Online modules and courses on effective writing can, therefore, offer opportunities for content instruction, meaningful feedback, and valuable peer collaboration to graduate-level writers in a format that is both convenient and appreciated by learners.

History of MHS 600 and Original Design

To prepare students adequately for the rigors of research-based writing typical for graduate-level education, especially the capstone projects at the end of the curriculum, the following learning outcomes were developed for MHS 600 in line with the Quality Matters (QM) framework:

1. Utilize the library website to locate resources and use the internet as a research tool;
2. Integrate the core concepts of information retrieval for finding, evaluating, analyzing, organizing, and presenting information;
3. Exercise critical thinking to evaluate information;
4. Develop a sustainable writing process that includes strategies for prewriting, drafting, and revision;
5. Create unified texts that engage and inform their intended audience;
6. Develop, evaluate, and improve academic writing skills; and
7. Apply format and citation guidelines based on style guides appropriate for the field.

The skills learned and practiced in this course are fundamental to subsequent courses in the MHS (MS in health science) program, all of which require a significant amount of reading and research. The entire program is delivered online. Some writing assignments in MHS courses are less formal, such as discussion boards or response papers, but many others are typical genres, such as literature reviews or annotated bibliographies. Overall, all courses in the curriculum require students to navigate the research process and produce organized and clear writing for a variety of audiences. As one of the first courses in the curriculum, MHS 600 lays the foundation for all these educational outcomes.

Redesign of MHS 600

Feedback from Previous Course Evaluations

In light of the existing literature on the academic literacies framework, information literacy curricula, graduate writing instruction, and online learning, we attempted to integrate these components when we were asked to redesign MHS 600 in the spring semester of 2017. The course had been taught for three consecutive summers, starting in 2014. The final course evaluations of the course taught in summer 2016 revealed that a significant number of the students enrolled in MHS 600 were dissatisfied with their experience.

Many questions of the final course evaluation that students complete are four-point Likert scale questions, where students are asked to indicate their level of agreement with various statements (ranging from "strongly agree" to "strongly disagree"). For example, almost a third of the respondents (23%, n = 26) disagreed/strongly disagreed that the assignments and activities (i.e., discussions, essays, interactive modules, etc.) facilitated learning. Also, 18% of all respondents (n = 26) did not feel that readings and other course materials facilitated learning. Out of the 88% who felt that course materials facilitated learning, only 11% strongly agreed. In addition to students' dissatisfaction with the course assignment and materials, close to half of the respondents (41%, n = 27) did not feel that instructor feedback on assignments was helpful. Much of this dissatisfaction stemmed from the course design, which gave students only one week to incorporate feedback on their previous draft. In the open-ended question on how this course could be improved, almost two-thirds of the comments (61%, n = 18) focused on the lack of timely feedback.

Based on student feedback, our priority was realigning the course design with learning outcome number 4: develop a sustainable writing process that includes strategies for prewriting, drafting, and revision. In the original course design, students spent the first three modules on writing process–related questions without starting to develop their own topic or research question. In a course that only lasts 8 weeks, we felt that selecting their topic and getting into the research literature needed to happen during the first 3 weeks. This change would also address the concerns about relevant course materials, assignments, and timely feedback voiced by so many students in the 2016 evaluations.

We observed another gap in the course design of MHS 600, as well as in the literature on course design of similar courses that drove our redesign: the lack of an effective combination between teaching information literacy skills (such as developing effective search strategies in health sciences databases) and writing skills (such as formulating a meaningful thesis statement and organizing a text effectively).[3,69] In the original course, the library faculty, for example, was not involved in any feedback on the students' writing assignments. The original design of the course presented three discrete units focused on research (modules 3–5), followed by three discrete units of writing (modules 6–8). However, finding useful and evidence-based research, generating and refining a research question, and organizing a research-based paper effectively go hand in hand. While we still felt some need for discrete units on research and writing, we also wanted to emphasize that the research and writing process are not separate processes; they intertwine throughout the entire research and writing process. We also made sure that our feedback on students' writing would come from both instructors and presented a coherent message.

Revision of the Course Centered on the Genre of the Research Review Essay

We structured our redesign process with the help of the QM framework, a framework that UMB's graduate school uses for its online courses. The QM framework originated among Maryland institutions in higher education and has gained immense popularity across the United States as a robust system of standards to evaluate online course designs, with the explicit goal that student learning outcomes, assignments, and course materials are aligned to ensure a high-quality student learning experience.[70,71] We organized our course modules following a backward-design approach that is a basic element in the QM framework. First, we used the already developed course-level learning outcomes and translated them into module-level objectives and assessments, followed by adding resources and activities that aligned with the course and module-level objectives and assessments. This phase-based approach pairs well with the method of scaffolded instruction, as it allows instructors to really think about how assessments and assignments connect to and build on each other.

Since our class was designed to be an introductory course, we decided that the more common genres of a literature review or research proposal would be beyond the capacity of an introductory one-credit course. Furthermore, our course was meant to prepare students for that task in the second half of their degree program, when they produce a literature review in their second year in a two-semester course on research methodology. As a result, we developed our own genre that we called the research review essay, which would allow students to practice the skills needed for a literature review but without the same pressure of needing to produce an exhaustive review of existing literature. Ultimately, our creation of this genre is meant to give students the permission to explore crafting an argument without feeling the pressure to be tested for their content knowledge at the same time.

The skills needed to produce a literature review in the health professions usually have to do with identifying a manageable research question based on the patient, intervention, comparison, outcome (PICO) framework to formulate clinical questions to inform evidence-based research,[72] searching existing literature on the chosen topic, navigating electronic databases successfully, selecting evidence-based research to answer the research question, writing a first draft of the lit review, revising their own writing, organizing a lot of information coherently for their audience, navigating the citation and referencing guidelines of the *Publication Manual of the American Psychological Association* (APA), and proofreading their own work. We redesigned the course so that its modules would reflect this process.

In Module 1, students participate in a discussion and review some handouts and literature on writing in the health professions and the writing process in general. Module 2 introduces the first writing assignment (a reflective assignment where students start to explore a topic that they select) of a total of four assignments due every 2 weeks, where each of these assignments builds on the next one. We felt that by having students select their own topic, we would increase their ownership of the writing process. Most students entering the PA program have experience in health-care settings (average hours of patient care prior to enrollment is 4,432 for cohorts from 2017–2019). They also complete a worksheet on developing thesis statements in Module 2, followed by another worksheet on their search strategy for relevant evidence-based research on their topic in Module 3.

In this worksheet, students are expected to complete a worksheet on effective database search strategies. They must also submit citations for at least four relevant papers. Detailed formative feedback on this worksheet allows them to adjust their focus, if needed, to prepare their second writing assignment. By finding and sharing relevant citations, students are better prepared to move on to the next module where they begin incorporating references into their essays. Module 3 also includes a discussion section where students discuss their challenges while searching the databases.

In Module 4, students revise their first reflective assignment and start exploring their chosen topic more deeply, including a description of their search process. This assignment emphasizes the shift from writing about a topic based on personal interest and some basic knowledge to presenting information based on evidence-based research. This assignment is also the last one where students are not required to use a certain citation style.

To prepare them for the next assignment in two weeks, which will be a draft of their formal essay, students complete a worksheet on the APA citations style in Module 5 and review material on how to incorporate sources into their writing.

Module 6 reviews some common stylistic choices typical for science writing, while students also work on their first drafts, which are due by the end of this module. Although we provide in-depth formative feedback on the first two assignments as well, students will most likely receive the most detailed formative feedback on this draft.

Module 7 continues the exploration of science writing conventions, while students continue revising their first drafts based on our feedback. In the last module, students learn about some basic revision strategies and submit their final version of the research review essay. The assigned points for each of the writing assignments also reflect the scaffolded nature of our writing assignment. With each assignment, the number of points that can be earned increases; this further emphasizes that each assignment builds on skills practiced in the previous assignment.

Lastly, we wanted to make this course as personal and interactive as possible. Online learning can at times feel very disconnected, and cognitive overload has been widely discussed as a barrier to successful online learning.[64] Key elements for this redesign were short targeted video lectures that we created, readings, other materials that cover relevant information, and other assignments that reinforced each course module's content, which was designed to equip students with the necessary skills to complete the final writing assignment. We wanted to include materials that would make the online learning experience as interactive as possible. In other words, we wanted to make sure that our students felt connected with us, even though we teach the class without any synchronous components. Since the focus of the class is creating the research review essay, all other instructional materials needed to direct students toward accomplishing that goal. We ensured that our video lecture would not be longer than 15–20 minutes.

Ideally, we tried to limit the lectures to 10-15 minutes, which was not always possible; this might be an area that we have to further revise, as shorter, more frequent videos prevent cognitive overload in online learning environments. In each of the videos produced for the course, we made sure to add interactive elements, such as drawings on the screen or visual components, added after recording, that highlighted key ideas. In the student course evaluations, students have frequently commented on appreciating the short videos and the fact that the videos—as well as the other course materials, such as websites, handouts, or articles—supported the course's learning objectives.

Results of the Redesign

Based on student course evaluations from the past three summers (2017–2019), our refocus on the research and writing process via a scaffolded assignment structure and formative feedback has been working. For example, compared to the 59% of respondents in the 2016 course evaluation (n = 27; 7% strongly agreed and 52% agreed with the statement) who felt that instructor feedback was useful, 96% of respondents in the course 2017–2020 course evaluations did (n = 93; 72% strongly agreed and 26% agreed with the statement). Students were also able to add comments to this question, and many of the respondents in the 2017–2019 course evaluations described the feedback they received as "helpful," "detailed," "useful," "excellent," "thorough," "relevant," "constructive," and "personalized." In the 2016 course evaluations, more than two-thirds of the comments (68%; n = 19) to this question mentioned that the feedback was too late for students to use for their revision process.

The layout of this 8-week course has also revealed what most one-shot information sessions typically conducted by research librarians are incapable of revealing, which is how students are searching for, retrieving, and using information. The course also allows for individualized feedback to each student including ideas for finding additional relevant literature, modifying database searches, and strengthening their overall searching skills; all things that will be required as students move through the curriculum, in addition to being critical skills for evidence-based clinical decision-making. For example, the week 3 discussion board prompt asks the students to discuss their literature search process and any challenges they encountered. An overwhelming theme was students' surprise at learning about database features for refining their search (e.g., age limiters, study design filters) and the use of alternate search terms to increase the number of results. Students found the module's embedded tutorials on basic database searching techniques to be helpful and illuminating.

Recommendations

Online learning presents a great opportunity for many students preparing for health professions, especially in areas that are more skill-focused than content-focused, such as a course on library research and scholarly writing. We firmly believe that an early introduction to these skills, followed by continuous practice through the remainder of the curriculum, leads to health professionals who are able to effectively use evidence-based medicine in their treatment decisions, as well as in writing and research projects. The academic literacies model, in combination with the existing literature on information literacy curricula, graduate writing instruction, and online learning (see Figure 9.1), provides a helpful framework for such introductory courses. Combining information literacy instruction with a scaffolded approach to course assignments and paired with regular, formative feedback, thereby emphasizing the socially and culturally constructed nature of genre and academic discourse (see also Chapter 2), can serve as a model for health professions training on the graduate level.

Consequently, based on our experience and the existing literature, we recommend six critical steps for developing introductory information literacy and writing courses in the health professions. One, identify partners in your institution's writing center and library who could serve as co-instructors/guest lecturers. Two, get support from instructional designers or someone at your institution who knows their way around your learning management system. Three, use the QM framework or similar backward-design frameworks for course design. Four, use a scaffolded approach to assess your students' work on the skills introduced in your course. Five, focus on formative feedback and other assignments that support students in practicing or testing knowledge relevant to producing their writing assignment. Six, create as many short, personalized videos as possible on topics that matter most to you. If crunched for time, use video material from other sources but include at least a few personal ones throughout the course. We are optimistic that recommendations like these can enhance "writing in the health professions" in digital spaces.

References

1. Cawley JF. Physician assistant education: an abbreviated history. *J Physician Assist Educ.* Published online 2007. doi:10.1097/01367895-200718030-00001
2. Cawley JF, Cawthon E, Hooker RS. Origins of the physician assistant movement in the United States. *J Am Acad Physician Assist.* Published online 2012. doi:10.1097/01720610-201212000-00008
3. Fasser C, Waters V, Erdman K, et al. Project-based learning for physician assistant students: a retrospective assessment of the master's paper project at the Baylor College of Medicine Physician Assistant Program. *J Physician Assist Educ.* Published online 2009. doi:10.1097/01367895-200920040-00002
4. Opacic DA, Roessler E. Defining scholarship in physician assistant education. *J Physician Assist Educ.* Published online 2017. doi:10.1097/JPA.0000000000000136
5. Ritsema TS, Cawley JF. Building a research culture in physician assistant education. *J Physician Assist Educ.* Published online 2014. doi:10.1097/01367895-201425020-00003
6. Hegmann TE, Axelson RD. Benchmarking the scholarly productivity of physician assistant educators: an update. *J Physician Assist Educ.* Published online 2012. doi:10.1097/01367895-201223020-00004
7. ARC-PA. Accreditation Manual Accreditation Standards for Physician Assistant Education. Accreditation Manual Accreditation Standards for Physician Assistant Education. Published 2018. Accessed May 6, 2020. www.arc-pa.org
8. Cipher DJ, Lemke H, Coleridge ST. Establishing a research agenda in master's-level physician assistant studies programs. *J Physician Assist Educ.* Published online 2003. doi:10.1097/01367895-200314020-00004

9. Bryant JE, Hurtt BC, Schultz K. Evaluation of the incorporation of an innovative writing assignment into a physician assistant basic biomedical course. *J Physician Assist Educ*. Published online 2010. doi:10.1097/01367895-201021030-00004

10. Tardy C, Buck RH, Pawlowski M, Slinkard J. Evolving conceptions of genre among first-year writing teachers. *Compos Forum*. Published online 2018.

11. Inoue AB. Classroom writing assessment as an antiracist practice. *Pedagogy*. 2019;19(3):373–404. doi:10.1215/15314200-7615366

12. Condon F, Young VA, eds. *Performing Antiracist Pedagogy in Rhetoric, Writing, and Communication*. The WAC Clearinghouse; 2017.

13. Gross M, Latham D. What's skill got to do with it? Information literacy skills and self-views of ability among first-year college students. *J Am Soc Inf Sci Technol*. Published online 2012. doi:10.1002/asi.21681

14. Koufogiannakis D, Wiebe N. Effective methods for teaching information literacy skills to undergraduate students: a systematic review and meta-analysis. *Evid Based Libr Inf Pract*. Published online 2006. doi:10.18438/b8ms3d

15. Kuh GD, Gonyea RM. The role of the academic library in promoting student engagement in learning. *Coll Res Libr*. Published online 2003. doi:10.5860/crl.64.4.256

16. Maughan PD. Assessing information literacy among undergraduates: a discussion of the literature and the University of California-Berkeley assessment experience. *Coll Res Libr*. Published online 2001. doi:10.5860/crl.62.1.71

17. Soria KM, Fransen J, Nackerud S. Library use and undergraduate student outcomes: new evidence for students' retention and academic success. *Portal*. Published online 2013. doi:10.1353/pla.2013.0010

18. Alkhezzi F, Hendal B. Information literacy among graduate students in Kuwait University's College of Education. *Educ Inf*. Published online 2018. doi:10.3233/EFI-170141

19. Conway K. How prepared are students for postgraduate study? A comparison of the information literacy skills of commencing undergraduate and postgraduate information studies students at Curtin University. *Aust Acad Res Libr*. Published online 2011. doi:10.1080/00048623.2011.10722218

20. O'Malley D, Delwiche FA. Aligning library instruction with the needs of basic sciences graduate students: a case study. *J Med Libr Assoc*. Published online 2012. doi:10.3163/1536-5050.100.4.010

21. Parramore S. Online active-learning: information literacy instruction for graduate students. *Ref Serv Rev*. Published online 2019. doi:10.1108/RSR-03-2019-0022

22. Mery Y, Newby J, Peng K. Why one-shot information literacy sessions are not the future of instruction: a case for online credit courses. *Coll Res Libr*. Published online 2012. doi:10.5860/crl-271

23. Belzowski N, Robison M. Kill the one-shot: using a collaborative rubric to liberate the librarian–instructor partnership. *J Libr Adm*. Published online 2019. doi:10.1080/01930826.2019.1583018

24. Daland HT. Just in case, just in time or just don't bother? Assessment of one-shot library instruction with follow-up workshops. *Lib Q*. 2015;24(3):125–139. http://liber.library.uu.nl/

25. Martin J. The information seeking behavior of undergraduate education majors: does library instruction play a role? *Evid Based Libr Inf Pract*. 2008;3(4):4–17.

26. Wang R. Assessment for one-shot library instruction: a conceptual approach. *Portal*. 2016;16(3):619–648. doi:10.1353/pla.2016.0042

27. Lee Roberts R, Taormina M. Collaborative co-design for library workshops. *Behav Soc Sci Libr*. Published online 2013. doi:10.1080/01639269.2013.755875

28. Moran C, Mulvihill R. Finding the balance in online library instruction: sustainable and personal. *J Libr Inf Serv Distance Learn*. Published online 2017. doi:10.1080/1533290X.2016.1223964

29. Contrino JL. Instructional learning objects in the digital classroom: effectively measuring impact on student success. *J Libr Inf Serv Distance Learn*. Published online 2016. doi:10.1080/1533290X.2016.1206786

30. Gall D. Facing off: comparing an in-person library orientation lecture with an asynchronous online library orientation. *J Libr Inf Serv Distance Learn*. Published online 2014. doi:10.1080/1533290X.2014.945873

31. Weightman AL, Farnell DJJ, Morris D, Strange H, Hallam G. A systematic review of information literacy programs in higher education: effects of face-to-face, online, and blended formats on student skills and views. *Evid Based Libr Inf Pract*. Published online 2017. doi:10.18438/B86W90

32. Ard SE, Ard F. The library and the writing centre build a workshop: exploring the impact of an asynchronous online academic integrity course. *New Rev Acad Librariansh*. 2019;25(2-4):218–243. doi:10.1080/13614533.2019.1644356

33. Napier T, Parrott J, Presley E, Valley L. A collaborative, trilateral approach to bridging the information literacy gap in student writing. *Coll Res Libr.* 2018;79(1):120–145. doi:10.5860/crl.79.1.120

34. Brooks-Gillies M, Garcia EG, Kim SH, Manthey K, Smith T. *Across the Disciplines A Journal of Language, Learning and Academic Writing Graduate Writing Across the Disciplines, Introduction*; 1997.

35. Micciche LR, Carr AD. Toward graduate-level writing instruction. *CCC.* Published online 2011.

36. Carter M. Ways of knowing, doing, and writing in the disciplines. *CCC.* Published online 2007.

37. Carter M, Ferzli M, Wiebe EN. Writing to learn by learning to write in the disciplines. *J Bus Tech Commun.* Published online 2007. doi:10.1177/1050651907300466

38. Russell DR *Writing in the Academic Disciplines: A Curricular History.* 2nd ed. Southern Illinois Press; 2002.

39. Rose M, McClafferty K. A call for the teaching of writing in graduate education. *Educ Res.* 2001;30(2):27–33. doi:10.3102/0013189X030002027

40. Bawarshi A, Reif MJ. *Genre: An Introduction to History, Theory, Research, and Pedagogy.* Parlor Press and WAC Clearinghouse; 2010.

41. Autry MK, Carter M. Unblocking occluded genres in graduate writing: thesis and dissertation support services at North Carolina State University. *Compos Forum.* Published online 2015.

42. Lea MR, Street B V. The "academic literacies" model: theory and applications. *Theory Pract.* Published online 2006. doi:10.1207/s15430421tip4504_11

43. Tardy CM. *Beyond Convention: Genre Innovation in Academic Writing.* University of Michigan Press; 2016.

44. Gordon-Handler L, Dimitropoulou K, Hassan L, Masaracchio M, Waldman-Levi A. Exploration of graduate health care student writing skills using a transformational learning approach to a literacy enrichment program. *J Allied Health.* 2019;48(3):201–208.

45. Vygotsky L V. *Mind in Society: The Development of Higher Psychological Processes.* Harvard University Press; 1978.

46. Cotterall S, Cohen R. Scaffolding for second language writers: producing an academic essay. *ELT J.* Published online 2003. doi:10.1093/elt/57.2.158

47. Riazi AM, Rezaiim M. *Teacher- and peer-scaffolding behaviors: effects on EFL students' writing improvement. CLESOR 2010 Proc 12th Natl Conf Community Lang ESOL.* Published online 2011.

48. Cardinale JA, Johnson BC. Metacognition modules: a scaffolded series of online assignments designed to improve students' study skills †. *J Microbiol Biol Educ.* 2017;18(1). doi:10.1128/jmbe.v18i1.1212

49. Yorke M. Formative assessment in higher education: moves towards theory and the enhancement of pedagogic practice. *High Educ.* Published online 2003. doi:10.1023/A:1023967026413

50. Frey N, Fisher D. *A Formative Assessment System for Writing Improvement*; 2013.

51. Wingate U. The impact of formative feedback on the development of academic writing. *Assess Eval High Educ.* Published online 2010. doi:10.1080/02602930903512909

52. Caffarella RS, Barnett BG. Teaching doctoral students to become scholarly writers: the importance of giving and receiving critiques. *Stud High Educ.* Published online 2000. doi:10.1080/030750700116000

53. Maher D, Seaton L, McMullen C, Fitzgerald T, Otsuji E, Lee A. "Becoming and being writers": the experiences of doctoral students in writing groups. *Stud Contin Educ.* Published online 2008. doi:10.1080/01580370802439870

54. Paltridge B. Thesis and dissertation writing: an examination of published advice and actual practice. *English Specif Purp.* Published online 2002. doi:10.1016/S0889-4906(00)00025-9

55. Ubell R. Advice for faculty members about overcoming resistance to teaching online (essay). *Inside HigherEd.* Published 2016. Accessed May 6, 2020. https://www.insidehighered.com/advice/2016/12/13/advice-faculty-members-about-overcoming-resistance-teaching-online-essay

56. Allen E, Seaman J. *2013—Grade Change: Tracking Online Education in the United States - OLC*; 2014. Accessed May 6, 2020. https://onlinelearningconsortium.org/survey_report/2013-survey-online-learning-report

57. Fain P. Master's degrees more popular, increasingly online. *Inside HigherEd.* Published 2018. Accessed May 6, 2020. https://www.insidehighered.com/quicktakes/2018/12/12/masters-degrees-more-popular-increasingly-online

58. Garret R. How Elite Universities are Changing the Online Master's Game. *Encoura.* Published 2018. Accessed May 6, 2020. https://encoura.org/how-elite-universities-are-changing-the-online-masters-game/

59. O'Callaghan FV, Neumann DL, Jones L, Creed PA. The use of lecture recordings in higher education: a review of institutional, student, and lecturer issues. *Educ Inf Technol.* 2017;22(1):399–415. doi:10.1007/s10639-015-9451-z

60. Kay R, Kletskin I. Evaluating the use of problem-based video podcasts to teach mathematics in higher education. *Comp & Educ.* 2012;59(2):619–627. doi:10.1016/j.compedu.2012.03.007

61. Scagnoli NI, Choo J, Tian J. Students' insights on the use of video lectures in online classes. *Br J Educ Technol.* 2019;50(1):399–414. doi:10.1111/bjet.12572

62. Miner S, Stefaniak JE. Learning via video in higher education: an exploration of instructor and student perceptions. *J Univ Teach Learn Pract.* Published online 2018; 15(2):2.

63. Sweller J. Cognitive load during problem solving: effects on learning. *Cogn Sci.* Published online 1988. doi:10.1016/0364-0213(88)90023-7

64. Mayer RE, Moreno R. Nine ways to reduce cognitive load in multimedia learning. *Educ Psychol.* Published online 2003. doi:10.1207/S15326985EP3801_6

65. Thomson A, Bridgstock R, Willems C. "Teachers flipping out" beyond the online lecture: maximising the educational potential of video. *J Learn Des.* Published online 2014. doi:10.5204/jld.v7i3.209

66. Link LR, Porter CL. Cross-campus collaboration to produce Camtasia-enhanced lessons to improve distance learning. *Internet Ref Serv Q.* 2014;19:245–253. doi:10.1080/10875301.2014.984820

67. Griffin J, Minter D. The rise of the online writing classroom: reflecting on the material conditions of college composition teaching. *Coll Compos Commun.* Published online 2013; 65:140–161.

68. Gonzalez M, Moore NS. Supporting graduate student writers with VoiceThread. *J Educ Technol Syst.* Published online 2018. doi:10.1177/0047239517749245

69. Kuntz S, Ali SH, Hahn E. Educational needs assessment highlights several areas of emphasis in teaching evidence-based medicine skills to physician assistant students. *J Physician Assist Educ.* Published online 2016. doi:10.1097/JPA.0000000000000078

70. Matters Q. About Quality Matters. Published 2020. Accessed May 6, 2020. https://www.qualitymatters.org/why-quality-matters/about-qm

71. Marlos Varonis E. Most courses are not born digital. *Campus-Wide Inf Syst.* 2014;31(4):217–229. doi:10.1108/cwis-09-2013-0053

72. Huang X, Lin J, Demner-Fushman D. Evaluation of PICO as a knowledge representation for clinical questions. *AMIA Annu Symp Proc.* 2006;2006:359–363.

10

ENHANCING COMMUNICATION COMPETENCIES

A Model for Pharmacy and Writing and Communication Center Partnerships

Janine Morris, Cynthia Moreau, and Kevin Dvorak

The Accreditation Council for Pharmacy Education (ACPE) Standards lists "professional communication" as one of its outcomes.[1] Upon completion of their graduate programs, students should be able to appropriately communicate with multiple populations verbally, nonverbally, and in writing. Being able to communicate effectively is closely tied to enhancing patient care,[2] displaying empathy and other soft skills,[3] and teamwork and collaboration,[4] which impact practitioner success and career satisfaction. Modeling and teaching students effective written, verbal, and nonverbal communication should begin immediately in pharmacy education and should continue being reinforced throughout the curriculum.[5]

One of the challenges of implementing a "writing in the health professions" curriculum is that programs that support students' written and verbal communication exist but are not very widespread or widely available at all institutions.[6,7] For institutions where writing in the health professions is not an explicit focus, we argue for the importance of health professions programs and writing and communication centers coming together to strategically integrate assignments and activities that enhance student writing and communication. The partnerships between writing and communication centers and graduate students across the health professions are of particular importance due to the unique writing challenges that graduate students often face.[8,9] This chapter thus describes a model of pharmacy and writing center partnerships to enhance student writing and presentation abilities. We describe a partnership that formed between the Writing and Communication Center (WCC) and the College of Pharmacy (COP) at Nova Southeastern University (NSU) and outline curricular changes that took place as a result. We begin by examining recent educational pushes for enhancing communicative competencies across pharmacy curricula and outline the development and outcomes of the partnership that took place at NSU. We end our chapter with recommendations for enhancing partnerships between writing centers and the health professions to support students in the health professions. (Other writing center partnerships are featured in Chapters 6 and 9.)

Writing and Communication in Pharmacy Education

In 1997, the World Health Organization report entitled "Preparing the Pharmacist of the Future: Curricular Development" outlined the 7 essential roles of the pharmacist, one of which was "communicator."[10] In recent years, the traditional role of the pharmacist has evolved from being

DOI: 10.4324/9781003162940-14

product-focused to patient-focused such that pharmacy graduates are being trained to provide patient-care services not directly associated with medication dispensing while working within interprofessional teams.[11] Also, as trends in the projected growth of the pharmacist profession now show a surplus of pharmacists entering the workforce, new graduates may seek careers in nontraditional pharmacy settings such as academia, the pharmaceutical industry, and managed care organizations, among others.[12] These changes mean that pharmacy graduates must be able to communicate and collaborate with a variety of audiences, including patients, caregivers, policymakers, physicians, nurses, and other health-care providers.[10]

A traditional doctor of pharmacy (PharmD) program consists of a 4-year curriculum, including 3 years of primarily didactic education followed by 1 year dedicated to pharmacy practice experiences or clinical clerkships, known as advanced pharmacy practice experiences. Pharmacy students also complete introductory pharmacy practice experiences in conjunction with the didactic curriculum during the first 3 years of the program. Providing instruction on and developing communication skills in pharmacy students can be complex, as there is a wide array of skills that are needed to deliver pharmaceutical care in a variety of settings. As medication experts, pharmacists are expected to communicate verbally and nonverbally with patients and other health-care professionals regarding drug therapy issues.[13] Many colleges and schools of pharmacy have dedicated communications courses in their curricula, as well as other activities that may be interspersed in other didactic courses and pharmacy practice experiences throughout the curriculum.

Wallman et al.'s systematic review of communications training in pharmacy education revealed that communication skills instruction in pharmacy curricula occurred through a variety of learning activities across the curriculum, and communication skills were mostly divided into two broad categories: oral communication skills and written communication skills.[10] Oral communication skills were divided into two subcategories: interpersonal communication and presentation skills. Interpersonal communication skills included patient-focused communication and interdisciplinary communication. Presentation skills involved formal presentations to an audience on a topic or idea. Written communication skills were further organized into three subcategories: academic, clinical, and reflective writing. Academic writing skills included research papers, essays, curriculum vitae, and letters of intent. Clinical writing skills included SOAP (subjective, objective, assessment, plan) notes, patient-care plans, written patient medical histories, and written patient educational materials. Reflective writing included self-reflective exercises and papers on student attitudes toward interdisciplinary teamwork and pharmacy practice experiences. Most educational interventions included in the review were designed to address multiple communication skills at once. For example, interpersonal communication skills were often taught alongside clinical writing or presentation skills. Also, reflective writing exercises were often used as a follow-up to a specific activity, such as a simulated patient interaction or interdisciplinary activity.

Hobson et al. also performed a review of writing tasks undertaken by pharmacy students during clerkship rotations, as mentioned in the introduction to this collection.[14] In this study, student writing samples were collected and coded to a rhetorical model to identify the four primary components of writing: message, audience, purpose, and occasion. Five categories accounted for 63.6% of the 198 documents obtained: in-service presentations, summaries (drug synopses, charts, reference information), patient case write-ups (pharmaceutical care plans), formulary reviews, and newsletters. The audiences for which students most frequently wrote included health-care providers (physicians, nurses, nutritionists, rehabilitation specialists) and other pharmacists. Most documents were identified as being intended to inform (73.2%) and less frequently intended to demonstrate (14.6%), persuade (9.1%), or reflect (0.5%). The authors concluded that most of the documents appeared to be linked to activities that students would be expected to complete in pharmacy practice settings upon graduation.

The available literature suggests that communication skills are taught in a variety of ways in pharmacy curricula and that the expectations of pharmacists with regards to oral and written tasks in pharmacy practice are diverse. Additionally, in the study by Hobson et al., the authors concluded that there was a gap between the writing tasks students were expected to complete during clerkship rotations and what is typically taught in college-level professional and technical writing courses.[14] Therefore, pharmacy students' writing skills need to be developed throughout the pharmacy curriculum. As such, we argue that colleges and schools of pharmacy can partner with writing and communication centers to help achieve these goals in a consistent manner throughout the curriculum.

Writing and Communication Centers and the Health Professions

More than a remedial service meant to support students on written communication alone, writing centers' roles have greatly expanded to support students with many kinds of communication-related projects.[15,16] According to Procter, writing centers are often positioned as important academic services that situate "writing as an intellectual activity … [that] contributes to the knowledge creation that is the core value of a university."[16(p416)] Writing centers often support writers across the disciplines, and their services have expanded from focusing on writing alone to helping students with communication across levels (including multimodal and visual projects and interpersonal communication).[17] As Jacob Herrmann writes, "For STEM students [and we argue, health professions students] especially, the connection between written and oral communication are irrevocably linked."[18] As we've argued earlier, the need for students to be able to deliver communication effectively to different audiences in multiple formats is particularly important for students in the health professions.

There are many benefits to establishing partnerships between writing and communication centers and the health professions. For example, Boquet et al.'s research highlighted the important interdisciplinary learning that took place between the School of Nursing, Writing Center, and Center for Academic Excellence at Fairfield University when those entities partnered together to support Nursing graduate students.[19] At their institution, the authors observed that "policy decisions affecting multiple stakeholders, too often made by one unit with little consultation, were put on the table for discussion, with needs of students, faculty, and programs all in consideration."[19(p9)] Seeking input from multiple stakeholders can ensure decisions are made that best assist students within specific programs.

Successful partnerships between various COP and writing centers have already taken place (e.g., Albany College of Pharmacy;[20] St. Louis College of Pharmacy[21]) and partnerships between writing and communication centers and health professions can prove useful for bringing together multiple stakeholders.[22,23] In Lerner's history of writing across the curriculum initiatives and partnerships between the Massachusetts College of Pharmacy and their Writing Center, he outlined important lessons for strengthening cross-disciplinary partnerships, including learning about professional values and how those align with the college, as well as understanding the institutional climate and needs.[22] As we demonstrate in the following section, the partnership that was developed between the NSU COP and NSU WCC was enhanced because of the time taken to build relationships among stakeholders and continue to reinforce communication skills across the curriculum.

COP and Writing Partnerships at NSU

The PharmD professional program at NSU consists of a traditional 4-year program, as well as an accelerated 3-year program for students who have previously earned a bachelor of science in pharmacy. The COP enrolls approximately 250 students annually across three campus sites: the main campus in Fort Lauderdale, Florida, and distance sites in Palm Beach Gardens, Florida, and San Juan, Puerto Rico. Course delivery primarily occurs synchronously via videoconferencing technology. In fall 2018, the PharmD program underwent significant curricular revision in an effort to align with ACPE Standards[1] to better prepare pharmacists for the evolving workforce. The new curriculum consists of a modular structure with an emphasis on team-based learning, applying content through active learning, and developing students' skills required to be successful in the pharmacy workforce. As new courses were being designed, it seemed like ideal timing to establish a partnership between the COP and the WCC to strengthen students' communication skills throughout the curriculum.

The WCC was developed in accordance with the university's Quality Enhancement Plan (QEP), which was a requirement for reaccreditation through the university's regional accrediting body. The primary goal of the QEP was to offer writing- and communication-related support to all students at the university, from first-year students to doctoral students, regardless of program, location, or modality. An additional goal was to develop and offer specific support structures for graduate and professional programs, acknowledging that such support programs are too often overlooked at these levels. Recognizing that NSU has eight colleges within its Health Professions Division (HPD), one critical early step in developing the WCC was to learn from HPD faculty about the types of writing- and communication-related projects assigned in these colleges, and the types of skills these students needed to be successful professionals. That way, the WCC team could build a strong rapport with their HPD colleagues and focus on providing discipline-specific assistance to students.

As the first semester of the revised PharmD curriculum was being designed, several opportunities were identified to begin integrating lectures and workshops to introduce students to various communication skills required for effective pharmacy practice. By introducing these concepts early in the curriculum, the goal was to create foundational skills students could continue to practice throughout the didactic and experiential curriculum. Throughout the year, the WCC worked with COP faculty to develop workshops to support the existing curriculum, focusing on things like reflective writing, professional communication, interpersonal communication, and visual presentation design. Through many conversations with faculty, the WCC learned about the programmatic objectives to ensure that the workshops supported skills that were being reinforced in other ways. To best support the multifaceted communication skills pharmacy students were learning, workshops took place within a sequence, with skills like professional communication and self-reflection building on one another over time.[24] Developing a strong partnership and ensuring faculty reinforcement was especially important for helping students learn the skills gradually and see them modeled in many ways by multiple people. Relying on faculty to reinforce workshop content throughout the year and curriculum served a similar function to repeating and having skills build on one another in different workshops.[24]

An additional opportunity to provide communication skills instruction occurred in the Pharmacy Applications I course, the first course in a five-course sequence. The Pharmacy Applications course sequence is intended to emphasize student application of content taught throughout the semester, with each course occurring over a 2-week period at the end of each semester. An activity was designed collaboratively by the Pharmacy Applications I course coordinator and WCC faculty to serve as a follow-up to material that had been presented during the incoming student orientation. During the first offering of the course in fall 2018, a workshop was designed to expose students to "best practices" for preparing written and oral presentations they would be expected to complete throughout the pharmacy curriculum and in pharmacy practice, including PowerPoint presentations, biomedical literature evaluations, and research poster presentations. During this session, the delivery of content occurred primarily through didactic lectures, with some active learning opportunities for students to practice their skills, including creating short presentations related to a drug therapy topic. The workshop appeared to be well received by students. However, student engagement appeared to be minimal to moderate, likely due to the fact that there was no graded activity or assignment linked to the workshop.

As the course coordinator prepared for the second offering of the Pharmacy Applications I course in the fall 2019 semester, the workshop was redesigned to increase student engagement and further encourage application and practice of written and oral communication skills. As such, the workshop was designed in conjunction with a graded team presentation assignment. Several days prior to the start of the course, preassigned student teams consisting of 7 to 8 students across all three pharmacy campus sites (31 teams total) were assigned a disease state as the topic of focus for their presentations. Disease state topics were chosen by the pharmacist course coordinator based on the Centers for Disease Control and Prevention data regarding the leading causes of death and disability in the United States,[25] as well as disease states that were expected to be taught in the following winter semester. The disease state topics included hypertension, dyslipidemia, heart failure, hypothyroidism, type 2 diabetes, chronic obstructive pulmonary disease, gastroesophageal reflux disease, urinary incontinence, osteoporosis, and benign prostatic hyperplasia. Also prior to the start of the course, students were provided with parameters to complete their presentations. Each team was tasked with creating a PowerPoint presentation consisting of no more than 20 slides and recording an audio-visual presentation that included all team members that was no more than 20 minutes in length. For each disease state, students were expected to cover the following: etiology, pathophysiology, risk factors, clinical presentation and diagnosis, treatment (including nonpharmacological and pharmacological options), goals of therapy and monitoring, and patient education/counseling points. Students were also responsible for including one slide with presentation objectives and one slide with appropriate references in American Medical Association format.

To assist students in completing their assignments, on the first day of the course, faculty from the WCC delivered a workshop on how to develop effective presentations, including how to plan, design, and deliver presentations while working in teams. As students were to record their presentations, considerations for completing recorded presentations were also discussed. Following the lecture, students were led through an exercise to aid in planning their presentations. In teams, students identified their presentation purpose and central ideas. Teams also created an outline of their presentations and were encouraged to use their outlines to divide workloads evenly among team members. During the workshop, WCC graduate peer consultants were available to students to practice presentations and receive feedback on their work in progress. During the remaining 2 weeks of the course, students were expected to meet with their teams to complete their PowerPoint presentations and recordings, and final presentations were due on the last day of the course. During this time, students also had the opportunity to make appointments with the WCC for additional assistance with their assignment, and 5 students on behalf of their teams took advantage of this offering. Dedicated self-study time was also built into the syllabus to allow for these activities to occur. The final presentations were graded by the course coordinator utilizing a rubric to evaluate the content, organization, and delivery of the presentation (see the Appendix for the rubric). The entire student team was given one grade for the content and organization of the presentation, while each student was evaluated individually for the delivery of their assigned portion of the presentation.

Successful completion of the presentation assignment by students required a combination of various oral and written communication skills. Students were able to practice academic and clinical writing skills by interpreting clinical information from various resources and producing a written presentation for a pharmacist audience. Students were also able to gain practice with proper citation formatting. These skills are important as pharmacy students and pharmacists are often asked to produce formal responses to drug information questions from health providers, which include a thorough review and evaluation of biomedical literature.[10] Students gained experience with oral presentation skills through recordings of their presentations while mastering the use of technology required to complete this task. Many students also acquired additional writing experience by preparing scripts for their verbal presentations. These skills are important, as pharmacists are increasingly involved in the provision of patient-care services via telehealth modalities.[26] Finally, interpersonal oral communication skills were emphasized as students needed to collaborate within their teams to complete the assignment. These skills can transfer to interprofessional practice settings in the future.

There are several challenges involved with the implementation and execution of communication skills instruction involving learning activities such as the one described. As previously discussed, a large class size of 250 students spread across multiple campus sites at NSU's COP makes it difficult to provide individualized instruction and feedback to students regarding their communication skills. In the team disease state presentation described, it would have been ideal if students had the opportunity to present in a live setting and gain immediate feedback from their peers and faculty members. This was further complicated by the short duration of the course that also included other content, assignments, and assessments during the 2-week time period. Given these challenges, the recorded presentation appeared to be the most feasible method to achieve the goals of the activity. Future iterations of this activity could also include a peer evaluation component such that students are required to evaluate their peers' presentations, which would allow students to receive additional feedback regarding their performance.

An additional challenge to implementation of the activity was ensuring all students had access to necessary technology to successfully complete their recorded presentations. Most teams utilized a video capture platform available through NSU (Kaltura Capture) on their personal computers to record. However, students at the Fort Lauderdale campus also had access to physical spaces, such as the Digital Media Lab and the WCC ground location, to practice and produce their recordings. These resources are not physically available at the distance sites in Palm Beach Gardens and San Juan. However, the WCC was available to work virtually with students at the regional campuses. Finally, the NSU COP has a diverse student population, with many students speaking English as a second language. These students may have felt especially challenged by the oral and written communication requirements of this assignment. While the WCC does support diverse language learners, one of the challenges is for students to self-identify as needing support and to seek out the resources.

During the fall 2019 semester when the group presentation activity was first implemented in the Pharmacy Applications I course, students performed well with a class average of 99%. Students were asked to complete a survey following the workshop that asked them to report on the usefulness of the workshop and likelihood of using WCC services. Of those that completed the survey, over 70% strongly agreed or agreed they "learned new writing strategies" in the workshop, and over 70% strongly agreed or agreed that "the content of the workshop may increase my ability to write effectively," emphasizing the interconnectedness of writing and verbal communication in developing presentations. Also of importance, close to 85% of participants strongly agreed or agreed that the workshop "content was practical to my academic needs," and 73% strongly agreed or agreed that the workshop "content was practical to my professional needs." These numbers illustrate that students immediately saw the relevance of the presentation to both their assignment and to their future as pharmacists.

The same activity was included as a graded component of the course again in the fall 2020 semester, and students achieved a class average of 98% on the assignment. The course coordinator noted it was apparent students had invested a lot of effort to prepare thorough and cohesive presentations that were appropriate for the intended audience. Of note, due to a modification in curricular structure at NSU COP, the course duration was increased from 2 weeks to 8 weeks during the fall 2020 semester, allowing students more time to complete their assignments. Also, during this semester, a reflective writing assignment regarding interprofessional education was added to the course syllabus, which further allowed students to reinforce reflective writing skills presented by the WCC during student orientation at the beginning of the semester. Finally, it is also important to note the delivery of the course in the fall 2020 semester was complicated as a result of the COVID-19 pandemic and NSU's transition to hybrid live/virtual education during this time. As such, all WCC-led workshops were held virtually, and many students worked with their teams remotely to complete the assignment. Some teams also utilized Zoom technology to record their presentations.

Institutionally, there still exists the challenge of providing systematic instruction and practice opportunities related to communication skills throughout the entirety of the pharmacy curriculum. This is complicated by the fact that courses in the revised NSU COP curriculum are still being designed as faculty and students adapt to the new curricular structure. However, in an effort to build upon the skills students developed in the Pharmacy Applications I course through completion of recorded disease state presentations, faculty members from the WCC were asked to lead another workshop on effective communication skills in the Pharmacy Application II course, this time emphasizing motivational interviewing techniques employed by pharmacists to empower patients to manage a variety of chronic disease states.

Conclusions and Recommendations

While we've outlined a specific example of how writing and communication centers can support students in the COP within a particular institutional context, we close the chapter with several takeaways for programs interested in strengthening partnerships for writing centers and health professions programs, and enhancing writing in the health professions:

Rely on institutional knowledge and expertise. As the COP began revising its curriculum, faculty across the college met often with the WCC to discuss curricular goals, student needs, and how to build those into courses across students' time in the program. By turning to the WCC, the COP began a dialogue about supporting their students and made connections with institutional resources that best supported them.

Build partnerships over time. The WCC is now entering its third year working with the COP. Each year, WCC and pharmacy faculty meet to discuss how the programs can be implemented or changed based on feedback from the previous year. As curricula are ever-evolving, it's important the partnership changes over time in response to student feedback. (For another perspective, see Chapter 4, which highlights institutional ethnography.) For instance, following the low student engagement in the 2018 Pharmacy Applications I course, subsequent workshops included additional pharmacy-specific examples and creative activities for students.

Build communication skills into the program at multiple levels. The written and interpersonal/interprofessional skills students need in order to be successful pharmacists are introduced and reinforced in different ways across the curriculum. For example, as an important practice for health professionals,[27] reflection is introduced in students' first-semester orientation. Students are given assignments asking them to reflect on their time in the program, and the reflective practices they learn during that first session are reinforced by multiple faculty in many classes.

Utilize writing and communication center services to help students professionalize. As the changing landscape of health professions necessitates strong communicators, students benefit from support not only with written assignments but also with other professional documents like resumes, CVs, and personal statements. Learning which institutional services (e.g., writing centers, career services) assist students with those types of writing and providing them ways to access those services can help set students apart once they begin entering the workforce.

As we've learned throughout our partnership, institutional and contextual structures will ultimately change and affect the kinds of programs and support services available for students in the health professions. We continue to emphasize the importance of seeing writing in the health professions as multifaceted and linked with other cognitive abilities (like design, reflection, and interpersonal exchanges). Recognizing that learning takes time, we argue writing and communication skills need to be an important curricular element—not a last-minute addition to a course. Building writing and communication skills into a curriculum takes time and constant reflection and work. What has been most successful for us as faculty partners is utilizing some of the skills we want our students to learn: open communication, willingness to listen, and ability to discuss needs, expectations, and desired outcomes.

References

1. Accreditation Standards and Key Elements for the Professional Program in Pharmacy Leading to the Doctor of Pharmacy Degree ("Standards 2016"). Accreditation Council for Pharmacy Education. https://www.acpe-accredit.org/pdf/Standards2016FINAL.pdf. Published February 2015.
2. Coomber P, Clavarino A, Ballard E, Leutsch K. Doctor–pharmacist communication in hospitals: strategies, perceptions, limitations and opportunities. *Int J Clin Pharm.* 2018;40:464–473.
3. Ratka A. Empathy and the development of affective skills. *Am J Pharm Educ.* 2018;82(2):1140–1143.
4. Planas L, Er N. A systems approach to scaffold communication skills development. *Am J Pharm Educ.* 2008;72(2):1–12.
5. Keller K., Eggenberger T., Belkowitz J., Sarsekeyeva M, Zito A. Implementing successful interprofessional communication opportunities in health care education: a qualitative analysis. *J Int Med Educ.* 2013;4:253–259.
6. Forsa C. Writing about health: a health writing course that emphasizes rhetorical flexibility and teaches for transfer. *Double Helix.* 2018;6:1–21.
7. Hobson H, Lerner N. Writing centers/WAC in pharmacy education: a changing prescription. In: Barnett RW, Blumner JS, Eds. *Writing Centers and Writing across the Curriculum Programs: Building Interdisciplinary Partnerships.* Greenwood Press; 1999.
8. Brady L, Singh-Corcoran N, Holsinger J. A change for the better: writing center/WID partnerships to support graduate writing. In: Lawrence S, Zawacki TM, eds. *Re/writing the center: Approaches to supporting graduate students in the writing center.* Utah State University Press; 2019.
9. Harrington S, Dinitz S, Benner R, et al. Turning stories from the writing center into useful knowledge: writing centers, WID programs, and partnerships for change. In: Myatt AJ, Gaillet LL, eds. *Writing Program and Writing Center Collaborations: Transcending Boundaries.* Palgrave Macmillan; 2017.
10. Wallman A, Vaudan C, Sporrong SK. Communications training in pharmacy education, 1995–2010. *Am J Pharm Educ.* 2013;77(2):1–9.
11. Urick BY, Meggs EV. Towards a greater professional standing: evolution of pharmacy practice and education, 1920–2020. *Pharmacy.* 2019;7(3):98.
12. Lebovitz L, Eddington ND. Trends in pharmacist workforce and pharmacy education. *Am J Pharm Educ.* 2019;83(1):4–11. doi:10.5688/ajpe7051.
13. Cipolle RJ, Strand LM, Morley PC. Chapter 10. Acquiring and applying the knowledge and clinical skills required to manage drug therapy. In: Cipolle RJ, Strand LM, Morley PC. eds. *Pharmaceutical Care Practice: The Patient-Centered Approach to Medication Management Services,* 3rd ed. New York, NY: McGraw-Hill; 2012.
14. Hobson EH, Waite NM, Briceland LL. Writing tasks performed by doctor of pharmacy students during clerkship rotations. *Am J Health-Syst Pharm.* 2002;59:58–62.

15. Mullin JA. Writing centers and WAC. In: McLeod S, Miraglia E, Soven M, Thaiss C. *WAC for the New Millennium: Strategies for Continuing Writing-across-the-Curriculum Programs.* WAC Clearinghouse; 2011.

16. Procter M. Talking the talk and walking the walk: establishing the academic role of writing centers. In: Starke-Meyerring D, Pare A, Aremeva N, Horne M, Yousoubova L. *Writing in Knowledge Societies.* WAC Clearinghouse; 2011.

17. Cheatle, J, Sheridan DM. Multimodal composing: Beyond the text. *WLN: A Journal of Writing Center Scholarship.* 2019;44(1–2):3–11.

18. Herrmann J. Divided communication: Oral and visual presentation in the writing center. *Praxis.* http://www.praxisuwc.com/praxis-blog/2019/6/27/divided-communication-oral-and-visual-presentation-in-the-writing-center?rq=presentation. Published July 2, 2019.

19. Boquet E, Kazer M, Manister N, et al. Just are: learning from and with graduate students in a doctor of nursing practice program. *Across Discipl.* 2015;12(3):1–14.

20. Center for student success. Albany College of Pharmacy and Health Sciences. https://www.acphs.edu/campuses/albany-campus/writing-center. Accessed 31 May 2020.

21. Norton writing center. *St. Louis College of Pharmacy.* https://www.stlcop.edu/campuslife/resources/norton-writing-center.html. Accessed 31 May 2020.

22. Lerner N. A history of WAC at a college of pharmacy. *Language Learning Across Disciplines.* 2001;5(1):6–19.

23. McGurr M. Writing centers, libraries, and medical and pharmacy schools. *J Med Lib Assoc.* 2020;108(1):84–88.

24. Autry MK, Carter M. Unblocking occluded genres in graduate writing: Thesis and dissertation support services at North Carolina State University. *Composition Forum.* 2015;31: http://compositionforum.com/issue/31/north-carolina-state.php.

25. Chronic diseases in America. National Center for Chronic Disease Prevention and Health Promotion. *Centers for Disease Control and Prevention.* https://www.cdc.gov/chronicdisease/resources/infographic/chronic-diseases.htm. Published October 2019.

26. Alvandi M. Telemedicine and its role in revolutionizing healthcare delivery. *Am J Accountable Care.* 2017;5(1):e1–e5.

27. King AE, Joseph AS, Umland EM. Student perceptions of the impact and value of incorporation of reflective writing across a pharmacy curriculum. *Curr Pharm Teach Learn.* 2017;9:770–778.

PART IV
Writing in Interprofessional Contexts

11

TEACHING CULTURALLY SENSITIVE CARE THROUGH REFLECTIVE WRITING

Cristina Reyes Smith

The United States is becoming increasingly diverse, and by 2045, it is anticipated that there will be no racial or ethnic majority.[1] In response, accrediting bodies for training in the health professions— including medicine,[2–4] dentistry,[5,6] nursing,[7,8] occupational therapy,[9,10] and physical therapy[11]— have assembled guides related to the topics of diversity, culture, and inclusion. However, the competencies identified in these guides may fall short of what local communities need from their care providers. Moreover, educators may struggle to prepare students for "culturally sensitive care" when courses are already full of foundational content. By one definition, it refers to "the ability to be appropriately responsive to the attitudes, feelings, or circumstances that share a common and distinct national, religious, linguistic, or cultural heritage."[12] Teaching culturally sensitive care can be a challenge for any educator.

As a start, I believe that training programs in the health professions can help students dive deeper into culturally sensitive care through elective courses, supplementing the required curricula. To provide one example, this chapter discusses an interprofessional elective course (IP 710) that I have taught at an academic health sciences center, highlighting an integral component of "writing in the health professions": reflective writing. (For additional models of reflective writing, see Chapters 7, 13, and 14.)

Background

To develop IP 710, we drew on several key areas of work: population health and cultural competence, interprofessional education, and Bloom's Revised Taxonomy.

Population Health and Cultural Competence

As a field of study, population health considers factors that make and keep individuals healthy outside of the health-care system, encourages health professionals to engage with local communities, and promotes collaboration between public health agencies, schools, businesses, and many others.[13] Those working in population health may run programs for individuals living with HIV/AIDS, analyze the outcomes of health insurance policies, study how the environment impacts activities of daily living, or advocate for positive changes in the health-care system, to suggest just a few ways.[14]

DOI: 10.4324/9781003162940-16

Population health has been repeatedly emphasized by international and national organizations, which have urged health professionals to more effectively address disparities related to race, ethnicity, geography, literacy, education, poverty, and other "social determinants of health." These organizations include the World Health Organization,[15,16] the Centers for Disease Control and Prevention,[17] the US Department of Health and Human Services,[18–20] the American Medical Association,[21] the American Hospital Association,[22] and the National Institutes of Health.[23] A milestone in these efforts has been the National Standards for Cultural and Linguistically Appropriate Services, or CLAS standards.[19,20] The CLAS standards (first proposed in 2000 and then updated in 2013) are designed to help health-care organizations provide effective, equitable, understandable, respectful, and quality care that, as the name suggests, is responsive to cultural and linguistic diversity (see Appendix 1). The Centers for Medicare and Medicaid Services has developed a tool kit to assist with implementation.[24]

Underlying the CLAS standards is the broader concept of cultural competence, which may be individual or organizational. Cross et al.[25] described cultural competence for organizations as a continuum from cultural destructiveness to cultural blindness, cultural awareness, cultural precompetence, and finally cultural proficiency. In explaining this framework, the researchers made several key points. First, health-care systems must incorporate cultural knowledge into how they do things. Second, to communicate well, health professionals must understand the client's concepts of health and family. Third, health professionals should have community contacts who can answer questions about culture. Fourth, health professionals must examine their own practices and find ways to improve, becoming more culturally competent.[25] While it may be impossible to become *completely* culturally competent, the framework has influenced health-care services, training, and additional frameworks over the years.

Marcelin et al.[26] recommended organizational and individual strategies to mitigate unconscious bias, a common barrier to cultural competence. Their strategies include diversity training that is meaningful, deliberation on personal biases, cultural humility and curiosity, and intentional experiences that bring exposure to greater diversity. These strategies lend themselves well to reflective writing, which as a form of reflection, can lead health professionals to greater thoughtfulness, precision, and opportunities for revelation and transformation, culturally or otherwise.

Interprofessional Education

The World Health Organization defines interprofessional education as occurring "when students from two or more professions learn about, from and with each other to enable effective collaboration and improve health outcomes,"[27(p7)] a theme in the introduction to this collection. Interprofessional education has been the subject of extensive study. In 2018, for instance, an integrative review of interprofessional education across the globe examined rural clinical learning environments in seven different countries. The results indicated that rural clinical learning environments provided meaningful experiences for students across the health professions: promoting students' respect for each other's roles and raising their awareness of how important it is to collaborate in delivering health care, especially in rural settings.[27]

Interprofessional courses described in the literature have included service-learning activities internationally[28–30] and in the United States. The latter have supplemented students' academic coursework by providing opportunities to serve vulnerable and underserved communities, such as those in palliative care[31] and those who are homeless.[32] These are only a couple examples from the large body of literature in this area. Yet, it seems clear that when courses are offered interprofessionally, students can benefit from interacting with students in other degree programs—particularly if some programs have more underrepresented students or more content on diversity, equity, and inclusion.

Bloom's Revised Taxonomy

You can think of Bloom's Taxonomy, mentioned in Chapters 9 and 12, as a pyramid: the bases are foundational skills in learning, such as remembering and understanding. Higher up are more sophisticated skills, such as applying, analyzing, evaluating, and at the very tip, creating.[33] Bloom's Revised Taxonomy conceptualizes transitioning students up the pyramid of learning from simple to more sophisticated integration of concepts—from remembering, understanding, applying, analyzing, evaluating, and then creating.[33] Krathwohl[34] described the development of three domains as originally categorized by Bloom and his committee: cognitive, psychomotor, and affective.

Cognitive learning relates to students transitioning from basic remembering to more complex levels of creating.[34] Psychomotor learning—or learning that involves "doing"—is addressed through practice and application through simulation and real-world scenarios such as students practicing motivational interviewing and counseling skills with patients with substance use disorders.[35] The affective domain provides a framework for values-based learning and has been utilized to introduce students to complex dimensions of professional roles related to beliefs and attitudes, facilitating critical thinking, adopting professional values, developing caring attitudes toward those served, and organizing values into their own personal philosophies.[36] The integration of cognitive, psychomotor, and affective domains of learning can lead to the best outcomes for positive interactions and quality care in future practice.[37]

The three types of learning are important for designing clinical experiences that promote culturally sensitive care. Students who have only cognitive knowledge of strategies, resources, and best practices may find themselves unable to apply what they know. Students who experience only cognitive and psychomotor learning may lack the empathy, emotional intelligence, and social awareness to successfully care for diverse and underserved communities. This limitation may be exacerbated when historic issues of mistrust, bias, or discrimination are present in the health-care organization or community. For example, 75% of people who took an implicit-association test demonstrated unconscious preference toward white race based on reaction times to words and pictures flashed in front of the participant.[26]

In assessments, therefore, instructors should consider all three types of learning, and in this regard, reflective writing can be very helpful, providing glimpses into what students have done, thought, and felt. But reflective writing can also enhance the learning experience for students, priming them for an interactive activity and increasing their depth of thought afterward, prompting them toward evaluating and creating. By creating space in our elective courses for reflective writing, we position students for optimal learning outcomes and success for all patients they may encounter.

Course and Program Development

IP 710: Cultural Sensitive Care had two forerunners at our academic health sciences center, which serves large numbers of rural residents in the US Southeast: a hybrid elective course for occupational therapy students (Cultural Caring: Service Delivery for Diverse and Under-Served Communities) and a fully online course for students in the bachelor of health-care studies programs (Culturally Sensitive Care). To further explore student perceptions, we conducted a survey in 2017.

The survey, focusing on occupational therapy students at the institution, revealed that 100% of the respondents (n = 20), as future practitioners, were interested in becoming more effective in cultural sensitivity. In addition, 67% of the respondents who did not take the hybrid elective course, mentioned earlier, reported that the primary constraint was time. Interestingly, many students who did not take the hybrid elective course strongly agreed that they were confident in their abilities to work with diverse and underserved groups, while only one student who took the course did. (This is consistent with a study by Halm, Evans, Wittenberg, and Wilgus,[38] which found that individuals may overestimate their cultural competence prior to training.) All but one respondent, who was neutral, reported that their personal experiences had positively impacted their perceived skills for working with diverse and underserved communities. Those who took the course agreed or strongly agreed that it had positively impacted their perceived skills for working with these communities.

Building on these findings, the first version of IP 710 was offered in 2018 as a 15-week lecture and discussion series that was open to students, faculty, and staff across colleges and programs. After a 20 to 30 minute lecture by a content expert, we divided participants into small groups for 15 to 20 minutes of discussion. All sessions were livestreamed, and close-captioned video recordings were provided on the center's training platform for ongoing use. Participants who completed all 15 weeks received a certificate of completion and were recognized at a reception with the center's leaders. There were over 75 participants in that first version of IP 710, including 19 students.

In the second and third years, the format was changed to a 2-day workshop, which was hybrid in 2019 and fully online in 2020 due to COVID-19. The workshop sessions featured subtopics that we addressed through the lens of the CLAS standards: addressing the opioid epidemic through interprofessional collaboration (2019) and interprofessional approaches to address mental health and well-being (2020). Students additionally participated in three class meetings: an overview, midterm, and wrap-up. During these meetings, I discussed the course schedule, assignments, and expectations, and students held small group discussions with guest speakers.

In the latest version of the elective (2020), the learning objectives were as follows:

1. Discuss interprofessional approaches to addressing mental health and well-being and the national CLAS standards as related to culturally sensitive care with individuals, communities, and populations.
2. Engage in clinical and/or community-based activities to apply strategies and further enhance learning about mental health and well-being.
3. Apply knowledge, skills, and awareness gained from course content and community-based experiences to develop a health education resource for a specific culturally diverse group.

Online modules with relevant videos, articles, and links to tools were posted to the course webpages. These included the following:

- Cultural Humility[39,40]: A lifelong commitment to self-evaluation and self-critique, acknowledging and addressing the power imbalances of the patient-physician dynamic, developing mutually beneficial and nonpaternalistic clinical practice and advocacy, and partnerships with communities on behalf of individuals and defined populations.
- Social Determinants of Health[41]: Environmental factors related to childbirth, living, learning, working, playing, worshiping, and age can impact health outcomes and risks related to daily function and quality of life.
- Unconscious/Implicit Bias[42]: Associations outside conscious awareness can lead to a negative evaluation of a person on the basis of irrelevant characteristics, such as race or gender.

Insights from Reflective Writing

Students engage with the course content largely through reflective writing (you can see some prompts we have used in the appendix). To guide students, we provide grading rubrics that include essential components listed in the assignment guidelines, including clear organization and content, as well as thoughtful analysis and critical thinking. These grading rubrics have helped students prepare reflective writings that both score well and generate deep and meaningful insights—sometimes drawing on their prior personal experiences. Students frequently share their reflections through written and verbal discussions before, during, and after the assignment, showing meaningful learning and growth.

Although students may choose to explore the literature as well, reflective writing assignments typically correspond to in-person learning; these activities have included client/caregiver interviews in in-patient hospitals, out-patient clinics, rural missions, senior centers, and community-based support groups. For many years, a primary activity was coordinated for the students. For example, one year, students attended a support group for Spanish-speaking families of children with disabilities and other special needs. This emerged from a long-standing partnership with a pediatric clinic, and a bilingual health worker was able to provide language and cultural interpretation between the English-speaking students and the attendees with limited English proficiency. One student wrote that the experience was a helpful reminder of how critical support systems are for clients, who may find encounters with the health-care system "new and scary," even if their provider has seen their child's condition many times before. The student also emphasized the importance of careful explanation and empathetic instruction.

In another coordinated experience, students received training from an academic hospital's patient and family education manager, who showed them how they might use an online video library that was created for educational purposes. The experience was tied to promoting pain management strategies to reduce patient discomfort and prevent opioid abuse for high-risk postsurgical patients. After receiving training, students could travel in pairs and interact bedside with in-patients at the hospital. Afterward, students were asked to complete a reflection of the experience, focusing on the cultural needs of the individuals they met and/or potential social determinants of health they could see in the interaction.

Some students chose to seek out experiences in the community or in their own clinical setting with culturally diverse individuals. The students wrote that the experiences opened their eyes to the challenges that many community members face due to language barriers, socioeconomic status, etc. One student wrote about an experience observing in a dental clinic where she discovered that what she had learned in her lecture class conflicted with the real-world choices faced by patients from a low socioeconomic background. The client selected tooth extraction and dentures for six teeth rather than paying for much more expensive crowns to save the teeth. She wrote that the learning experience provided an opportunity to "see first-hand" the impact of social determinants of health. She went on to provide ideas to increase health-care education, improve access to care in lower-income communities, and emphasize the importance of patient-centered care.

However, students were also given the option to coordinate their own experiences, provided they met the course guidelines. For example, students may volunteer in a pro bono clinic with culturally diverse clients numerous times, working to improve their communication skills, establish rapport, and make recommendations that are sensitive to social determinants of health and the needs of their clients. Some students chose to investigate the needs of rural and/or lesbian, gay, bisexual, transgender, queer/questioning, intersex, ally/asexual + (LGBTQIA+) individuals. One student who completed a pediatric rotation at a local children's hospital described an experience with an 18-year-old patient from a rural community. The patient struggled with both a congenital heart defect and chronic mental illness. In addition, the patient had recently come out as part of the LGBTQIA+ community. The student described how the patient had limited access to support systems due to his geography and the potential long-term adverse effects of minimal social interaction, limited physical activity, and poor nutrition. The student reflected that the patient, and others like him, needed continuous support from a "comprehensive and culturally sensitive healthcare team" to promote healthy growth and development.

In addition to these first-person encounters with clients, reflective writing assignments may require students to engage interprofessionally, learning from practitioners from other disciplines. For example, students can attend an interprofessional workshop panel, interview a health-care provider in a different discipline, or attend an interprofessional grand rounds. The reflection assignment cues the student to consider the roles of the health professionals involved, compare and contrast their own roles, and discern the variety of approaches needed to meet the needs of culturally diverse populations. Following a panel discussion held during a class meeting, a student wrote of the many challenges facing effective and efficient delivery of health care across professions. The student noted that, by listening to the panel, he had come to better understand how a trusting, healthy patient/provider relationship can "help eliminate bias" and "better address [the patient's] needs," including during national crises such as the opioid epidemic.

These examples illustrate how learning activities can help students transition from passive to active learning about culturally sensitive care, emphasizing new or common clinical experiences. Students may have engaged in these experiences multiple times. Even so, reflective writing before, during, or afterward can provide structure, support the learning competencies in the uppermost part of Bloom's pyramid, and provide critical feedback for their future practice.

Conclusion and Recommendations

While interprofessional courses may provide accessibility for students across a variety of academic years and schedules from multiple academic programs, it is important to provide flexibility, course requirements, and clear expectations for participation. It is also helpful to provide the schedule at the start of the semester so that students may plan accordingly and be set up for successful participation. Students may feel compelled to immerse themselves in a course elective related to this topic due to personal or professional goals. However, the demands of simultaneous core coursework may be challenging and will need to be prioritized. Students may be engaged in didactic and/or clinical coursework throughout the semester. Having all content provided asynchronously (including video recordings of any live content for students unable to attend) can provide continuity of the learning experiences, a structure to provide realistic student expectations, and an inclusive experience for all students.

Barriers to implementation may include limited time and resources for faculty to coordinate course activities. Many institutions may have limited expertise in this area. Establishing evidence-based knowledge and practice in this area may take substantial amounts of time. However, faculty members may enjoy learning alongside their students through interaction with community partners, collaboration with content experts locally and/or nationally, and from students' prior experiences and knowledge. An additional potential barrier is that cultural diversity is a vast and potentially infinite topic. This may feel overwhelming to educators. However, educators can prioritize content based on local communities being served and areas of desired growth (i.e., underserved, rural, global, etc.).

Underrepresented individuals are most likely to serve the diverse communities from which they came, and they may be able to provide valuable insights. Academic institutions that prioritize community needs can seek to develop faculty recruitment pipelines, recruit faculty from diverse backgrounds for potential leadership and expertise, and develop teams of collaborators to reduce burnout of underrepresented faculty working in this area. Programs can also engage current practitioners and clinicians to learn alongside students—leading to the potential development of faculty and student pipelines. Lastly, funding may be limited for interprofessional initiatives and coursework. Educational and/or community-based grants may be available to lay the groundwork for courses and programs that can be offered on an ongoing basis from year to year.

Ultimately, as the United States continues to grow more diverse and global connectivity becomes more commonplace (see also Chapter 3), it will become ever more important to train and prepare a generation of health-care practitioners who are competent and effective in-service delivery with culturally diverse clients across a spectrum of unique needs and characteristics. Future health professions education should continue to provide opportunities for culturally sensitive care both within the core curriculum and elective course offerings for students who wish to explore this topic further. Writing in the health professions can provide opportunities for engaging today's learners to promote culturally sensitive care, help learners advance to more complex levels of growth, and prepare students for careers across real-world communities both domestically and abroad. Engagement in writing can help health professions students progress to optimal learning and preparation for entering the workforce and improve outcomes in providing culturally sensitive care for all patients and communities they may encounter.

Appendix 1: CLAS Standards

Principal Standard

1. Provide effective, equitable, understandable, and respectful quality care and services that are responsive to diverse cultural health beliefs and practices, preferred languages, health literacy, and other communication needs.

Governance, Leadership, and Workforce

2. Advance and sustain organizational governance and leadership that promotes CLAS and health equity through policy, practices, and allocated resources.
3. Recruit, promote, and support a culturally and linguistically diverse governance, leadership, and workforce that are responsive to the population in the service area.
4. Educate and train governance, leadership, and workforce in culturally and linguistically appropriate policies and practices on an ongoing basis.

Communication and Language Assistance

5. Offer language assistance to individuals who have limited English proficiency and/or other communication needs, at no cost to them, to facilitate timely access to all health care and services.
6. Inform all individuals of the availability of language assistance services clearly and in their preferred language, verbally and in writing.
   "Ensure the competence of individuals providing language assistance, recognizing that the use of untrained individuals and/or minors as interpreters should be avoided."
7. Provide easy-to-understand print and multimedia materials and signage in the languages commonly used by the populations in the service area.

Engagement, Continuous Improvement, and Accountability

8. Establish culturally and linguistically appropriate goals, policies, and management accountability and infuse them throughout the organization's planning and operations.
9. Conduct ongoing assessments of the organization's CLAS-related activities and integrate CLAS-related measures into measurement and continuous quality improvement activities.

10. Collect and maintain accurate and reliable demographic data to monitor and evaluate the impact of CLAS on health equity and outcomes and to inform service delivery.

11. Conduct regular assessments of community health assets and needs and use the results to plan and implement services that respond to the cultural and linguistic diversity of populations in the service area.

12. Partner with the community to design, implement, and evaluate policies, practices, and services to ensure cultural and linguistic appropriateness.

13. Create conflict and grievance resolution processes that are culturally and linguistically appropriate to identify, prevent, and resolve conflicts or complaints.

14. Communicate the organization's progress in implementing and sustaining CLAS to all stakeholders, constituents, and the general public.

Appendix 2

Prompts we have used to guide students' reflective writing

Cultural Considerations Reflection: Review the literature related to the health-care needs of a chosen cultural group. Submit a brief reflection incorporating course concepts. For example, conduct a PubMed search about the health-care needs of clients from a religious minority group

Client/Caregiver Reflection: Participate in a client/caregiver interview or meeting to learn more about the needs of families from an underserved community. Submit a brief reflection within one week of experience. For example, attend a support group for Spanish-speaking families of children with special needs to learn about language and cultural barriers

Interprofessional Interview Reflection: Participate in an interprofessional interview or meeting to discuss needs. Submit a brief reflection within 1 week of the experience. For example, meet with health-care providers who provide services to homeless populations

Community-Based Health Education Presentation: Apply knowledge learned to conduct a community-based health education activity for an underserved community. Submit a brief reflection within one week of experience. For example, conduct a health education presentation for families of children in foster care.

Interprofessional Workshop Summary: Select an interprofessional panel session from the Mental Health and Well-Being Workshop. Submit a brief reflective summary related to the various roles of professionals and approaches to meeting client needs. Students might attend a session on technological approaches for access to care in rural communities

Health Education Resource: Work with a partner to review literature related to the health-care needs of a chosen cultural group. Create a health education resource for a targeted community by applying knowledge learned from the literature and course sessions. Post a 1- to 3-minute video on Harbor/Moodle demonstrating your health education resource. For example, create a one-page flyer for sexual and gender minorities about HIV prevention and awareness

Client Clinical Summary: Participate in a clinical session under the supervision of a clinician or interview a client who is at risk for mental health issues. Submit a brief reflective summary that considers cultural factors and social determinants of health that may impact client risk and outcomes. Students might participate in a clinical visit with postsurgical veterans who may be at risk for opioid dependence.

References

1. Vespa J, Medina L, Armstrong D. Demographic turning points for the United States: population projections for 2020 to 2060. Census.gov. https://www.census.gov/content/dam/Census/library/publications/2020/demo/p25-1144.pdf. Published February 2020.

2. Diversity and Inclusion. *Association of American Medical Colleges*; 2021. Accessed April 10, 2021. https://www.aamc.org/what-we-do/diversity-inclusion

3. Health Equity Research and Policy. Association of American Medical Colleges. https://www.aamc.org/what-we-do/mission-areas/medical-research/health-equity. Accessed April 14, 2021.

4. Teaching hospitals' commitment to addressing the social determinants of health. *Association of American Medical Colleges*. https://www.aamc.org/download/480618/data/aamc-teaching-hospitals-addressing-sdoh.pdf. Accessed April 10, 2021.

5. 2020-2025 diversity and inclusion plan: advancing inclusion while growing membership diversity. *American Dental Association*; 2019. Accessed April 20, 2021. https://www.ada.org/~/media/ADA/About%20the%20ADA/Files/ADA_Diversity_Inclusion_Plan.pdf?la=en

6. Feinberg M. Minority oral health in America: despite progress, disparities persist. *2015 Kelley report: health disparities in America*. 2015. http://www.ada.org/~/media/ADA/Advocacy/Files/160523_Kelly_Report_Dental_Chapter.pdf https://www.ada.org/~/media/ADA/About%20the%20ADA/Files/ADA_Diversity_Inclusion_Plan.pdf?la=en

7. Cultural competency in nursing education. *American Association of Colleges of Nursing*. https://www.aacnnursing.org/Education-Resources/Tool-Kits/Cultural-Competency-in-Nursing-Education. Accessed April 10, 2021.

8. Diversity, equity, and inclusion in academic nursing. *American Association of Colleges of Nursing*; March 20, 2017. https://www.aacnnursing.org/Portals/42/News/Position-Statements/Diversity-Inclusion.pdf. Accessed April 10, 2021.

9. Hansen RH, Hinojosa J. Occupational therapy's commitment to nondiscrimination and inclusion (edited 2004). *Am J Occup Ther*. 2004;58(6):668.

10. Hildebrand K, Lewis LJ, Pizur-Barnekow K, Schefkind S, Stankey R, Stoffel A, Wilson LS. Frequently asked questions: how can occupational therapy strive towards culturally sensitive practices. The American Occupational Therapy Association; 2013. https://miota.org/docs/FAQCulturalSensitivity.pdf

11. Commission on Accreditation in Physical Therapy Education. Position papers: accreditation handbook; November 2015. https://www.capteonline.org/globalassets/capte-docs/capte-position-papers.pdf. Accessed April 10, 2021.

12. Office of Minority Health. 2001. *National Standards for Culturally and Linguistically Appropriate Services in Health Care*. Washington, DC: US Department of Health and Human Services.

13. Institute of Medicine. 2014. *Population Health Implications of the Affordable Care Act: Workshop Summary*. Washington, DC: The National Academies Press. https://www.nap.edu/read/18546/chapter/1#ii

14. Braveman B. Health policy perspectives—population health and occupational therapy. *Am J Occup Ther*. 2015;70(1). doi:10.5014/ajot.2016.701002

15. Gender, equity, and human rights: Social determinants of health. *World Health Organization*. https://www.who.int/gender-equity-rights/understanding/sdh-definition/en/. Published 2021.

16. Health inequities and their causes. *World Health Organization*. https://www.who.int/news-room/facts-in-pictures/detail/health-inequities-and-their-causes.

17. Health Equity—Office of Minority Health and Health Equity—CDC. *Centers for Disease Control and Prevention*. https://www.cdc.gov/healthequity/index.html. Published March 11, 2021.

18. Social Determinants of Health. US Department of Health and Human Services Office of Disease Prevention and Health Promotion. https://health.gov/healthypeople/objectives-and-data/social-determinants-health.

19. National Standards for Culturally and Linguistically Appropriate Services in Health Care: Executive Summary. US Department of Health and Human Services Office of Minority Health. https://minorityhealth.hhs.gov/assets/pdf/checked/executive.pdf. Published March 2001.

20. National Standards for Culturally and Linguistically Appropriate Services in Health and Health Care: A Blueprint for Advancing and Sustaining CLAS Policy and Practice. US Department of Health and Human Services Office of Minority Health. https://thinkculturalhealth.hhs.gov/assets/pdfs/EnhancedCLASStandardsBlueprint.pdf. Published April 2013.

21. Reducing disparities in health care. *American Medical Association*. https://www.ama-assn.org/delivering-care/patient-support-advocacy/reducing-disparities-health-care.

22. Eliminating health care disparities: implementing the national call to action using lessons learned: AHA. *American Hospital Association*. https://www.aha.org/ahahret-guides/2012-02-01-eliminating-health-care-disparities-implementing-national-call-action.

23. Health disparities and inequities. *National Institutes of Health*. https://www.nhlbi.nih.gov/science/health-disparities-and-inequities#:~:text=Differences%20in%20health%20among%20population,%2C%20blood%2C%20and%20sleep%20disorders.

24. A practical guide to implementing the National CLAS Standards: for racial, ethnic and linguistic minorities, people with disabilities and sexual and gender minorities. *U.S. Centers for Medicare & Medicaid Services*. https://www.cms.gov/About-CMS/Agency-Information/OMH/Downloads/CLAS-Toolkit-12-7-16.pdf. Published December 2016.

25. Cross TL, Bazron BJ, Dennis KW, Isaacs MR. Towards a culturally competent system of care: a monograph on effective services for minority children who are severely emotionally disturbed. *ERIC*. https://files.eric.ed.gov/fulltext/ED330171.pdf. Published February 28, 1989. Accessed April 6, 2021.

26. Marcelin JR, Siraj DS, Victor R, Kotadia S, Maldonado YA. The impact of unconscious bias in healthcare: how to recognize and mitigate it. *J Infect Dis*. 2019;220(220 Suppl 2):S62–S73. doi:10.1093/infdis/jiz214

27. Framework for action on interprofessional education and collaborative practice. *World Health Organization*. https://www.who.int/hrh/resources/framework_action/en/. Published December 21, 2015.

28. Johnson AM, Howell DM. International service learning and interprofessional education in Ecuador: findings from a phenomenology study with students from four professions. *J Interprof Care*. 2017;31(2):245–254. doi:10.1080/13561820.2016.1262337

29. Velez R, Koo LW. International service learning enhances nurse practitioner students' practice and cultural humility. *J Am Acad Nurse Pract*. 2020;32(3):187–189. doi:10.1097/jxx.0000000000000404

30. Coffin D, Collins M, Waldman-Levi A. Fostering inter-professional education through service learning: the Belize experience. *Occup Ther Health Care*. 2021 19;1–11. doi:10.1080/07380577.2021.1877862

31. Boucher NA. Direct engagement with communities and interprofessional learning to factor culture into end-of-life health care delivery. *Am J Public Health*. 2016;106(6):996–1001. doi:10.2105/ajph.2016.303073

32. Pierangeli LT, Lenhart CM. Service-learning: promoting empathy through the point-in-time count of homeless populations. *J Nurs Educ*. 2018;57(7):436–439. doi:10.3928/01484834-20180618-10

33. Armstrong P. Bloom's taxonomy. Vanderbilt University Center for Teaching. 2016 May. https://programs.caringsafely.org/wp-content/uploads/2019/05/Caring-Safely-Professional-Program-Course-Development.pdf. Accessed April 10, 2021.

34. Brown LP. Revisiting our roots: Caring in nursing curriculum design. *Nurse Educ Pract*. 2011;11(6):360–364. doi:10.1016/j.nepr.2011.03.007

35. Hanson J. From me to we: Transforming values and building professional community through narratives. *Nurse Educ Pract*. 2013;13(2):142–146. doi:10.1016/j.nepr.2012.08.007

36. Krathwohl DR. A revision of Bloom's taxonomy: an overview. *Theory Practice*. 2002;41(4):212–218. doi:10.1207/s15430421tip4104_2

37. Muzyk AJ, Tew C, Thomas-Fannin A, et al. Utilizing Bloom's taxonomy to design a substance use disorders course for health professions students. *Subst Abus*. 2018;39(3):348–353. doi:10.1080/08897077.2018.1436634

38. Seaman, M. (2011). Bloom's taxonomy: Its evolution, revision, and use in the field of education. *Curric. Teach. Dialogue*, 13: 29.

39. Halm MA, Evans R, Wittenberg A, Wilgus E. Broadening cultural sensitivity at the end of life: an interprofessional education program incorporating critical reflection. *Holist Nurs Pract*. 2012;26(6):335–349.

40. Tervalon M, Murray-Garcia J. Cultural humility versus cultural competence: a critical distinction in defining physician training outcomes in multicultural education. *J Health Care Poor Underserved*. 1998;9(2):117–125.

41. US Department of Health and Human Services, Office of Disease Prevention and Health Promotion. Social determinants of health; 2018. https://health.gov/healthypeople/objectives-and-data/social-determinants-health

42. FitzGerald C, Hurst S. Implicit bias in healthcare professionals: a systematic review. *BMC Medical Ethics*. 2017;18(1). doi:10.1186/s12910-017-0179-8

12

COMMUNICATING "PATIENT-CENTERED CARE"

A Case Study for Collaborative Writing in the Health Professions

Susan E. Thomas

What does it mean to build a health-care organization from the ground up? What kinds of writing and communication, what discursive and rhetorical forms, what material and symbolic practices are significant as professionals come together to realize an alternative vision of a health-care environment? These were the questions posed to Dr. Anne Surma and me by the executive of the Chris O'Brien Lifehouse, an integrative cancer treatment center in Sydney, Australia. From the center's inception in 2009, we had followed its development with great professional interest, but in 2012, this relationship became more formal, as we were invited to join the research team and contribute to the task of theorizing, analyzing, interpreting, and ultimately writing the center's "story," as it unfolded—a story that was becoming as much about communication as medical innovation. For three years, we followed Lifehouse's development through four distinct phases, discussed later, interviewing executive, clinical, and administrative staff through critical transitions in the organization's history and documenting our findings. While both Dr. Surma and I have spent our careers as scholars of writing and communication and independent consultants, this was our first experience of observing firsthand as researchers the ground-up development of an integrative, world-class health-care organization and the constitutive role of writing and communication within it. As our own views of writing in the health professions were challenged, expanded, and transformed by our collaboration with Lifehouse, we became increasingly convinced that students exposed to the Lifehouse story would have a similar experience.

Like Opel and Hart-Davidson,[1] I argue for the primary care clinic as a writing space, drawing on shared findings from the Lifehouse project, used here with Dr. Surma's permission. Our study presents diverse perspectives of professionals participating in the initiative. Here, I draw on their insights to capture the challenges of realizing an alternative hospital model and the significance of these challenges as a model for understanding writing in the health professions, including in interprofessional contexts. (See Chapter 8 for another perspective on workplace research in the health professions.)

Case studies are particularly beneficial for teaching writing in the health professions, as they draw on actual scenarios to demonstrate some of the common challenges and consequences of writing and communicating in clinical contexts. They allow students to consider diverse, often conflicting, perspectives by putting themselves in the positions of affected staff members and discovering through these lenses the importance of recognizing the primary care clinic as a writing space.

DOI: 10.4324/9781003162940-17

Case-based learning (CBL) has long been used in medical, law, and business schools and has more recently gained popularity within undergraduate education, especially STEM disciplines.[2] CBL involves guided inquiry and is grounded in cognitive and social constructivism, enabling students to create new meaning by interacting with their existing knowledge and the situation being presented.[3] Implementing CBL in the classroom yields a number of benefits. Williams[4] maintains that CBL utilizes collaborative learning, facilitates the integration of learning, develops students' intrinsic and extrinsic motivation to learn, encourages self-reflection and critical reflection, allows for scientific inquiry, integrates knowledge and practice, and supports the development of a variety of learning skills. Versatility, creativity, and self-guided learning are inherent in CBL.[5] The stories encompassed in a case study framework contribute directly to CBL's success.

Jonassen and Hernandez-Serrano[6] explain that storytelling is a method of negotiating and renegotiating meanings that allows us to enter into other's realities through their stories, a theme in the next chapters. This helps students find their place in a culture by encouraging them to explain, interpret, and attain vicarious experience, and ultimately distinguish between positive and negative models of practice. Storytelling, which sees the story as the product of the inquiry and invites the reader into the story to engage at both emotional and rational levels with the narrator's experience,[7] is particularly pertinent as a method of empowerment. The researcher-as-storyteller understands the story itself as containing analytical techniques, theory, and dialogical structures[8,9] which can speak for themselves:

> In a narrative analysis, storytellers emphasize that participants' stories of the self are told for the sake of others just as much as for themselves. Hence, the ethical and heartfelt claim is for a dialogic relationship with a listener…that requires engagement from within, not analysis from outside, the story and narrative identity. Consequently, the goal and responsibility are to evoke and bear witness to a situation … inviting the reader into a relationship, enticing people to think and feel *with* the story being told as opposed to thinking *about* it.[10(p185)]

Thistlethwaite et al.[5] identify several benefits of using CBL in health professions education, including student engagement and learning enhancement. Other studies[11–14] have demonstrated the role of CBL in attaining desired learning outcomes. Their findings suggest that CBL can be useful for cultivating a participatory and experiential learning environment that assists students in analyzing and evaluating information to create meaning, thereby reflecting the top three goals of Bloom's Revised Taxonomy of educational objectives.[15] (Chapter 11 addresses Bloom's Revised Taxonomy in greater detail.).

Lifehouse Case Study Background

In the late 1990s, the Sydney Cancer Center Board and clinicians committed to setting up a comprehensive cancer treatment center at the Royal Prince Alfred Hospital, the largest in Sydney. In 2006, Professor Chris O'Brien, a consultant head and neck surgeon, and his colleague Professor Michael Boyer presented a report to the local health authority recommending the establishment of an integrated cancer center. Soon afterward, O'Brien was diagnosed with an aggressive brain tumor. His own cancer treatment motivated him to secure the monetary, political, and community support to build the center he and his colleagues had proposed. Believing that cancer-related services and treatment were fragmented and ill-suited to addressing the complex medical, social, and emotional needs of individual patients and their families, O'Brien and Boyer's aim was to amalgamate cancer treatment and research activity to provide patients with comprehensive clinical care, emotional support, and complementary therapies within a single facility.

Central to the philosophy behind the center's development and commitment to holistic practice was the building's design. The nine-story glass, aluminum, and terracotta-tiled structure is an architectural landmark built around a central atrium, allowing natural light to pour through and exposing the interconnectedness between the clinical, research, integrative, and public areas of the facility. Inside, the building's public spaces are inviting and spacious, with several of them communal—a large café, a lounge arranged around the atrium, and the Living Room, a space dedicated to counseling services, complementary therapies (such as acupuncture, massage, exercise classes, and yoga), and education for patients, carers, and families. The project, funded by state and federal governments and corporate and community fundraising, was several years in the making, and the purpose-built, nonprofit cancer center was opened to ambulatory patients in November 2013. A year later, day surgery facilities were opened. In March 2015, 96 in-patient rooms, eight operating rooms, and an intensive care unit were also opened. From a staff of 120 in mid-2013, the center has grown to over 600 staff.

Lifehouse values were publicly articulated as follows:

Our people experience a culture that is underpinned by our values. Just as we strive to create a place of sanctuary for our patients, we aim to create an environment that actively involves and inspires our people. Our values drive our culture, represent what we stand for and guide how we take action and make decisions.

Collaboration—Working together driving excellence

Respect—Honoring dignity, embracing diversity

Empowerment—Enabling independence and confidence

Nurture—Cultivating compassionate support

Discovery—Innovative research, inspiring hope

These values resonate with what Alvesson and Thompson[16(p487)] describe as "the paradigm of the post-bureaucratic organization"—that is, one that "operates on the basis of horizontal and vertical networking, and mutual adjustment, and…guided by visions and shared values rather than command and control." However, our study found a disconnect between the published descriptions of Lifehouse's values and mission and the experiences of individuals and groups working across different professional domains within the facility. We were primarily interested in the challenges involved in devising and articulating "new" approaches to "patient-centered" cancer treatment and introducing a more holistic care model. Our study investigated how such tensions sustain the complex human, social, and ethical underpinnings of communication and mitigate the effects of instrumentalist approaches to working in a contemporary hospital environment. This investigation also has considerable pedagogical value, as practical, in-depth studies of how writing in various genres is operationalized in real-world settings have much to offer students.

Writing as a Socially and Professionally Productive Practice

A number of scholars argue that not only is communication constitutive but also it is constitutive of an organization.[17–20] In other words, for human subjects, the activity of communicating is a meaning-making process, a significant activity through which we build, reinforce, adapt, or change our social worlds and our relationships with others. Central to this position is that in communicating, we enact a fundamental dimension of what it is to be human. As Robyn Penman[21] points out, drawing on Martin Heidegger's position that we are situated interpreters[22] and on John Stewart's that "the person is irreducibly relational not individual, social not psychological,"[23(p27)] it is the relational process of communicating that ensures a collaborative and creative process of constructing the world we inhabit. However, this process is not without its conflicts, dissonances, and setbacks, as our interviews with Lifehouse staff demonstrate.

Research and practice in the health professions, both in Australia and internationally, have found that an integrated, patient-centered approach results in better quality care and improved outcomes for patients, staff, the health-care system, and the community at large.[24–26] Communication is pivotal to the success of this approach,[27–29] as is the participation of patients in the design of the communication processes and practices informing their cancer journey.[30,31] But how do health-care professionals themselves perceive their and others' roles as writers and communicators in building an organization oriented to patient-centered care, and in carrying out their professional responsibilities? We aimed to capture staff insights into how communication is articulated and understood in actively developing an innovative comprehensive cancer care environment, how staff members make sense of the relationship between their communicative activities and patient-centeredness, and how staff reflect on and evaluate their own and others' communication practices at the new center. Above all, we aimed to understand how all of these things eventually come to bear on writing in the health professions.

The center's executive gave us full access to any staff members willing and available for interview. The first participants were members of the executive, and from those initial interviews, we relied on snowball sampling to extend our interview participant base. Our study comprises 31 semistructured interviews with staff (executive, clinical, integrated medicine, and administrative), carried out in four phases and informed by a review of publicly available material, various reports, and internal documents (including completed staff questionnaires) supplied to us by Lifehouse.

The Interviews

The first phase of interviews was carried out in October 2013, just before the facility was opened; the second in January and February 2014, post-opening; the third in July and August 2014; and the fourth in February 2015, just before the opening of in-patient facilities. We phased the interviews this way to accommodate the time constraints of staff and to capture participants' snapshot perspectives at specific moments in the organization's early operational history.

Interviews lasted between 45 minutes and an hour and were audio-recorded and professionally transcribed. We asked participants for their insights into their professional roles, their perspectives on their work as employees of the cancer center, and their ideas about the current and future state of the organization. We framed all discussions by a focus on communication-related activities, which was maintained in our analysis of the interview material. In evaluating the interview transcripts, we took a critical and interpretive stance, reading and rereading them closely and analyzing them according to key ideas that emerged across interviews and within and between interview phases. As we interpreted the data, we also noted patterns, resonances, and conflicts with other organizational texts. As patterns and themes emerged, we looked to relevant existing literature to reread our findings in light of secondary material, making inferences and drawing conclusions.

Interviews with members of the executive revealed a palpable sense of stress, nervousness, excitement, and trepidation about the imminent launch of the facility but also a collectively confident and imaginative sense of the organization's purpose and distinguishing features. More than one member drew on the center's key promotional literature (composed by the executive) to talk about how the new facility was to be dedicated to delivering "uncompromising care" through offering a comprehensive and integrated range of services organized around patient needs and preferences.

They also referred to the "empowerment" of the patient in relation to their treatment and care and to the "collaborative" approach to building the organization.

However, one participant drew attention to the unknowability, uncontrollability, and "ambiguity" of what the unfolding organization would *do* and *become*, as the project transformed from a concept into an operational facility. Here, we see how the material and symbolic worlds are intertwined in the process of building, envisioning, and imagining the emerging organization: "What is treated as material is constitutively entangled with, and never ontologically distinct from, the symbolic."[32] This observation is particularly significant when considering writing in the health professions, which is almost always collaborative.

A clinical member of the executive team reflected on the importance (and challenge) of communicating the facility's vision to prospective staff:

> Is this just a shiny building, or is there something more important behind it than the shiny building? And the answer is of course, yes, there's something much more important than a shiny building.... That [communication] is often also to clinical teams, because I think that we will have failed in this project if all we succeed in doing is a really fancy removal job from an old building into a new building. That will be a complete failure. It will have cost us...whatever million dollars in order to move some people across the road. And that's dumb. So getting across what's special, what do we want to do differently is another really big communication task. And that's much harder than the technical stuff, because it's a mix of communication, and actually getting people to buy into a vision and buy into a way of doing things.

In contrast to the overall cohesiveness of the center's vision and ethos reported in interviews with the executive, the comparatively diverse set of participants interviewed in the second phase of the study shed light on a perceived lack of leadership due to the gap between the departure of the inaugural CEO and the arrival of a new CEO, and staff perceptions of a relatively disconnected and isolated executive team. Comments such as "we've been a bit of a headless organization for quite some time," and "you kind of wouldn't mind knowing what [the executive team's] plans are," as well as "not all staff in leadership roles support the [center's] vision," further suggests a disconnect between the executive team and the rest of the organization. For some, there was a strong sense that communication had become "siloed" as Lifehouse transformed into an operational facility. A member of the administrative team commented,

> Well, I think it's pretty siloed. I mean...when we were all on one floor it was much easier to grab people...there was a lot of team-building stuff that was done before....You can't spend all day rah-rah-ing but we have to really be careful we don't lose that because you can see people starting to blame others for things that are going on.

"Rah-rah-ing" seems shorthand for the numerous structured team-building activities, formal and informal conversations, and negotiations involved in developing a cohesive workforce, which preceded the facility's opening (but only involved a relatively small number of the center's now large staff). With the center becoming a working hospital, and with the number of staff and the size of organizational units growing exponentially, siloing manifests itself in a perceived distance between the executive and other staff. In another participant's view, "It's a bit of a mystery...the communication between the levels doesn't really happen very freely.... I think at each level people are communicating well but the communication between [levels], no." It seems that the operational demands of running a rapidly expanding hospital weaken the impetus to overturn traditional hierarchies and strengthen flexible staff-led, context-sensitive work practices. This, in turn, has had an impact on how—or how well—staff members communicate with one another across all levels of the organization.

Four months into the center's opening, these more dispersed, decentered processes of communicating were also having an impact on the development of the center's vision, according to one participant:

> Hopefully, I think in the future we'll have much more targeted meetings…where we get better…information on the strategic direction of the organization. I think most of us are in the dark about some of the things that are going on around the place right now.

And in the view of another participant,

> I don't think we have a kind of a really decided version of how we want to be different and what we stand for. I know there are values floating around and stuff, but they don't particularly speak to me.

These participants' comments indicated their sense of a lack of orientation or anchoring in how the organization is being represented in writing and how that representation strikes a chord with their own professional concerns.

According to several interviewed staff members, the opening of the center, with all the pressure to treat patients, integrate new teams, adopt new information technology (IT) systems, and adapt to changes in the executive team, the broader aims of the center had been sidelined. For example, one interview participant, a clinician and member of the executive, commented "there's still a significant disconnect between operations—between the coalface, between the happiness of the workforce—and the organization's vision."

In considering the ways values might be integrated into practice rather than merely "floating around" in promotional literature, it became clear that communicating the culture of an organization cannot be achieved by circulating a written set of slogans or center-specific information through online staff training modules. This can result, observed one person, in "a loss of culture and cultural awareness." Rather, such communication should be *embedded in* ongoing professional practice and direct interaction with staff about what concerns them. The interview participant who commented on the happiness of the workforce noted, for example, that written definitions of "engagement" are far less useful than "talk[ing] *to people* about what *their* issues are and what *their* problems are…and us[ing] that as a strategy to engage [them]" (italics added). Here, through a lexical and syntactical recasting of the practice of communicating, this participant explains eloquently and succinctly the resistance of clinical staff to managerial writing that ignores staff members' specific professional concerns in situated contexts and obscures the ethical dimensions of staff relationships within the facility.

Tensions Surrounding "Patient-Centered Care"

Perhaps the most contentious aspect of the center's start-up was the use of the term "patient-centered care," so closely associated with the cancer center's ethos and explicit commitment to its patients. Much of the impetus in setting up the facility had been to develop an alternative "infrastructure," as initially represented on the center's website:

> Everything we do at [the center] has its foundation in and is designed around the concept of "patient-centered care" The voice of the patient has been at the heart of the design and

development of [the center]. This starts from the way we greet and speak to patients and our respect for different cultures. It extends to our hospital executive, the development of information technology and patient information, the layout and design of the building, the close collaboration between clinicians and members of our patients' care teams and our commitment to clinical trials.

But for some participants, the focus on "patient-centered care" as a new approach implied that staff, many with considerable experience in the health-care sector, did not practice patient-centered approaches in their previous positions. This clearly antagonized certain individuals: as one clinical staff member remarked, "We're always patient centered…we've always been patient-centered"; while another observed, "It's what we've always tried to do." Nonetheless, in the view of some participants, the practices of certain staff did not have the patient as the primary focus: "We've inherited people [who] have very strong opinions about the way things are done and they're not necessarily prepared to go the extra distance for the patient, which is really disappointing." In addition, several participants in administrative roles identified the traditional hospital hierarchy, where, according to one participant, "everyone bows to the doctors," as inhibiting the whole-of-organization shift to a patient-centered approach. Another highlighted the problem, particularly in relation to some doctors' mode of "behav[ing] and communicating the same way" as they did before joining the center, as showing a lack of respect for others, particularly nonclinical staff.

Harnessing the term as shorthand for the different, intersecting, and sometimes contradictory ways the center's model is imagined as unique provoked resentment, as well as extended discussion about how the term is relevant to the ways individual professionals focus on patients. Less frequently articulated, however, were the complex relational connections between clinical and nonclinical staff, between the hospital executive and staff, between administrative and other professional roles, and, importantly, between infrastructural (IT and other) systems, tools, and spaces and the relative strength of those connections in improving the capacity to deliver patient-centered care. "Patient-centered care" is not just the quality or the commitment devoted to the one-on-one relationship between clinician and patient but also the intricate network of relationships between patient and the range of professionals she or he encounters during her or his cancer journey. A clinical member of the executive commented that patient-centered care in the mainstream health-care setting is not happening because "the physical infrastructures or the human resource infrastructure doesn't let it happen." Another participant commented,

> So while individual clinicians in the existing system will provide great care, the overall patient experience may not be great and we need to explain that to potential employees. And that is, yes you provide great care today, and we really want you to continue to do that, but we need to ensure that you understand that when patients move to another department that you're working with them, or with the other department to share information, and you're working with new systems and procedures to ensure that there's a very seamless flow of information.

The objectives to reduce layers of bureaucracy, to transform the conventional hospital structure that currently serves, according to one staff member, "neither the patients nor clinicians…well"; to provide an integrated approach to holistic cancer care in a single facility; and to demonstrate how patient-centeredness is an active and iterative process—and "is every interaction that a patient has, whether it's finance, billing, admin, clinical, whatever"—seem to have been lost in the deployment of "patient-centered care" as a catch-all slogan. Nevertheless, despite early setbacks, the very *process* of staff grappling with these tensions and complexities, identifying conflicts, and working toward resolution is precisely what has shaped the cancer center as an organization constituted by communication.

Discussion

Two key issues emerge in the interviews that are directly relevant to teaching writing in the health professions. First, negotiation over contested versions of "patient-centered care" will likely be compromised when both the patient and the professional are perceived solely as atomistic individuals, rather than as complex relational beings whose experiences and responsibilities are understood as interdependent with other individuals and teams, as well as other systems and contexts. These individual complexities must be considered in any collaborative writing situation where multiple personalities and viewpoints converge.

Second, in this complex organization, the many (often competing) discourses representing its myriad dimensions as a hospital seem to jostle for primacy. However, instead of prioritizing one discourse over another—i.e., concluding that the economic dominates the social, or the managerial trumps the clinical, a space for critical reflection needs to be created, where the tensions and contradictions between discourses and their contexts are explicitly and carefully debated and negotiated by staff and patients. How do we balance, combine, or disentangle our individual, professional, social, and organizational interests and obligations in response to specific others, situations, and practices? In their diverse commentary quoted earlier, interview participants highlight the communicative and rhetorical challenges involved in doing so. These human connections, rather than empty slogans, are what define, contextualize, challenge, modify, and make purposeful the primary care clinic as a writing space.

Case Study Development

Using the anonymized staff interviews described previously, I have developed a case study group assignment for my graduate-level WRIT6000 Professional Writing class, which attracts students from the health professions. Assigning pseudonyms to Lifehouse and its employees, I have devised a series of staff profiles based on interview data to help students assume these personas in order to consider more carefully the importance of inclusive, purposeful, ethical writing and communication within a health-care setting. Students are asked to focus particularly on how the term "patient-centered care" is used in a range of publicly available organizational documents, including websites, informational literature, press releases, surveys, and advertising material. Students are asked to form small groups, with each group member assuming the persona of one of the following: a hospital staff member, an external stakeholder, a patient, or a patient's family member, with each group containing as many different personas as possible. Groups are then asked to choose an organizational document from those provided, with each member analyzing it from the perspective of their persona and evaluating it for clarity, logic, inclusiveness, and ethics. Students are also asked to anticipate the potential of the document to generate a range of responses (understanding, agreement, confusion, misunderstanding, etc.) among hospital staff members, depending on their roles and perspectives.

Once the groups have drawn their own conclusions about the issues surrounding the term "patient-centered care," they are presented with anonymized staff comments from the Lifehouse interviews to determine how their impressions compare with those of actual staff members. Students then revise their chosen document for improved clarity, inclusiveness, and ethical considerations, considering issues around sole authorship versus collaborative authorship, audience awareness and analysis, focus groups and feedback, and usability testing. Along with the revised documents, each group completes a post-assessment memo, addressed to me, outlining the problems they identified, the approach they took in revising the document, and their rationale for each change made.

According to comments on student satisfaction surveys, students in health professions have responded to the case study in the following ways:

- They begin to recognize the primary care clinic as a writing space.
- They learn that the most effective writing is collaborative and inclusive, with multiple authors and perspectives and carefully implemented processes of feedback and usability testing.
- They learn that writing in the health professions has consequences—particularly in relation to staff morale and job satisfaction.
- They learn the value of problem-based learning. Rather than merely reading textbooks and writing about hypotheticals, students put themselves in the positions of actual health professionals and grapple with real problems that demand creative solutions.
- They learn the value of teamwork and developing empathy for others' perspectives.
- They learn that even the best intentions in writing can result in texts that are offensive, inflammatory, or confusing.
- They learn that different audiences will bring a diversity of experiences, cultural backgrounds, and social conditioning to their reading of documents—and that a range of responses should be anticipated and respected.

Faculty teaching writing in the health professions benefit from using the case study in the following ways:

- They are better able to demonstrate the theoretical and practical considerations of writing in the health professions by immersing students in a real-world context that transcends the limits of course readings and more traditional assignments.
- They are better able to gauge students' ability to apply what they have learned by observing their approaches to "solving" the case study.
- They are able to bring research and teaching together in a meaningful context that benefits both students and research partners and demonstrates the power of research-led teaching to strengthen students' learning experiences.

Student feedback on the case study has been positive, with 85% of students in the 2019 Professional Writing cohort indicating on course satisfaction surveys that the case study was their favorite aspect of the Professional Writing class. Some commented that skills learned through the project had also helped them "reason through" other assignments—and prepare better for assignments in other classes—largely by discussing objectives with peers and "workshopping" drafts together. Other students commented that they had dreaded collaborative work due to negative past experiences, but the case study had "changed their mind" due to its practical grounding in an actual context with clear objectives—rather than "more arbitrary" approaches to group work that "often feel like little more than busy work." One student wrote that the case study allowed them to "stand in someone else's shoes" and learn from their mistakes and insights without having to make the same mistakes on the job.

Implications for Practice

While building effective case studies for teaching can be time-consuming, the outcomes will usually justify the effort. Since most institutions of higher learning around the world are now encouraging research-led teaching, community engagement, and experiential, participatory learning, case studies provide an effective means of achieving all of these in the classroom.

Writing Case Studies

A logical first step for identifying a possible case study is considering how your research is incorporated in the curriculum and reading materials for your course(s). It is also a good idea to consider the benefits for the research partner (if there is one), as well as the university. As my case study demonstrates, collaborating with a community organization that is also a research partner makes sense for the benefit of both and can make the case study easier to incorporate into the course curriculum.

If such a partner is not available, there are open resources and databases containing public cases that instructors can download and make accessible in the classroom. These include the National Center for Case Study Teaching in Science,[33] a database featuring hundreds of accessible STEM- and social science–based case studies, and the Johns Hopkins Medical Center.[34]

If open access cases do not appeal or are irrelevant to their subject matter, instructors might opt to write their own. There are several resources instructors might consider, including the helpful guidelines under the "how-to" tab on the Canadian National Center for Biotechnology's website.[35]

Introducing Case Studies in the Classroom

While I am aware of entire courses (especially in the health professions) based on case studies, instructors new to case studies may be best served by implementing them gradually on a smaller scale, perhaps including a single case in their curriculum and building on it at their desired pace, ideally in response to student feedback. It might also make sense for those new to teaching with case studies to introduce them in small classes—perhaps graduate-level courses—to gauge student responses and also to fine-tune based on usability testing. Case studies create a classroom learning environment distinctly different from the traditional teacher-centric setting, with a "buzz" emanating from increased conversation, collaboration, and even laughter. Unconventional seating arrangements and creative timetabling may also be necessary to achieve a case study–friendly environment; therefore, smaller classes will make it easier for instructors to pilot case studies and adapt them gradually within a course framework.

While case studies can be assigned as individual assignments, they present an excellent opportunity for encouraging collaborative problem solving and exposing students to diverse teams and a variety of perspectives that can help them solve the case, in harmony with the tenets of inter-professional education. When forming groups, instructors should encourage as much diversity as possible, regardless of whether groups are self-selected or allocated by the instructor. In the case study detailed in this chapter, for example, I found it useful to group mature-age students with considerable industry experience with younger students lacking such experience, and to make each group as gender and culturally diverse as possible. The combination of honed expertise and fresh enthusiasm and ideas made for creative and thoughtful solutions for solving the case. If more than one case study is assigned in a single course, it can make sense (provided things are going well) to keep the same groups together for the duration of the course, to capitalize on established rapport within the group.

In a case study situation, instructors become facilitators of student learning, walking around the classroom to monitor student progress and offering support to any struggling groups. When using case studies in class, instructors might consider starting class with a large group discussion to clarify key concepts and answer common questions before splitting into groups. An online discussion board (on Blackboard or Canvas, for example) is helpful for keeping track of common concerns, problems, or sections of the case study that need clarification. It can also be useful to have groups mentor each other, especially when some groups work faster than others to "solve" the case.

Assessing case studies will depend on how they are used in class—as a formal (graded) assignment or as a means of discussion. In either case, it is important to devise a group contract that sets out the expectations of how the group will function and what is expected of each group member. It is also a good idea to have groups report back to the class on a regular basis to help them stay on track and keep them accountable. Cases (or excerpts) can also be included on exams or in other formal assessment scenarios where students are asked to apply their knowledge. Thus, CBL has great potential for enriching "writing in the health professions."

Notes

1. Ethics approval (Murdoch University Reference Number 2014/146) was obtained for the Lifehouse study according to who uses it, in what contexts, and for what purposes (with research publication being an approved purpose). Each study participant gave full, informed consent before their interview (and on each subsequent occasion if we interviewed them more than once). In two instances, employees were interviewed twice, in different phases; one staff member was interviewed three times in three different phases.

2. Interviews with patients themselves did not form a part of this study.

3. Dr. Anne Surma has kindly given written consent for the findings of our mutual research project with Lifehouse to be included in this chapter. I acknowledge Dr. Surma's considerable contribution to this work and am grateful for her professional generosity.

4. I would also like to acknowledge the professional generosity of Associate Professor Chris Milross, director of radiation oncology and medical services at Lifehouse, who served as our academic liaison throughout the duration of our study. This work would not have been possible without his advocacy, insights, and encouragement.

References

1. Opel DS, Hart-Davidson W. The primary care clinic as writing space. *Writ Commun.* 2019 Jul;36(3):348–378.
2. Herreid CH. Case studies in science: A novel method of science education. *J Res Sci Teach.* 1994;23(4):221–229.
3. Lee V. What is inquiry-guided learning? *New Dir Learn.* 2012;129:5–14. Print.
4. Williams B. Case-based learning—a review of the literature: is there scope for this educational paradigm in prehospital education? *Emerg Med.* 2005;22(8): 577–581. Print.
5. Thistlethwaite JE et al. (2012). The effectiveness of case-based learning in health professional education. A BEME systematic review: BEME Guide No. 23. *Med Teach.* 2012;34(6): e421–e444.
6. Jonassen DH, Hernandez-Serrano J. Case-based reasoning and instructional design: using stories to support problem solving. *Educ Technol Res Dev.* 2002;50(2):65–77.
7. Frank AW. The standpoint of storyteller. *Qual Health Res.* 2000;10(3):354–365. Print.
8. Bleakley A. Stories as data, data as stories: making sense of narrative inquiry in clinical education. *Med Educ.* 2005;39(5):534–540.
9. Ellis C. Compassionate research: interviewing and storytelling from a relational ethics of care. *The Routledge International Handbook on Narrative and Life History.* Goodson I, Andrews M, Antikainen A, eds. New York: Routledge;2016 Oct 4:431–446.
10. Smith B, Sparkes AC. Narrative inquiry in psychology: exploring the tensions within. *Qual Res Psychol.* 2006;3(3):169–192.
11. Bonney KM. Case study teaching method improves student performance and perceptions of learning Gains. *Microbio Biol Educ.* 2015;16(1):21–28.

12. Breslin M, Buchanan R. On the case study method of research and teaching in design. *Des Issues.* 2008;24(1):36–40.

13. Herreid CF, ed. (2013). *Start with a Story: The Case Study Method of Teaching College Science.* Originally published in 2006 by the National Science Teachers Association (NSTA); reprinted by the National Center for Case Study Teaching in Science (NCCSTS) in 2013.

14. Krain M. Putting the learning in case learning? The effects of case-based approaches on student knowledge, attitudes, and engagement. *J Excell Coll Teach.* 2016;27(2):131–153.

15. Armstrong, P. "Bloom's taxonomy." *Vanderbilt University Center for Teaching.* https://cft.vanderbilt.edu/guides-sub-pages/blooms-taxonomy/. Accessed January 31 2021. Web.

16. Alvesson M, Thompson P. "Post-bureaucracy?" In: Ackroyd S, Batt R, Thompson P, Tolbert PS, eds. *The Oxford Handbook of Work and Organization.* Oxford: Oxford University Press;2005:485–507.

17. Cooren F, Kuhn T, Cornelissen JP, Clark T. Communication, organizing and organization: an overview and introduction to the special issue. *Organ Stud.* 2011;32(9): 1149–1170.

18. Putnam LL, Nicotera AM, eds. *Building Theories of Organization: The Constitutive Role of Communication.* New York: Routledge;2009.

19. McPhee RD, Zaug P. The communicative constitution of organizations: a framework for explanation. *Electron J Commun.* 2000;10. http://www.cios.org/EJCPUBLIC/010/1/01017.html.

20. Taylor JR, Van Every EJ. *The Emergent Organization: Communication As Its Site and Surface.* Mahwah, NJ: Lawrence Erlbaum;2000.

21. Penman R. On taking communication seriously. *Aust J Commun.* 2012;39(3): 41–64. Print.

22. Heidegger M. *Being and Time.* (J. Macquarrie & E. Robinson, Trans.). Oxford: Blackwell;1962.

23. Stewart J. One philosophical dimension of social approaches to interpersonal communication. *Commun Theor.* 1992;2(4):337–347.

24. *What is Patient-Centered Healthcare? A Review of Definitions and Principles.* 2nd ed. London: IAPO;2007.

25. *Patient-Centered Care: Improving Quality and Safety through Partnerships with Patients and Consumers.* Sydney: ACSQHC;2011.

26. Mead N, Bower P. Patient-centerdness: a conceptual framework and review of empirical literature. *Soc Sci Med.* 2000;51(7):1087–1110.

27. Sarangi S. Other-orientation in patient-centered healthcare communication: unveiled ideology or discoursal ecology? In: Garzone G, Sarangi S, eds. *Discourse, Ideology and Ethics in Specialized Communication.* Bern: Peter Lang;2007:39–71.

28. Epstein RM, Street RL. *Patient-Centered Communication in Cancer Care: Promoting Healing and Reducing Suffering.* Bethesda, MD: National Cancer Institute;2007.

29. Iedema R, Manidis M. *Patient–Clinician Communication: An Overview of Relevant Research and Policy Literatures.* Sydney: Australian Commission on Safety and Quality in Health Care and UTS Center for Health Communication;2013.

30. Tsianakas V, Robert G, Maben J, Richardson A, Dale C, Wiseman T. Implementing patient-centered cancer care: using experience-based co-design to improve patient experience in breast and lung cancer services. *Support Care Cancer.* 2012;20(11):2639–2647.

31. *The Patient Centred-Care Project: Evaluation Report.* London: The King's Fund;2011. Retrieved from http://www.kingsfund.org.uk/sites/files/kf/field/field_publication_file/patient-centerd-care-project-evaluation-aug11.pdf.

32. Kuhn TR. & Putnam LL. Discourse and communication. In: Adler P, Du Gay P, Morgan G, eds. *The Oxford Handbook of Sociology, Social Theory and Organization Studies: Contemporary Currents.* Oxford: Oxford University Press;2014:414–446.

33. National Center for Case Study Teaching in Science. https://sciencecases.lib.buffalo.edu/. Accessed January 31, 2021.

34. Johns Hopkins Medicine. https://www.hopkinsmedicine.org/gec/studies/. Accessed January 31, 2021.

35. National Center for Biotechnology Institute. https://www.ncbi.nlm.nih.gov/pmc/articles/PMC2597880/. Accessed January 31, 2021.

13

GRAPHIC MEDICINE

Theory, Utility, and Practice in Interprofessional Contexts

Kathryn West and Brian Callender

As a novel form of writing in the health professions, graphic medicine is a notable contribution to the use of narrative in medicine. Simply defined as the "intersection of the medium of comics and the discourse of healthcare,"[1] graphic medicine relies on comics' characteristic properties, broadly defined: a combination of words and images to tell a story in a time-and-space-oriented way. While participants should seek to improve their word choice and artistic ability, simple stick-figure drawings and small words can be just as effective in communicating story as expertly drawn figures and poetic turns of phrase. In recent years, graphic medicine has been increasingly integrated into traditional scholarly spaces, notably in the *Annals of Medicine*'s Graphic Medicine web-section, as well as the *New England Journal of Medicine*'s "Graphic Perspectives"; as a medium, comics are also being utilized as a research methodology.[2–6]

In our communities, we have developed several series of workshops focused on comics as a form of self-reflective storytelling. Several of these workshops have taken place at our home institution, the University of Chicago: one was for providers and patients in a comprehensive health-care program; the other was for frontline providers responding to the COVID-19 pandemic. A third series took place at a local nonprofit dedicated to those affected by a cancer diagnosis. Professionally, our health-care backgrounds, our professional values, and our experiences in interprofessional contexts inform our approach to creating a workshop environment that is open-minded, open-ended, and responsive to changing needs for patients and providers to reflect on their experiences.

In this chapter, we will outline the theoretical background and practical considerations for using graphic medicine as a form of writing in the health professions. Taking an autoethnographic approach, which emphasizes self-reflection and close observation,[7] we will also share examples of graphic medicine activities that we have developed, along with considerations for adjusting them based on the setting. While there are challenges to collecting robust data and quantifying the efficacy of such humanities-based approaches, to the extent that we can, we will offer examples of the work created and anecdotal data that demonstrate the impact of these activities on participants.

Graphic Medicine in Interprofessional Contexts

The basic professional values of social work and medicine include service, social justice, dignity and worth of the person, importance of human relationships, competence, and integrity.[8] These values align well with the principles of graphic medicine and are enhanced by this novel way

DOI: 10.4324/9781003162940-18

of interacting with oneself, patients, and other health professionals. Moreover, graphic medicine dovetails with various modes of mental health treatment, such as expressive arts therapies, narrative therapies, and cognitive behavioral therapies. By increasing our collective understanding of a variety of health and illness narratives, we have the potential to impact how institutions and, ultimately, society are organized around the topics of health and illness.

Graphic medicine is, at its core, a way to tell stories to ourselves and others through the medium of comics. This attention to story is relevant across the spectrum of clinical and nonclinical experiences. In our own observations, we have found the principles of *the worth of the person* and *the importance of human relationships* especially lacking—and, thus, highly needed—in the world of health care, where patient-provider relationships can be fraught: these relationships should be simultaneously respectful and evidence-based, close and yet adherent to boundaries, and grounded in expertise from both sides, fostering shared decision-making. The tensions within these relationships are, of course, predicated on the medical and emotional complexity of the care being discussed; thus, expectations for the parameters of the relationship are variable and dynamic.

Recognizing challenges like these, Rita Charon described how providers might "closely read" their patients, akin to how students of literature closely read passages of novels or poems. Charon coined the term "narrative medicine" to broaden how providers might listen to their patients and reflect on their stories, not just on their symptoms. This kind of listening and reflecting can apply to graphic medicine as well. Though Charon had clinical medicine in mind, narrative medicine is broadly applicable across the health professions (for an additional example, see the "teacherless writing groups" described in Chapter 14). As Charon says,

> Our bodies age, but they also exist simultaneously in all times.... Our bodies are texts, then, clerking the records of what we have been through, hoarding evidence of past hurts, remembering as only bodies can the corporeal stabilities that keep us alive.[9(p122)]

Graphic medicine also borrows from narrative therapy in its desire to externalize and examine problems as separate from the people who experience them.[10] In our workshops and in graphic medicine practice more generally, participants externalize the "problem" by putting it down on paper, creating an exterior space in which it can live.

Additionally, we pull from the field of cognitive behavioral therapy, which focuses on the connections between thoughts, feelings, and actions.[11] The intentional act of self-reflection that is enacted through graphic medicine offers a way for practitioners, patients, and students to examine more closely their thoughts and feelings about health, illness, and healing. In slowing down the reflection process—something that happens naturally when using such a hands-on form—assumptions about what it means to be healthy or ill can become more apparent. Emotional "space" is created so that participants more closely inspect what they think and feel.[12]

In art therapy, there is a "concept of a triangular relationship, with art forming a vital third component" and the clinician and patient each as the other two components.[13] Applying this concept, it is necessary in graphic medicine to honor the comic being created as its own entity: both of the person who made it and also as a stand-alone piece. In our workshops, participants can but are not obligated to share their own work. They are encouraged to share thoughts about the work created by others—seeing the pieces, once completed, as capable of relaying multiple messages, even ones unintended by the creator. This triangular relationship is also helpful in reassuring participants that the comic is capable of communicating important messages about their health and illness, even if they struggle to see themselves as an "artist" or worry about their artistic ability.

In acknowledging the importance of telling, listening to, and seeing stories, we must recognize the different media through which these stories are created, including how visual methodologies' unique properties enhance the storytelling experience. We live in a highly visual culture where comics are both valued and accessible. We believe that the medium of comics is particularly adept at capturing narratives of illness and health from both "phenomenological" and "narrative-construction" perspectives.

First, phenomenology calls attention to how important space and time are in the illness experience.[14–16] Indeed, illness impacts how we perceive time and interact with our surroundings (space/place), sometimes in dramatic ways, which is well suited to depiction in comics. As a medium, comics depict space and time through the sequencing of images and text that tell a story. Some comics consist of a single panel that captures a moment in time. In others, time unfolds as the reader's eyes move from panel to panel. Thus, by creating the text and images within a panel, as well as between panels, participants can manipulate crucial aspects of space and time within their own illness narrative.

For many participants, an illness experience often involves multiple narratives that intersect. The visual and spatial layout of comics allows multiple narratives to simultaneously exist while showing how they are connected and important to a participant's own telling of their illness experience. The ability of comics to layer narratives like this allows for a more nuanced, true-to-life telling of an illness history, showing how each strand impacts the others.

Second, creating a story through comics is relatively simple and likely something that we have all done as children. Regardless of participants' artistic abilities, they can create basic images (figures, places) and text (dialogue, numbers) that are central to their narrative and that express perspective, ideas, and emotion. The activities described next are based on these premises. In combining the properties of comics with the principles of narrative medicine, graphic medicine provides a unique way to construct, read, and share narratives of health, illness, and well-being. (For additional perspectives on the value of narratives, see the other chapters in Part IV.)

In graphic medicine, as in all the fields that inspire it, the essentials are constant: a requisite understanding of other humans through the stories they tell and the way they tell them, a desire to cocreate a reality upon which a helping and caring relationship can be built, an attention to both the "text" (what participants create visually) and the "subtext" (underlying meanings, sometimes verbalized during postcreation discussions and sometimes left unsaid), and a belief that the stories a person may tell can be expansive, unlimited, and changing. In our workshops, we encourage modes of creation and cocreation that are culturally relevant, broadly accessible, and based in an inherent honoring of each person's unique ability to self-reflect and contribute to our collective ideas of health and illness. We thus ground this work in the same principles of justice, relational importance, and dignity of personhood that workshop facilitators must consider at all times.

Graphic Medicine Workshop Examples

There are many ways in which graphic medicine can be enacted in the training of future and current health professionals.[17–19] In utilizing graphic medicine as a tool for training health professionals, creating space for self-reflection, it is necessary to consider the audience and goals of the activity. Here, we provide several workshop examples that we have adapted to a variety of settings. In addition to each example, we provide sample questions we used and considerations for modifying the workshop content based on where it will be run.

Our workshop series was initially developed for use in the University of Chicago's Comprehensive Care Program,[20] which caters to those in the hospital's catchment area who are Medicaid/Medicare dual eligible and have at least one chronic health condition. The workshops were then adapted for use at a local branch of Gilda's Club,[21] where those living with cancer and their loved ones have access to community programming and support. They were adapted once more at the University of Chicago for health-care faculty who served on the front lines of the COVID-19 pandemic. The first two versions of this workshop series were led in-person prior to the pandemic; the last one was held virtually.

For us, an important consideration was sequencing the activities, as this order can impact the participants' overall experience. We conceived the aforementioned three-part series of workshops as a movement from self to community, creating connection through sharing about health, illness, and well-being. While the focus of the workshops was on positive aspects of each participants' body, life, and community, this focus was balanced with some reflection on personal negative aspects of these entities in order to foster dialogue and recognize hardships as a way to move toward healing and receiving help.

We tried to emphasize the importance of art in the physical and emotional space of any graphic medicine activity by the way the workshop space is set up.[22] This required thoughtful selection of materials and locale and had to be adaptable to both in-person and virtual setting options. When we met in person, we provided a variety of media, including crayons, colored pencils, pencils, pens, and markers so that participants could choose the writing implement(s) and color palette that best suited their expression. It was important to provide supplies that are accessible; this meant both thick and thin versions of supplies when possible so that grip and mobility wouldn't be barriers to comic making. We also wanted participants to be able to spread out their materials in a way that makes sense for them.

When meeting in person, we made sitting in a circle a priority so that workshop participants were facing inward toward each other and none had their backs to anyone else. In a virtual space, we provided instructions for participants to collect art supplies ahead of the workshop and suggested a variety of materials, including the option to create comics on a computer if that was more comfortable. For both in-person and virtual workshops, we found a group size of five to ten participants was ideal in order to have a robust conversation with time for each participant to share.

At the start of our workshops, we set appropriate group expectations, which included language about assuming best intentions, volunteering commentary that is constructive and curious rather than directive, and acknowledging the vulnerability and openness demonstrated by each participant just for showing up and sharing their work. When power differentials were most apparent—for example, if providers and patients are participating together in a workshop—even more care was needed.

For all workshops, we explained the purpose and format. We also invited participants to introduce themselves briefly. When time allowed, we led a mindfulness activity to help group participants focus on their own physicality.

While we encouraged participants to use a combination of text and images in response to the questions and prompts, we allowed participants to respond to the prompts in ways that were most meaningful to them. In setting the tone for the workshops, we found that it can also be helpful to play music while participants are creating. Workshops can be adapted based on time constraints, but generally required about 45 minutes to complete thoroughly and need be no longer than 75 minutes. For each, the facilitator may choose to save all discussion and sharing until the end of the session or to pause throughout for reflection and sharing. In the following sections, we introduce body-mapping, life-mapping, community-mapping, and other activities.

Body-Mapping

Body-mapping was typically the first activity used in our workshops since it prompted participants to look inward and focus on how they understand their health and illness as physical phenomena. So often, the medical model of care focuses on a patient's symptoms and bodily limitations instead of strengths and abilities. Thus, the goal of body-mapping was for participants to reconnect more deeply with their physical selves; our hope was to reintegrate the physical self that is the primary focus of the medical establishment with the full, holistic self of each participant.

We provided an agender person outline as a template upon which to create. However, for workshops with the physical space and time, and for participants who are comfortable and able to do so, butcher block paper could be used to trace a life-size outline of each person. This outline can be filled in during the workshop.

Instructions and questions we have used:

1. Draw that part of your body you are thinking most about today.
2. Draw something that represents how you are feeling today. Where are these feelings living? How can you depict them?
3. Draw your favorite body part; why is it your favorite body part?
4. Draw your least favorite body part; why is it your least favorite body part?
5. Draw a physical scar; can you depict how you obtained that scar?
6. Draw an emotional scar; can you depict how you obtained that scar?
7. Draw a tattoo that you have; if you don't have a tattoo, what imagery feels like it should be part of your body?
8. Which part of your body are you most concerned about and why? What part of your body feels the best today? What part feels the worst? Which part of your body do you associate with illness? Which do you associate with health?
9. Fill in features that define your physical body; fill in features that define your non-physical body (mind/soul). Fill in anything that isn't here yet that you think should be.

Example:

This image depicts some of the ways in which words and images can be utilized in this activity and how both emotionality and physicality can exist in the artistic rendering of the self.

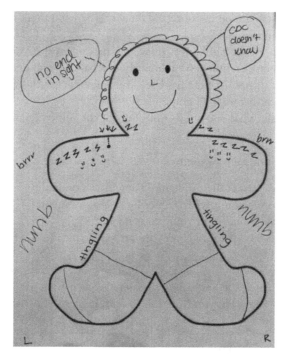

FIGURE 13.1 A body map depicting an adverse response to a vaccine and the process of healing and feeling grateful for the positive effects of the vaccine-accrued immunity

Life-Mapping

The goal of life-mapping was to look at participants' lives in a more comprehensive way, contextualizing their illnesses within their overall well-being. In this activity, participants were asked to reflect on specific illness experiences, perhaps cancer or COVID-19. They were also asked to consider high and low points in other parts of their lives. We plotted all this on time lines (x-axis) according to how participants defined their own well-being (y-axis; Figure 13.2). We believed this could help participants to see life as an ever-changing progression in which feelings of wellness—psychological, emotional, spiritual, physical, social—aren't fixed. Rather, they are part of a greater whole.

This activity needed to be approached carefully to avoid ending the workshop with feelings of hopelessness if an illness or other circumstances were causing participants a downward wellness trajectory. As a result, we ended with participants setting goals, prompting them to look forward with a growth mindset.[23]

We found the SMART goal[24] format useful, which can help participants establish feelings of control over realistic goals, in line with strengths-based psychological approaches, such as positive psychology.[25] When possible, we used a larger piece of paper to tape smaller drawings onto so that things can be moved around as needed during the workshop. However, if space or materials are limited, this could be modified to fit onto standard printer paper and done directly on the paper. This could also be adapted to a virtual environment by encouraging prompts to be drawn onto one large paper.

Instructions and questions we have used:

To begin, draw a simple graph with an x- and y-axis. The x-axis should be labeled "time" and the y-axis should be labeled "well-being." For each of the following prompts, draw right on the graph in the spot where it best fits, or draw in a separate comic square and then place/tape it on the graph where it best fits.

1. Think about your current state of well-being and draw what is contributing to that state.
2. Think of a significant childhood memory and draw it; when you think of your childhood, what three things are most memorable?
3. Draw one or several personal high points; draw an achievement that you are proud of.
4. Draw one or several personal low points; think about a past loss and draw that.
5. Draw the moment of diagnosis; what has been your medical/health-care low point? What has been your medical/health-care high point?
6. Draw your goals. Draw what you are fearful of about the future. Draw what you are hopeful about for the future.

Pandemic-specific questions we have used:

1. When did you first hear about the pandemic? Draw that moment.
2. When did the pandemic first impact your life? Draw that moment.
3. Draw something that you miss from your pre-pandemic life.
4. Draw something that you don't miss from your pre-pandemic life.
5. What are you hopeful for?
6. What are you fearful of?
7. Imagine you've just turned 100 and your grandchild asks what the pandemic was like and what you learned from it. Draw what you would share with them.

Example:

Figure 13.2 is an example of a pandemic map depicting a decline in well-being as the pandemic has gone on, using the now-ubiquitous imagery of the surgical mask floating downward. The provider who created this also noted that they

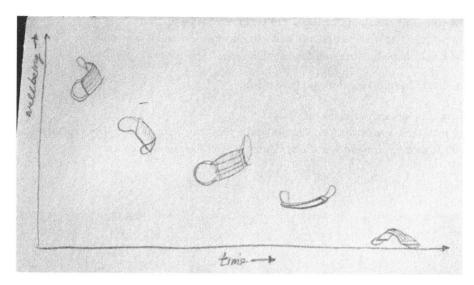

FIGURE 13.2 A pandemic map depicting current health, health-related goals, and the incident that pre-ceded many current health challenges

noticed early signs of burnout in the drawings that presaged an increase in my ProQOL [Professional Quality of Life Measure] burnout scores. I thought that was interesting when I found them last week while on vacation. They were darker than I remembered! I was just making fast automatic sketches during the two sessions and didn't reflect as much on them in the moment.

Community-Mapping

The purpose of community-mapping was to explore how participants understand the meaning of "community," starting at home and emanating outward. We considered health care as a part of a community, influencing the lives of both patients and providers, and thus we asked about it specifically.

The participants were then asked to think about how various elements of community are connected to one another. In our workshops for faculty members, we found that this activity could be adapted to address specific questions of equity and access. These workshops occurred just after the murder of George Floyd, and thus, we found it necessary to raise questions about racial disparities, peace, and safety. For this activity, we partnered with our Office of Diversity and Inclusion[26] to set prompts that met the specific moment. The disparities in access to resources and safety were put at the forefront of the activity. These topics became fodder for further conversations and also reminded participants that every community has its own strengths, regardless of the struggles that many concurrently exist within it. This activity took advantage of the visual nature of comics to create a map of one's community.

General instructions and questions we have used:

1. Draw your current home; draw your favorite location in your home; draw your least favorite location in your home; create a short comic about one of your favorite moments in your home.
2. Draw a portrait of those who live with you; now include close friends and where they are in relation to you physically and emotionally.
3. Think of positive locations in your community and map them on your community map; draw your favorite place in your community.

4. Draw your least favorite place/a place of harm in your community.
5. Draw an aspect of your community that was once present and is now missing.
6. What is your hope for your community? Draw a wished-for place.

Pandemic/social justice questions we have used:

1. What spaces are uncomfortable or chaotic?
2. How have these spaces changed because of the pandemic and/or the police brutality protests?
3. What places have changed as a result? For the better? For the worse?

Example:

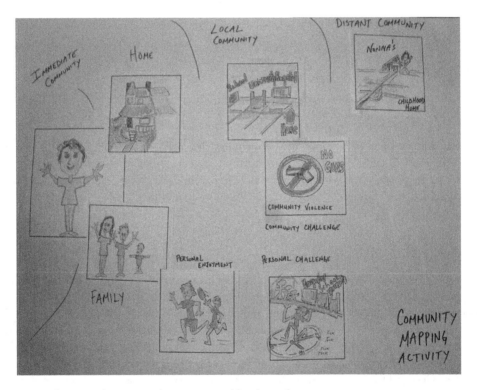

FIGURE 13.3 An example community map created by the authors

This depicts the idea of community, especially as it has changed as a result of the pandemic

Other Activities

We have also had success with other workshops activities, including jam comics; "before, during, after"; and graphic journaling.

Jam Comics

This activity is built on the childhood staple, the exquisite corpse/jam drawing, where one person begins a drawing, passes it along to a friend who adds to it, who then passes it along, etc., with each person adding a bit to complete the full picture. In this health care–specific rendering, the focus was on a general clinical experience. Categories have included getting to the doctor, having a yearly physical, getting a diagnosis, or having surgery, and should be applicable to the full group in the room. Depending on group size, facilitators could pass the template around the full group or break into smaller groups of three to four people. Each participant began in the upper leftmost square, with however they define the beginning of the chosen experience.

After a short time—3 to 5 minutes was usually best—the template was passed along, and the next part of the experience was created in the adjacent panel. The goal was to share the totality of experience—however that is defined—in the multiple panels provided in the template. Additionally, this activity helped participants see the shared elements of various health-care experiences but also to see where individual experience differs and how that might impact how the encounter is perceived. A six-box panel is usually sufficient and can be easily recreated in any basic document-producing software. Ours was created in the Office Suite.

During, Before, After

In this activity, participants focused on a specific clinical encounter and created a basic multi-panel comic. The goal of this activity was to help participants process encounters that are meaningful to them, moving beyond the moment and understanding it in a fuller context. By doing so, participants might see a better "after" that could emerge.

Participants first drew or place a box in the middle of their paper where they draw the "during" of the encounter: whatever the crux of their story is. Any encounter could be chosen, but it was often valuable for them to choose one that is "sticky," which is to say, one that has stayed with the participant, comes to mind quickly, and brought on strong emotions at the time. After the "during" has been drawn, we moved to the "before," wherein the participant was asked to share what happened before the heart of the encounter.

To do so, they drew a square to the left of the "during" image. If the participant knew what happened, this could be drawn. If they didn't know, they were asked to imagine what might have led to that moment. This could be done in just one box, or other boxes can be added to depict a series of moments which led to the "during" moment. The participant could then move to the "after," where they depicted what happened after the "during." This could be real or imagined based on the participant's access to that information and could be done in one square to the right of the "during" or in multiple squares. Additionally, we explored time and perspective by asking participants to view the encounter from the perspective of other characters (physician, nurse, caregiver, loved one) in the narrative.

Graphic Journaling

A less formalized graphic medicine activity we have found helpful—especially for trainees or students—is a graphic journal. The idea is to set up a regular practice of drawing an image or short (three to four image/panel) sequence from a clinical experience. It's possible to use any of the previously mentioned activities as a form for the journaling, but we have encouraged participants to freely draw as well. This practice helped participants process their day through comic making and encouraged this way of thinking for patients or providers who are regularly interacting in the health-care world. Graphic journaling also encouraged participants to focus on the day-to-day work of being in the world of health care, helping them create meaning from their daily interactions.

For us, it has been helpful to put a time frame in place—say, a weekly graphic journal during a specific clinical rotation in medical school or a journal entry from a patient at each chemotherapy appointment. That way, we could ensure the graphic journal was not an overwhelming prospect, but our hope was that it would become a habit. (For another kind of reflective journaling, see Chapter 7.)

Challenges

Though we believe strongly in the power and importance of graphic medicine as a modality, there are, as ever, challenges with its implementation. Based on an autoethnographic look at our own workshop experiences, these challenges can be broken down into two categories: those that are logistical to the workshops we conducted and those which are inherent to the modality of graphic medicine in and of itself.

The first category, the logistics of a workshop or workshop series, is easier to address and will vary by institution and environment. Simply put, we believe that these workshops are most impactful when they can be available to both providers and to patients in the same setting where they can harness key aspects of narrative to medicine to learn about and understand one another. However, neither being a medical provider nor being a patient is imbued with a sense of extra time and energy. For providers, just getting to the room for an activity like this can be a challenge when there are competing interests of patient care, administrative tasks, research activities, and other meetings, it is hard to find a time in the day that is conducive to having providers sit down to do these activities. For patients, often a barrier to attendance was the illness they want to process with these workshops. For many of our patients, their continued care and multiple medical appointments mean they are short on time and energy to join an activity like this one. Resource-related barriers could also prove challenging if patients needed to find and pay for transportation to participate. While technological barriers may also exist in terms of access to videoconferencing software, we anticipate that one benefit of virtual workshops will be that they are more easily attended and may reduce barriers to participation for patients, providers, and students. Thus, we emphasize that it is necessary to consider the audience and the means by which the workshops can be made most accessible.

The second category, challenges inherent to graphic medicine itself, are more difficult but also have more universal opportunities for being addressed. First is the consideration that through these activities, negative experiences and emotions are going to surface. In fact, some of the questions suggested earlier ask participants to actively engage with these emotions in order to process them differently and see them in a new context. Facilitators of these activities—and any done under the auspices of graphic medicine—must make clear the purpose and potential to help participants, working to avoid "narrative iatrogenesis," which can be defined as emotional harm or trauma resulting from the act of creating or recreating a narrative. Therefore, it is important to bring each activity to a conclusion that is focused on empowerment. This means validating concerns that are raised, while also focusing on the power that can be found in better knowing ourselves and in sharing our stories. All this can help us reorient toward our goals and strengths.

Lastly, there is a need for strong empirical, data-driven evidence to indicate the short- and long-term effects and impacts of either this or similar graphic medicine workshops, particularly with patients and providers. This remains an area in need of well-designed research to answer questions about the benefits of these activities, though that has been challenging given the relatively limited number of participants and the often informal flow and structure that may be hard to duplicate from session to session. While collecting data has been a challenge, we are hopeful that future iterations of these workshops will be conducted under the auspices of a robust research study.

However, we are confident in the utility of these workshops and the field of graphic medicine as a whole, both because it is a field built on strong, evidence-based practices—as described earlier—and because our experiences in the field and anecdotal data demonstrate the power of these workshops. In a small quality improvement survey of four participants from the Comprehensive Care Program graphic medicine programming, all participants surveyed "agreed" or "strongly agreed" that the workshops helped them connect with their doctor/other health-care provider and "agreed" or "strongly agreed" that it enhanced their health/well-being. In response to the two-part workshop COVID-19 series, one participant shared that they

> found the sessions extremely helpful for enabling me to slow down, reflect on the turbulent and soul-sucking effects of COVID-19 and systemic racism, and simultaneously recognize great sources of strength and support. Drawing pictures simplifies and prioritizes my thoughts. Helps me identify the core and essence of what has influenced me and is important to me, and helps me understand my own personal story.

We hope that future studies will allow for what we have seen in our workshops to bear out in the data. Thus, the future of these workshops may lie in conducting them in a framework of traditional quantitative and qualitative research methodologies.

Looking Forward

Graphic medicine is an expanding field of study and one which serves and is served by its implementation in the process of teaching writing to future health professionals to use for themselves and for their patients. While the field was founded by those with dual knowledge and expertise in both medicine and art, there is no level of understanding or ability required prior to utilizing graphic medicine in practice.

While we shared a curated set of graphic medicine activities, this expansive field has more to offer. You can, and should, imagine new activities that will best meet the needs of your students, clinicians, or patients. As you adapt these activities for your clinical and/or educational environment and needs, the goal should always be to incorporate both words and images, to think about form and function as you create, and to find ways to bring people into the process of creating and sharing their narratives. Accessibility should always be at the forefront of devising graphic medicine workshops: Which activities best suit your audience of participants? How can you give image/ text examples from a diverse group of creators? How can you provide templates which are neutral enough for everyone to be able to put themselves onto the page equally (for example, a gender-neutral body map)? What writing instruments might you need so that everyone can see, hold, and use them? How can you word your prompts to be inclusive?

There are several areas of the health-care world that would be especially well-served by graphic medicine into which we, the authors, hope to expand our work and hope you will do the same. Mental health care is too often deemed separate from the rest of health care, and graphic medicine offers an opportunity to reunify the body and mind and their connection via drawing. Even in the act of drawing and writing, the mind and body must work in harmony. Additionally, the experience of living with mental illness is one that often exists beyond words, and thus those who live in that space deserve both words and images to share how they are experiencing their minds. In this sense, it is not surprising that one of the more expansive subgenres of graphic pathography focuses on mental health, and there are several fantastic examples of graphic memories that deal with mental illness. Another area we hope to continue to expand our work in is cancer care—where one workshop series took place and where many published graphic novels focus. (Cancer care is a focus in Chapter 12.) And, in light of the COVID-19 pandemic, which has overtaken so much of our world, and which has led to so much social isolation, we look to graphic medicine as an important tool for redeveloping or deepening patient-provider connections in addition to reflecting on the importance of community. It is an opportunity to share the medical world from within during a time of uncertainty, change, loss, and innovation.

References

1. Czerwiec, MK et al. *The Graphic Medicine Manifesto.* The Pennsylvania State University Press; 2015.
2. Al-Jawad M. Comics are research: graphic narratives as a new way of seeing clinical practice. *J Med Humanit.* 2013;36(4):369–374. doi:10.1007/s10912-013-9205-0
3. Galman S. The truthful messenger: visual methods and representation in qualitative research in education. *Qual Res.* 2009;9(2):197–217. doi:10.1177/1468794108099321
4. Kuttner P, Weaver-Hightower M, Sousanis N. Comics-based research: the affordances of comics for research across disciplines. *Qual Res.* 2020:146879412091884. doi:10.1177/1468794120918845
5. Kuttner P, Sousanis N, Weaver-Hightower M. How to draw comics the scholarly way: creating comics-based research in the academy. In: Leavy P, ed. *Handbook of Arts-Based Research.* 1st ed. New York: The Guilford Press; 2018:396–422.
6. Flowers E. Experimenting with comics making as inquiry. *Vis Arts Res.* 2017;43(2):21–57.
7. Chang, H. *Autoethnography as Method.* London: Routledge; 2016.
8. Code of Ethics. National Association of Social Workers. https://www.socialworkers.org/About/Ethics/Code-of-Ethics/Code-of-Ethics-English https://www.acponline.org/about-acp/who-we-are/mission-vision-goals-core-values; 1996, rev. 2017.
9. Charon R. *Narrative Medicine: Honoring the Stories of Illness.* New York: Oxford University Press; 2008.
10. Freedman J, Combs G. *Narrative Therapy: The Social Construction of Preferred Realities.* New York: Norton; 1996.
11. Institute for Quality and Efficiency in Health Care. Cognitive Behavioral Therapy. *InformedHealth.* 2013. https://www.ncbi.nlm.nih.gov/books/NBK279297/. Accessed January 23, 2021.
12. White M, Epston D. *Narrative Means to Therapeutic Ends.* Auckland, NZ: Royal New Zealand Foundation of the Blind; 1990.
13. Case C, Dalley T. *The Handbook of Art Therapy.* London: Routledge; 2014.
14. Carel H. *Phenomenology of Illness.* Oxford University Press; 2016.
15. Toombs SK. Illness and the paradigm of the lived body. *Theor Med.* 1988;9:201–26.
16. Toombs SK. The temporality of illness: four levels of experience. *Theor Med.* 1990;11:227–41.
17. Anand T, Kishore J, Ingle GK, Grover S. Perception about use of comics in medical and nursing education among students in health professions' schools in New Delhi. *Educ Health.* 2018;31:125–9.
18. George DR, Green MJ. Lessons learned from comics produced by medical students: art of darkness. *JAMA.* 2015;314(22):2345–6.
19. Green MJ. Comics and medicine: peering into the process of professional identity formation. *Acad Med.* 2015; 90:774–779.
20. Comprehensive Care Program. (n.d.). Retrieved from https://ccpprogram.uchicago.edu
21. Gilda's Club Chicago. (n.d.). Retrieved from https://gildasclubchicago.org
22. Case C, Dalley T. *The Handbook of Art Therapy.* New York: Routledge; 2006.
23. The Science & Psychology of Goal-Setting 101. PositivePsychology.com. https://positivepsychology.com/goal-setting-psychology/.
24. S.M.A.R.T. Goals. *Psychology Today.* https://www.psychologytoday.com/us/blog/in-the-face-adversity/201705/smart-goals.
25. What Is Positive Psychology & Why Is It Important? [2020 Update]. PositivePsychology.com. https://positivepsychology.com/what-is-positive-psychology-definition/. Published 2020. Accessed January 24, 2021.
26. BSD Diversity | The University of Chicago Biological Sciences. *Voices.uchicago.edu.* https://voices.uchicago.edu/bsddiversity/.

14

PROMOTING WRITING THROUGH TEACHERLESS WRITING GROUPS

Lucy M. Candib, Stacy Potts, Katharine Barnard, Jill Tirabassi, Lisa S. Gussak, Henry DelRosario, and Daniel Lasser

People from all walks of life may ultimately enter employment in the health professions. They come to this work with variable training and experience in writing—from high school, technical school, college, medical or nursing school, graduate education in the sciences, social sciences or humanities, from other educational environments, or from previous professions. They may be called upon to write in their health professions, bringing back the history of joys—or frustrations— resonating from their past efforts. While no single strategy fits to guide people toward effective and rewarding writing experiences, writing groups are one method flexible enough to meet the needs of many interprofessional groups of health-care providers whose work settings do not support their growth and development as writers.

Writers in the health professions may experience a variety of obstacles to writing: first, writing for publication may be an expectation because of their role in professional or academic hierarchies, but the institutions themselves may not support the necessary time and resources. Moreover, the expectations to publish for advancement or success may not match personal aspirations. For many clinicians, their work with patients may be a higher priority in terms of time and sense of accomplishment. Time is short—for everyone—but shorter for people with small children, busy clinical lives, and dependent family members, as well as for those responsible for students, learners, or trainees at multiple levels. Moreover, self-doubt may plague a person: internalized assumptions about abilities based on gender, class, race, or choice of career may limit personal expectations about the worth of anything that person may write. Thus finding ways to manage time and self-doubt are two of the key issues in fostering writing; coming to see writing as something essential for the work or for oneself is a third. So the question arises: How can busy health professionals foster their own ability to write—for example, scholarly work, position papers, other technical work, or humanistic pieces—once they are out of school and in the workplace for the long haul?

While some chapters in this book address teaching writing to health professionals as an academic pursuit, in reality, many individuals working in health-related fields do not view writing as a serious goal, at least in the initial stages of their careers. Writing is seen as useful for daily documentation and administrative tasks necessary to *do their work*. At some point, they are expected to write *about the work*, which is a new task and, for many health professionals, a difficult one. Writing groups are a partial answer to the challenge they face.[1,2] Paul Silvia, the psychologist-author of *How to Write a Lot*,[3] noted "flavors" of writing groups: goals and accountability groups, write-together groups, and feedback groups.

DOI: 10.4324/9781003162940-19

In the first kind of group, the members meet regularly to report on their goals from the previous meeting and to state their goals for the next period of time, with one member keeping track of the commitments. Such groups may be combined with the second type, write-together groups, wherein members spend much of the time together working on their individual projects. He sees the third kind, feedback groups, as potentially the most problematic since he sees giving and taking feedback in constructive ways as not something that comes naturally. He opines that the feedback process can become conflictual, leading easily to the dissolution of a group.

Silvia is not sanguine about writing groups in general, preferring his own recommendation of a behavior change model based on scheduling writing time individually. However, he does state, "A good writing group will reinforce one's writing schedule, make writing feel less solitary, and stave off the darkness of binge writing."[3(p47)] What does he mean by the "darkness of binge writing?" This may involve the tyranny of midnight when, after much procrastination, the task has to be done by the next day. In the urgency of the moment, the writing does get done, but it is a grim process that feels best when it is over and done with. In contrast to Silvia's attempt to dismiss writing groups as a strategy, in this chapter, we will review the history of writing groups and describe our experience with a long-running Teacherless Writing Group as a method to strengthen and support an interprofessional group of writers over several years. (For an "environmental scan" of additional methods, see Chapter 3.)

Historical Perspective and Literature Review about Writing Groups

But first, some history. Writing groups, in the form of people writing and reading their work to others, were popular institutions in the United States in the nineteenth century. As early as the 1830s, the Lyceum movement emerged outside of elite academic institutions as a setting where young men of limited means might get experience with writing and reading their work to others. The Chautauqua movement in the latter part of the century reinforced this function. With the development of colleges and academies of higher education for women in the mid-nineteenth century, women, who previously had only attended Lyceum meetings with a male family member, now began getting together in women's clubs to write. Women's clubs were an example of American mutual improvement societies typical in the late nineteenth century and were linked to the widespread development of public libraries across the country in the early twentieth century. Writing groups using peer pairings and group feedback finally entered the classroom at the elementary school level in the 1930s when education reformers introduced the idea of children writing for their peers in order to have an audience who will give them feedback. Yet it was not until the 1960s and '70s that high school and college classrooms took up the model of the group as a way to learn how to write. Students and teachers found benefits in this method. Conducting education in writing as a peer group process opened the possibility for students to develop skills in writing without the negative judgment of the teacher's authority and offered teachers relief from the tedium of grading unending piles of student papers.

As the model of teaching writing in a group format took hold in college classrooms in the 1970s, there was concomitant development of theory in rhetoric and composition. Peter Elbow was one of the key educators in this sea change; he then took his strategy out of the college classroom into the community. His book, *Writing Without Teachers*, is a classic in how to start a Teacherless Writing Group.[1] The National Writing Project, growing out of the Bay Area Writing Project, emerged as a nationwide training program for composition instructors that required participants themselves to engage in writing groups. Thousands of teachers were trained in the model of writing groups for education in the classroom, while Elbow's book, honed within his classroom but explicitly aimed at writers outside school walls, was highly successful and published as a trade book, with hundreds of thousands of copies sold over the years. (The summary of the history of writing groups in this chapter is drawn from Gere's book *Writing Groups: History, Theory, and Implications.*[4])

Separate from educational developments within universities focused on composition and rhetoric, writing groups in medicine and nursing in particular also became popular over the past 50 years. Primarily stimulated by the professional need to write and subsequently publish both for members' career goals and for promoting the status of their department or field in the institution, such groups have historically focused on the process of writing, editing, and preparing manuscripts suitable for publication. The focus of attention within groups may range from healthy writing habits and supportive feedback for authors, all the way to the development of the structure of a scientific article and identification of the requirements for publication in relevant journals. Typically, writing groups have been composed of health professionals from a variety of academic locations in nursing, medicine, dentistry, pharmacy, and other health fields. Both individual and collaborative writing efforts may be featured. These groups mostly fall into Silvia's category of "goals and accountability" groups. Some groups are linked with formal instruction, such as seminars or courses, with specific attention to attributes of quality scientific articles in relevant fields—e.g., appropriate literature review, explicit methods and statistics, review of limitations, writing clarity, and avoidance of jargon and verbosity.[5,6] Some include mentors and more junior faculty in the same groups, with explicit partnering for some research papers, leading to ongoing mentoring relationships;[7–12] others are composed primarily of peers who come together to support each other and provide feedback in the writing process.[13–16] In one community hospital-based model, physicians established a collaborative writing group in which the members agreed to research and write papers together, dividing up the tasks, with good success in publication and in spreading their writing group model to others within the hospital system.[17] Within hospitals, academic institutions, and medical research centers, the placement of designated mentors within writing groups has been successful in generating research projects and publications in nursing, pharmacy, and dentistry,[11,18–20] some with joint authorship but eventually with authorship by the more junior author.

The evidence base for strategies to improve and increase writing for publication is more experiential than systematic. A 2015 review by Galipeau et al.[2] presents the available data. Most studies looked at outcomes of publication rates from specific interventions measured by the number of articles published prior to and after the writing intervention. Most of the strategies to promote writing—such as writing coaches, individual mentoring by faculty members, both online and in-person workshops, and independent study—focused on teaching individual writers. Those strategies involving groups with an emphasis on group process ranged from writing courses of varying intensity, faculty development programs, group meetings with faculty advisors, writing retreats, recurring writing workshops of several days' duration, and peer writing groups. Galipeau et al.[2] found descriptive evidence that writing interventions of various types were usually followed by an increase in publication[7,21] by individuals and by groups of individuals who worked together across time.

An impressively robust ongoing example of an interdisciplinary writing group is the course which has been running for over 30 years at the University of Rochester School of Medicine and Dentistry, with faculty from the Family Medicine and Psychiatry Departments.[5] This group, composed of physicians, nurses, psychologists, family therapy trainees, and others, is required for postdoctoral fellows in primary care psychology, family therapy, and family medicine, as well as junior faculty in family medicine. It is also open to faculty in various departments of the medical center but is most commonly attended by faculty in family medicine and psychiatry. Participants are expected to submit two pieces of work over the course of a 9-month period, and trainees are expected to rotate the role of chief discussant of others' submissions. Two papers are discussed at each session, often drafts of articles for journals in various fields but also articles prepared from dissertations, case reports, and 55-word stories, poetry, or other reflections related to working as a health professional. The presenters must provide the other participants with their manuscript one week ahead of time, along with the questions they have and where they may wish to submit the work for publication. The chief reviewer facilitates the group discussion, focusing first on the authors' concerns. This format shows commitment at an institutional level, as it involves multiple faculty from several disciplines who are committed to graduate education, with sanctioned time on a monthly basis. All participants, as well as the leader who is a psychologist on the faculty in family medicine and psychiatry, review every submission and provide oral and written feedback to the presenting writer. This level of commitment is unusual among medical writing groups that usually coalesce around members' needs rather than an academic commitment. As an interdisciplinary mix of faculty and graduate learners, the Rochester group has not exactly functioned as a peer writing group, but its egalitarian, trainee-led structure offers a more nonhierarchical atmosphere typical of peer writing groups. The family physicians, family therapists, and their learners share a vision of writing as part of their academic careers. Over the years, the group members have derived substantial support from the institutional commitment of their university toward the development of the writing and publication accomplishments of the engaged educators and leaders in their fields.

How Do Writing Groups Work? Why Are Writing Groups Useful?

Many articles and books on writing groups in the health professions identify the challenges of writing itself: time (as in, perceived time[22]), self-confidence,[23] discipline, habit, poor preparation from prior educational experiences,[12] unfamiliarity with how to get published, and so on.[6,24] Race,[12,16,23,25] specialty, and specific dynamics of hospitals and other health organizations[26] may pose specific challenges that limit their members' ability to identify confidently as writers. Historically, women have faced this challenge for centuries and continue to struggle for professional equity in educational settings,[27] including medical schools where, ironically, women students now outnumber men.[28] Although women physicians' publications may actually exceed men's after mid-career, nevertheless, leadership and authorship in publication in the realm of medicine in particular remain firmly in men's hands[29,30] across many fields, including internationally.[31,32] The number of publications in the United States by women in cardiology, surgery, neurology, and even breast imaging radiology[33–36] continue to lag behind those by men at the same academic rank. In obstetrics and gynecology, where women now outnumber men in both faculty and residencies, women have taken the lead in first authorship, but they continue to lag in the seniority of last authorship.[37] In women-majority pediatrics, men continue to dominate the opinion-shaping key authorship of editorials and perspective pieces.[38]

Family medicine[15,39] and nursing[24,40–42] are both fields where academic departments identify the need for increased publications. Perhaps because both these fields focus on the caring relationship (rather than the power derived from science), these clinicians share the difficulty of finding their own sense of *authority* to write professionally. One particular challenge is that providers who have chosen to be clinically focused (including physicians, nurses, family therapists, or other kinds of psychotherapeutic clinicians) may not identify as researchers or writers and may face greater challenges to define their work as worthy of being written up. When they find themselves in an academic setting, they may struggle more with the requirement to publish when their own promotion or the promotion of their field within the institution depends on it. Likewise, faculty members in medically related fields including dentistry and pharmacy[11,20] face similar challenges when their advancement depends on publications. Individuals from less prestigious groups, such as nurses, including nurse practitioners, primary care physicians, physician assistants, and health-care professionals from underrepresented minorities may also be more self-critical and explicit about not feeling qualified to write, much less to publish.[8,12,13,16,23]

Emerging out of Johns Hopkins University, Writing Accountability Groups are specifically designed to counter the writing challenges encountered by health professionals. These groups, (informally known as WAGS), functioning with far more limited resources than the robust educational strategy of the Rochester course described earlier, are now becoming common-place in medical settings.[43] Their goal is explicit: the production of publications. The subtitle of Skarupski's book says it all: "Bootcamp for increasing scholarly productivity." The model demonstrates that time itself can be snatched—in small planned segments—from busy days and weeks, without getting up at the crack of dawn or burning the midnight oil. Sixty minutes once a week for 10 weeks at a convenient place and time in one's workweek does not seem too hard. At the opening of a WAG session, members spend 15 minutes sharing whether they met their goals from the previous week and what they plan to do during that writing session. They spend 30 minutes writing, and in the final 15 minutes, they share *when* they will write during the following week, with plans to reconvene the following week and report back. Realistic short writing sessions are recommended. This structured group strategy shows promise in promoting the frequency and duration of writing, especially for researchers committed to grant writing and generating publishable articles.[12]

Accountability in such writing groups has three aspects. First, it is built into the statements members make in their group about how they will use time in the moment and going forward for a week. A second aspect of accountability is the commitment—putting intention into words. That statement taps a deeper level of responsibility. People in the health professions are accustomed to following through with commitments and showing up when they have agreed to do so, lest they risk letting someone down. Really, in this case, they would be letting themselves down not to use the time as described, but verbalizing the commitment reinforces it. A third aspect of account-ability has to do with the relationships that develop. Something happens in a group when people talk about their writing, even briefly, together. Even a group of two, getting together as "writing buddies," serves the group function of accountability. Think of this as a parallel to consistent physi-cal exercise with a friend or group of friends. Candib[44] has called this phenomenon "writing-in-relation." This connection may be particularly useful for women health professionals, as it builds on culturally familiar patterns around responsibility and caring.

Not all groups pay explicit attention to the relational foundation of the writing that can be fostered in their setting, but the dynamic is undoubtedly in play anyway. Quite often, after several years of meeting, writing support groups have jointly published research articles on their degree of success with publication and on meeting members' professional needs for recognition.[10,15] In some groups, particularly those in settings where research is prioritized, members who might be fel-lows or residents gain support through collaboration on articles, sometimes splitting responsibility based on availability during certain challenging clinical months.[21] Most articles about long-running groups comment on the nonjudgmental support members gain that facilitates their writing, but they also expand on the way camaraderie, acceptance, appreciation, intellectual nourishment, and growth of mutual respect all play a role in how such groups work for the benefits of their mem-bers.[5,6,10] In articles on writing groups, much of the success, measured in numbers of publications, is attributed to this positive relational environment.

Apart from the "productivity" groups, or even at some of the productivity groups, health profes-sionals put forward "creative writing" because of their strong desire to express the powerful feelings and insights they experience from their work. Such contributions, which now garner some recog-nition academically within the medical humanities arena, would not have previously been consid-ered "professional" writing. Today, dozens of medical journals have a section for poetry, personal narratives of illness, and descriptions of authors' responses to clinical experiences. Admittedly, success in such writing does not capture big grants or propel promotion in obvious ways, but faculty or trainees winning poetry prizes garners prestige for departments, and students are drawn to faculty who foster the experiential aspect of their emerging professional identities. Family medicine may be particularly inclined to recognize this need because of the emphasis on the relational aspect of our work and our recognition of the need to foster the personhood of the doctor him-herself in the work. Writing groups may be able to play a role for health professionals in other health fields by providing support for writers whose projects may not be what is traditionally considered "professional" writing.

Our Teacherless Writing Group

On the initiative of one of the authors (LC), and with the support of the then-department chair (DL), our group convened in 2016–2017 as a Teacherless Writing Group in the spirit of Peter Elbow's *Writing Without Teachers*.[1] In most respects, our group follows Elbow's organizing scheme. Each writer may bring a piece of writing to share with the group, reads his or her work two times with silence in between, and then awaits commentary. Listeners are asked to provide feedback in a variety of ways, addressing primarily how the piece seemed to them, using "I statements." Elbow has very specific instructions for how listeners should provide this feedback and how authors should consider it. The group always includes a 12-minute period of free writing that allows time for people either to let flow whatever may be going on for them or to use the time to try to get to the kernel of something they have been chewing on. Many health-care professionals have severe internal editors; free writing can serve as one way to shut down that editor, at least temporarily, which can be very liberating. For this reason, our group, from its inception until the present, has included a short free writing period in every meeting, adapting another of Elbow's strategies for our professional needs.

Our group is now in its fourth year. It is composed of writers from the Department of Family Medicine and Community Health at every level of education and training beyond residency, as well as in various life stages: three now senior or emeritus/a (these faculty have adult children and are already grandparents); four with teenage children, mid-career; two with very young children, born since they joined the writing group. The group is now stretching to admit two family doctors, new to our department, just starting both their families and professional lives. Although the group started with professionals from a variety of health fields beyond medicine itself (behavioral health, social work, pharmacy), these members did not stay for the long term for individual reasons. Now, all but one are family doctors, including a hospitalist, a laborist (someone who works primarily on the labor/maternity floor), several at a federally funded community health center, others at the university-based family medicine or preventive medicine practices. One member of the group is active in preventive health research, and the majority have continuity primary care practices. The other member is a nonclinical medical geneticist with a career in medical editing. All write for themselves primarily, although several have worked on pieces that have ultimately been published over the course of the group's existence.

On the whole, our written work fits within narrative medicine, the term developed by Rita Charon, who founded the graduate program by the same name at Columbia University, a program for health-care professionals pursuing further education in how narrative informs work in the healing fields.[45] This genre has also been called "medical humanities," fostered by medical schools for the personal growth of medical students into physicians. The creative work by our predominantly clinical group of authors often draws inspiration from our medical practices, as well as at times from nature or personal life experiences. (See also Chapter 13.) While our group has not focused on polished products, some participants have used the group to receive feedback on specific pieces of writing they hope to submit for publication. Poetry and prose emerging from our group have been published in various electronic forums dedicated to medical writing.

After various attempts to meet at the hospital, our group settled on a weeknight dinnertime at a small Ethiopian restaurant. (During the pandemic, we met virtually.) We free write while waiting for the food to be prepared and then eat, followed by reading and responding. Elbow recommends a group size of 8, which requires about 2.5 hours, but our slightly smaller quorum usually meets for 2 hours. Night call and shift work in health care make a regular schedule difficult. People who all work in one institution may be able to build their group meetings into the beginning or end of the workday, but people coming from different locations, as we do, may have to identify a day and time that will work for the most people for each subsequent meeting. Likewise, the frequency of sessions will depend on the levels of professional and family commitments of prospective members. Elbow suggests that groups commit to weekly meetings for 12 weeks, but overnight call and small children make weekly meetings untenable for our physician members. We have settled on Tuesday evening meetings monthly, with the subsequent meeting date arranged at the end of each meeting or by an electronic poll.

Reflections of Group Members

To give an experiential sense of our Teacherless Writing Group for this chapter, members agreed to provide some individual reflections about the group's importance in their growth as writers and as doctors. As each member shared her/his own perspective, some common themes emerged. Members joined for their own reasons but came together to develop skills and to have a safe space that allowed vulnerability.

> There is a sense of respect for our shared vulnerability when we share our work. Writing is personal, and as such, sharing it means bearing a bit of our tender inner selves.
>
> (KB)

> Putting yourself forward, having a voice that can be heard.
>
> (DL)

> [T]he group itself is important to me. The connection and trust in each other is really what mattered to me.
>
> (JT)

> The goal of joining (the group) was to push past my vulnerabilities and be brave. What I have learned in time is that I am not alone, but also that I have more fears than I thought. The raw nature of sharing my writing is still incredibly challenging for me.
>
> (SP)

The common sense of vulnerability in the reflections of the individual members highlights how the writing group builds skills that enable writers to share more fully in this trusted environment. Trust takes time to build and having a stable core group of members has been critical to the development of the group.

The various stages in life and career of the members weave an intricate fabric of support similar to a multigenerational family serving different needs for each member. The relationships between the individuals in the group provide the support and safety that nurture our developing skills.

> It helps that I know and trust the members of our Department's writing group. Some have been my mentors for 20 years, some are friends and all are colleagues.... On one occasion, when [feedback] did not work well, the affected writer had the courage to bring her hurt to the group, and to share her writing again; I believe this made the group stronger and made us all more attentive to how we listen.
>
> (KB)

> I have been in the group since the start and enjoyed watching it grow and evolve into a committed group of attendees. Often, I do not have anything to read at our meetings, having pushed off writing in favor of other activities that take precedence. Nonetheless, I love hearing what my colleagues have written and value the discussions that veer towards process, origination, or context. My decision to attend each month is never based on if I have got something to share or not. With time, I have become more comfortable giving and receiving feedback.
>
> (LG)

> It was enlightening to meet with fellow faculty members at various points in our careers and realize that there are not such big differences between us. I appreciated that we all were self-conscious or struggled with self-expression at times, but decided to commit to be in the group together.
>
> (JT)

The support offered by members from different points in their career allows an openness to different perspectives. The common experiences provide reassurance about the importance of the writing and encourage dissemination. Our experience is consistent with the role of Teacherless Writing Groups as conceived of by Peter Elbow; he suggests that groups rely on the nonjudgmental support that members cherish from their colleagues.

The group allows for exploration of our writing in a different way from writing alone. Reflecting on the power of our group process of reading the piece twice, our members share,

> Reading a piece twice is a very powerful experience. As the listener, you hear the piece differently the second time; as the writer, you feel truly listened to and cared for.
>
> (KB)

> Reading it aloud (twice) helps me to consider where to work on next. I push myself to accept that this is not a final product I am sharing but an opportunity to get invaluable feedback and make my writing better. Reading my work aloud is so different from just sharing the text. Hearing myself share the writing aloud expands it for me also. I can find the cadence differently, and I can see where there are gaps that my mind might have been filling in when I read it silently.
>
> (SP)

The group process allows individual members to reflect on their experience with the reading. Hearing it twice, the listeners have slightly different experiences the second time through. Elbow's read-aloud strategy has been adopted in programs for advanced practice nurses as well.[46,47]

Questions raised through discussion of the writing provide valuable feedback and improve the final product and future writing.

Time for free writing during our meetings is another routine element. Our members have different views of this exercise:

> Interesting that free writing is the technique that is purported to be central to the writing group, and to getting people un-stuck with their writing. Maybe I have not given free writing enough credit, but for me, the free writing feels divorced from the process I go through when writing on my own. Free writing conjures the feeling of journal writing in middle school, just taking whatever is in my mind and putting it on paper, usually the events of the day, the good the bad the ugly, in whatever messy and stream-of-consciousness form they tumble on to the page. It conjures images of Dumbledore pulling a cottony memory from his temple and dropping it into a vial. But, different from the magical stored memories, what I put on paper during free writing is not writing that I return to, it is just a means of clearing the cobwebs.
>
> (KB)

> Free writing has given me an effective tool to use when I want to write but do not have any form or structure to my work. It also allows me to capture thoughts that have come into my head, and likely gone out again just as quickly. It is a form of muscular and cognitive training similar to the gym or Scrabble. It also allows me to capture bits of a bigger story I have been writing over time.
>
> (LG)

> Free writing allows me to commit to just writing without editing. The practice of keeping the pen moving warms those writing muscles and prevents my inner critic from paralyzing my thinking. Free writing allows freedom, I can skip over a word I cannot think of, I can move on from a thought that meets a dead end. I know that no one will hear it, no one will see it. I know that it is just allowing me to practice getting the ideas out on paper.
>
> (SP)

Free writing plays an important role in our writing group process. Though it is used differently by individual members, each finds it useful. Although we free write as individuals, doing the activity during group time with a common timer running creates a sense of accountability and togetherness in the work.

Although all members feel that the group encourages them to write more, academic productivity has not been a focus or stated goal of the group. Our members have varied experiences with the group's impact on their productivity.

> I cannot say the group has gotten me motivated to expand my writing toward more scholarly efforts, as I largely write as a creative outlet. I appreciate that there are no set goals for our group, particularly related to output or publication. For me, this is a more comfortable place as creative/narrative writing is an adjunct to my work, not a primary function or focus of my work.
>
> (LG)

> The writing group stimulates me to think about broadening the scope of my academic writing by putting writing and editing at the forefront of my mind. It commits time and helps the

writing muscles practice. I am a runner. I know that it will hurt to run if I have not done it in a while. It will be harder than when I get into a rhythm. If I think about the "writing muscles" needing regular exercise, it makes sense to build it into my regular schedule. The writing group helps to do that, even if I am sharing narrative at the group, the academic writing will come more easily.

(SP)

My enjoyment of academic research and writing has also flourished during this time. I now write with much greater capacity since I joined the group. It helped me overcome occasional writing paralysis, as coming to the group with a piece felt better than showing up with nothing to share. Free writing was a wonderful tool for me to create a starting point for writing, even if it was a pitiful one. The group has helped me to be a more productive writer, even though what I bring to the writing group has no relation to my academic writing. In fact, I usually write poetry about my dogs, nature or (now) my son.

(JT)

The scheduled writing group gives members a structure to think about writing, write, and share their work. It encourages more frequent writing and serves to make writing more comfortable.

One member had been our department chairperson for more than two decades. Despite his historic leadership position, he sits in the group as an equal member. The group has been important to him and his reflections echo those provided earlier. He additionally provided a reflection on his experience as a leader demonstrating the importance of the writing group in a formula for department success.

From my perspective as a former Department Chair, there are several reasons to provide a Teacherless Writing Group for the faculty. First, participation in a TWG improves one's writing, as well as one's comfort with the process of writing. Second, group involvement provides a starting point for written materials that progress to presentation and/or publication. Third, participation in a group serves as a source of emotional support: Writing and sharing provide an outlet for stress and anxiety. Participants have written about long and difficult days, working within highly stressful environments, responding to loss, grief and trauma. During the COVID pandemic, participants wrote about waiting for their own test results and fears of serving as a vector for patients or families.

Writing helps experienced clinicians reflect and gain insight about their patients. Sharing their thoughts provides comfort for others as they listen to stories about members' experiences with patients, with their careers, and with being doctors. It is heartwarming to recognize that members come to an evening meeting of the TWG even if they have not found the time to write since the last meeting. Being present with other doctors writing and reading their writing is a way of helping oneself become a better doctor.

The narrow definition of writing as an academic purs+2 uit—writing for publication—is inadequate for the skill set required of today's clinical educator. Activities like a TWG can help faculty members to serve as role models for clinical documentation, teaching, publication, advocacy and narrative writing, while they gain personal and emotional support from the group.

(DL)

Having a respected leader as a member of our group serves to support the group in a unique way. His writings reveal his own vulnerabilities and identity as a family physician in ways that we would not otherwise see. His humble engagement with other members' writings provided a perspective of experience, as well as conveying respect for members of the department. His unpressured support of the group, as well as his engagement with it, was a foundational and encouraging component to the group's formation and ongoing success.

For our group of medical writers, implicit in our work is an understanding that writing is a direct, accessible way to reflection. One step removed, we recognize that such reflection is key to professional development,[48] a kind of development that is not measured by productivity. Writing helps us know what we think; it is an avenue into reflection about what we do and how we experience it. Health-care work makes serious demands on people; our writing group offers us the possibility to expand our human capacity, as persons and as doctors. Writing and reflecting together in a group involved in parallel work builds a small community of peers with whom we can redress our misgivings about our ability to write and share the joys and sorrows of the work—as well as those successes when our written work is recognized in the broader forums of health care. Over the more than 3 years of its existence, the overall sense of our writing group is that the support of the group encouraged more writing and allowed the strengthening of our writing skills, including sharing our work, despite our vulnerability, and accepting each other's responses.

Implications for Practice

For educators interested in the practical aspects of starting a Teacherless Writing Group, the first step is to read Peter Elbow's book *Writing Without Teachers*. With his instructions clear in mind, the next step is to recruit potential members who can commit to a longitudinal group process for writing. Calling it "teacherless" means that it is not a passive class and that each participant is in charge of their own learning. The organizer is not the teacher. Having some official blessing from a senior faculty or administrator, as we did, may be helpful in certain settings. Once people are recruited, and before they assemble, the key step is that they too read Elbow's book. The initiator of our group (LC) gave every participant a copy of the book (available secondhand online for only postage) and asked each person to read at least Chapter 4 on reading and responding in the group. Peter Elbow's recommendations about how to read one's work to others and how to respond to others' work are foundational in setting up a thoughtful and supportive setting for both writers and responders who will soon be in the other position. It also helps if members read Elbow's work on free writing (in other chapters) as a strategy for getting into their own writing with fewer struggles, to reinforce the value of free writing as a strategy and as a part of the group process. Having consistent membership, longevity, and demonstrating careful listening have all helped foster a sense of trust, which has been foundational to allowing members to share vulnerability and give and receive feedback. Meeting in a small restaurant has also been key: it creates a sense of community, enjoyment, ritual (eating *and* writing together), and removes us from the intrinsically time-pressured and judgment-prone setting of our primary work.

Different kinds of writing groups have different formats, may have some internal hierarchies, and may serve specific professional purposes depending on career stage and setting (academic or not). It is clear that dedicated "productivity" groups or "writing accountability groups" can have a significant impact on writing confidence and publication rates for group members who enter the group process with specific goals. Nevertheless, underlying the contrasting goals of increased publication for some groups versus mutual support and reflection for others, all writing groups that prosper share certain commonalities: an ongoing commitment emerging from an inherent sense— as health-care professionals—of responsibility toward and for others; some form of accountability among group members; changes in writing practices (such as free writing and use of short writing times); the building of trust among the group members, enabling them to show vulnerability; a freeing up from internal self-criticism and paralysis; and, over time, a deepening sense of human connection. These values are a continuing source of sustenance to our members, and we expect that other groups would find this energy sustaining as well.

References

1. Elbow P. *Writing without Teachers*. New York: Oxford University Press; 1973.
2. Galipeau J, Moher D, Campbell C, et al. A systematic review highlights a knowledge gap regarding the effectiveness of health-related training programs in journalology. *J Clin Epidemiol*. 2015;68(3):257–265.
3. Silvia PJ. *How to Write a Lot: A Practical Guide to Productive Academic Writing*. 2nd ed. Washington, D.C.: American Psychological Association, 2019.
4. Gere AR. *Writing Groups: History, Theory, and Implications*. Carbondale and Edwardsville: Souther Illinois University Press; 1987.
5. Piercy FP, Sprenkle DH, McDaniel SH. Teaching professional writing to family therapists: three approaches. *J Marital Fam Ther*. 1996;22(2):163–179.
6. Steinert Y, McLeod PJ, Liben S, Snell L. Writing for publication in medical education: the benefits of a faculty development workshop and peer writing group. *Med Teach*. 2008;30(8):e280–e285.
7. Files JA, Blair JE, Mayer AP, Ko MG. Facilitated peer mentorship: a pilot program for academic advancement of female medical faculty. *J Women Health*. 2008;17(6):1009–1015.
8. Jackson D. Mentored residential writing retreats: a leadership strategy to develop skills and generate outcomes in writing for publication. *Nurse Educ Today*. 2009;29(1):9–15.
9. Klimas J. Optimizing writing schemes for addiction researchers. *J Subst Use*. 2017;22(4):454–456.
10. Kulage KM, Larson EL. Implementation and outcomes of a faculty-based, peer review manuscript writing workshop. *J Prof Nurs*. 2016;32(4):262–270.
11. Oakley M, Vieira AR. The endangered clinical teacher-scholar: a promising update from one dental school. *J Dent Educ*. 2012;76(4):454–460.
12. Thorpe RJ, Jr., Beech BM, Norris KC, Heitman E, Bruce MA. Writing accountability groups are a tool for academic success: the obesity health disparities PRIDE program. *Ethn Dis*. 2020;30(2):295–304.
13. Brandon C, Jamadar D, Girish G, Dong Q, Morag Y, Mullan P. Peer support of a faculty "writers' circle" increases confidence and productivity in generating scholarship. *Acad Radiol*. 2015;22(4):534–538.
14. Chai PR, Carreiro S, Carey JL, Boyle KL, Chapman BP, Boyer EW. Faculty member writing groups support productivity. *Clin Teach*. 2019;16(6):565–569.
15. Grzybowski SC, Bates J, Calam B, et al. A physician peer support writing group. *Fam Med*. 2003;35(3):195–201.
16. Martinez MA, Alsandor DJ, Cortez LJ, Welton AD, Chang A. We are stronger together: reflective testimonios of female scholars of color in a research and writing collective. *Reflective Pract*. 2015;16(1):85–95.
17. Salas-Lopez D, Deitrick L, Mahady ET, Moser K, Gertner EJ, Sabino JN. Getting published in an academic-community hospital: the success of writing groups. *J Gen Intern Med*. 2012;27(1):113–116.
18. Van Schyndel JL, Koontz S, McPherson S, et al. Faculty support for a culture of scholarship of discovery: a literature review. *J Prof Nurs*. 2019;35(6):480–490.
19. Bodenberg MM, Nichols K. Time for an "upgrade": how incorporating social habits can further boost your writing potential. *Curr Pharm Teach Learn*. 2019;11(11):1077–1082.
20. Franks AM. Design and evaluation of a longitudinal faculty development program to advance scholarly writing among pharmacy practice faculty. *Am J Pharm Educ*. 2018;82(6):6556.
21. Lukolyo H, Keating EM, Rees CA. Creating a collaborative peer writing group during residency. *Med Educ Online*. 2019;24(1):1563421.
22. Candib LM. Making time to write? *Ann Fam Med*. 2005;3:365–366.
23. Sonnad SS, Goldsack J, McGowan KL. A writing group for female assistant professors. *J Natl Med Assoc*. 2011;103(9):811–815.

24. Rickard CM, McGrail MR, Jones R, et al. Supporting academic publication: evaluation of a writing course combined with writers' support group. *Nurse Educ Today*. 2009;29(5):516–521.

25. Wilmot K, McKenna S. Writing groups as transformative spaces. *High Educ Res Dev*. 2018;37(4):868–882.

26. Yancey NR. The challenge of writing for publication: implications for teaching-learning nursing. *Nurs Sci Q*. 2016;29(4):277–282.

27. Chen ST, Jalal S, Ahmadi M, et al. Influences for gender disparity in academic family medicine in North American medical schools. *Cureus*. 2020;12(5):e8368.

28. AAMC AAoMC. The majority of U.S. medical students are women, new data show. December 9, 2019. https://www.aamc.org/news-insights/press-releases/majority-us-medical-students-are-women-new-data-show

29. Reed DA, Enders F, Lindor R, McClees M, Lindor KD. Gender differences in academic productivity and leadership appointments of physicians throughout academic careers. *Acad Med*. 2011;86(1):43–47.

30. Nocco SE, Larson AR. Promotion of women physicians in academic medicine. *J Women Health*. 2020;14:14.

31. Fridner A, Norell A, Akesson G, Gustafsson Senden M, Tevik Lovseth L, Schenck-Gustafsson K. Possible reasons why female physicians publish fewer scientific articles than male physicians—a cross-sectional study. *BMC Med Educ*. 2015;15:67.

32. Chauvin S, Mulsant BH, Sockalingam S, Stergiopoulos V, Taylor VH, Vigod SN. Gender differences in research productivity among academic psychiatrists in Canada. *Can J Psychiatry*. 2019;64(6):415–422.

33. Blumenthal DM, Olenski AR, Yeh RW, et al. Sex differences in faculty rank among academic cardiologists in the United States. *Circulation*. 2017;135(6):506–517.

34. Mueller C, Wright R, S G. The publication gender gap in US academic surgery. *BMC Surg*. 2017;17(1):16.

35. McDermott M, Gelb D, Wilson K, et al. Sex differences in academic rank and publication rate at top-ranked US neurology programs. *AMA Neurol*. 2018;75(8):956–961.

36. Khurshid K, Shah S, Ahmadi M, et al. Gender differences in the publication rate among breast imaging radiologists in the United States and Canada. *AJR Am J Roentgenol*. 2018;210(1):2–7.

37. Metheny W, Jagadish M, Heidel R, et al. A 15-year study of trends in authorship by gender in two U.S. obstetrics and gynecology journals. *Obstet Gynecol*. 2018;131(4):696–699.

38. Silver J, Poorman J, Reilly J, Spector N, Goldstein R, Zafonte R. Assessment of women physicians among authors of perspective-type articles published in high-impact pediatric journals. *JAMA Netw Open*. 2018;1(3):e180802.

39. Sommers PS, Muller JH, Bailiff PJ, Stephens GG. Writing for publication: a workshop to prepare faculty as medical writers. *Fam Med*. 1996;28(9):650–654.

40. Sanderson BK, Carter M, Schuessler JB. Writing for publication: faculty development initiative using social learning theory. *Nurse Educ*. 2012;37(5):206–210.

41. Thomas SP. Nurturing the novice writers in psychiatric-mental health nursing. *Issues Ment Health Nurs*. 2017;38(9):685–686.

42. Shellenbarger T, Gazza EA. The lived experience of nursing faculty developing as scholarly writers. *J Prof Nurs*. 2020;36(6):520–525.

43. Skarupski KA. *WAG your Work—Writing Accountability Groups: Bootcamp for Increasing Scholarly Prouctivity*. Columbia, South Carolina: WAGYourWork.com; 2018.

44. Candib LM. Writing troubles for women clinicians: turning weakness into strength using writing-in-relation. *Fam Syst Health*. 2006;24:302–317.

45. Narrative Medicine. https://sps.columbia.edu/academics/masters/narrative-medicine. Published 2020. Accessed May 23, 2020.

46. Rohan A, Fullerton J. Effects of a programme to advance scholarly writing. *Clin Teach*. 2019;16(6):580–584.

47. Rohan A, Fullerton J. Developing advanced practice nurse writing competencies as a corequisite for evidence-based practice. *J Am Assoc Nurse Pract*. 2020;32(10):682–688.

48. Mann K, Gordon J, MacLeod A. Reflection and reflective practice in health professions education: a systematic review. *Adv Health Sci Educ* 2009;14(4):595–621.

Conclusion

THE "PROGNOSIS" OF WRITING IN THE HEALTH PROFESSIONS

Michael J. Madson

The contributors have covered a lot of ground, sharing experiences as teachers, course designers, scholars, and writers. While each of their chapters has offered distinct perspectives, we share the purpose of strengthening the emergent interdiscipline of "writing in the health professions" practically and advancing it conceptually. No collection, of course, can represent every health profession or genre, and thus, we had to be selective. In this collection, we chose to make our main focuses (1) clinical, reflective, and scholarly writing; (2) instruction tailored to current and future health professionals; and (3) graduate and professional settings. These, we believe, are areas of significant need, and we hope that the chapters provide helpful instructional models, supporting faculty development.

In the four parts, each chapter concluded with practical takeaways for teachers or administrators. This final chapter turns the discussion more fully to scholarship, outlining several overlapping possibilities for future study.

Health Professions and Genres

Maintained by the US Department of Labor Statistics, the *Occupational Outlook Handbook* reports data on more than 40 health professions, which span from athletic training and audiology to veterinary technology.[1] The International Standard Classification of Occupations (2008 revision) recognizes a similar number.[2] The majority of these health professions have received little attention from writing researchers, creating wide gaps in "writing in the health professions" literature.

In recent years, instructional scholarship on writing has become more visible in public health,[3–8] social work,[9–14] pharmacy,[15–20] and dentistry, among other health professions.[21–25] Still, the lion's share likely belongs to nursing and medicine, where there remains much work to be done. In 1988, Yanoff and Burg observed that the genres of medicine "have never been comprehensively classified and analyzed. Many types are taken for granted, although some, particularly the published kinds, are acknowledged as difficult for physician–writers."[26(p35)] This observation appears no less valid today. Although comprehensive classification and analysis is a lofty goal, additional scholarship on health professions genres, medicine certainly included, can enhance the teaching of writing. These genres may include mutt genres[27] and intermediary genres,[28] which Lillian Campbell illuminated, as well as genre sets, systems, repertoires, and ecologies.[29]

As Kathryn West and Brian Callender showed, genres are more than words. They can also be highly visual, and future studies might evaluate how visual literacy is taught in the health professions.

DOI: 10.4324/9781003162940-20

Places

"Writing in the health professions," as an emergent interdiscipline, needs broader coverage of the places where writing is done. Institutionally, these places include not just classrooms but also out-patient surgical facilities, blood banks, medical laboratories, insurance offices, and hospice homes. They include centers specializing in radiology and imaging, dialysis, diabetes education, physical rehabilitation, and addiction treatment, to name only a few. In the collection, Susan E. Thomas analyzed how staff members communicate at an integrative cancer treatment center, fleshing out tensions in the notion of patient-centered care. Elizabeth L. Angeli reported her efforts to create data-driven writing curricula for fire cadets, applying ideas from numerous bodies of scholarship: writing across the curriculum, writing in the disciplines, technical communication, first-year writing, workplace learning and adult education, situated learning, and community engagement. Given their richness, these chapters may serve as a springboard for further institutional research.

Geographically, writing scholars have highlighted instructional practices in China, Croatia, the Netherlands, Iran, and Japan,[30] as well as Latin America, where the interdiscipline is "barely emerging" according to Elizabeth Narváez-Cardona and Pilar Mirely Chois-Lenis. Future studies should give special attention to regions where health-care systems are facing alarming shortages in staff, exploring how writing instruction may assuage burnout, increase facility efficiency, and prepare the next cohort of health professionals.

Languages

The collection has focused on English language writing, reflecting international trends in scientific and medical publishing. Salager-Meyer[31] noted that by the year 2000, journals in medicine, nursing, and dentistry were already publishing more than ten million peer-reviewed papers annually. Of these, over 80% were written in English. Succumbing to pressure, journals that originally published in national languages have switched to English, such as the *Croatian Medical Journal*, *Mexican Medical Journal*, and *Saratov Journal of Medical Scientific Research*, which had started as a Russian language publication.[31]

In the Francophonie, questions linger over the status of French language journals, which have come to a crossroads: "Are they going to become vehicles of teaching, of popularization, of liaison between members of medical societies, of general public information contributing to decision-making in the field of public health? Or will they maintain their scientific status?"[32(p475)] The answers will impact writing instruction, especially at graduate and professional levels.

Amid these trends, many second language writers publish scholarship in English, including several of the contributors here. Thus, future studies should examine, in greater detail, how health professionals attain advanced proficiency in English as a second or foreign language, how they overcome barriers in the research and publication process, and how institutions can provide effective assistance, which may include editing, statistical, and bibliographic services. Questions like these fall within the orbits of second language writing, English for medical purposes, and related bodies of scholarship. (Though a mouthful, "second language writing in the health professions" would be a significant development.)

Future studies should not be limited to the English language. Scholarship is needed on additional languages, including translation.

The Third (and Fourth) Industrial Revolutions

The third industrial revolution, centering on digital technologies, has had a deep influence on writing instruction, and several chapter contributors have highlighted online and hybrid formats. In their chapter, Isabell C. May and Emilie M. Ludeman referred readers to Quality Matters, a framework developed by the MarylandOnline consortium.[33] In addition, readers may benefit from the *Position Statement of Principles and Example Effective Practices for Online Writing Instruction*, which was commissioned by a leading organization for writing teachers.[34] Frameworks like these can guide scholarship that investigates the affordances and challenges of teaching writing in digital spaces.

Future scholarship should also parse how writing instruction in digital spaces affects writers themselves, including their professional identity formation. Empathy, in particular, is a critical attribute of health professionals across specialties, and studies have begun to explore "digital empathy": caring and concern for others that is expressed through computer-mediated communication.[35] As in offline settings, reflective writing online can likely promote empathy, along with clinical judgment, critical thinking, leadership, and observational skills, but more data are needed.[36]

Questions of professional identity may assume even greater importance during the current industrial revolution, the fourth. In the typical, elevated rhetoric of futurisms, Schwab has stated,

> The Fourth Industrial Revolution…will change not only what we do but also who we are. It will affect our identity and all the issues associated with it: our sense of privacy, our notions of ownership, our consumption patterns, the time we devote to work and leisure, and how we develop our careers, cultivate our skills, meet people, and nurture relationships. It is already changing our health and leading to a "quantified" self, and sooner than we think it may lead to human augmentation.[37]

This is because the fourth industrial revolution involves a fusion of physical, digital, and biological spaces, making it all the more personal. As yet, cutting-edge technologies have had little discernable impact on the practices of medical writing and editing, according to the survey study by Rebecca Day Babcock and her colleagues. But things may be different in the near future.

Theories and Methods

The aforementioned research areas will require a wide array of theories and methods.

Theories

Several contributors illustrated the usefulness of adapting theories that originated in other fields. Threshold concepts are a good example, appearing in two chapters in the nursing section. As Deborah E. Tyndall explained, threshold concepts originated in engineering, and they have since been applied in writing studies and nursing education. Through threshold concepts, we can better understand how health professions students and trainees grow as writers, attending to "liminal spaces" where they can get stuck.

A long-standing concern in "writing in the health professions" is materiality, the physical properties tangled up in the processes and artifacts of writing. For instance, a well-regarded textbook from the mid-nineteenth century advised readers that, when writing a prescription, the "first care" is to use the proper materials: sturdy paper and a pencil, if not an ink pen. The textbook further counseled against the bad habit of writing prescriptions on a scrap of newspaper, the flyleaf of a schoolbook, or another flimsy material, which indicates profound carelessness.[38(p575)]

Lingard points to a more contemporary example: the booking sheet for a hospital's operating room. How, Lingard asks, does the booking sheet shape the surgical team's communication strategies? How might a miswritten booking affect the team? To better account for materialities like these, she recommends an alliance between genre theory, activity theory, and actor-network theory.[39] While her recommendation is an intriguing one, there are additional possibilities. It may be useful to incorporate linguistic landscaping[40–42] and geosemiotics,[43] which theorize writing displayed in public, such as clinic signage. There is also immense potential in sociocultural theories.

More broadly, theoretical work can create crosswalks between disciplines, as Kenzie and McCall showed. These authors developed an undergraduate writing course ("writing for the health professions") informed by the rhetoric of health and medicine, the medical humanities, and disability studies. In their descriptions, they explained how the three disciplines have appreciable differences but also complement each other. For example, the medical humanities supply "attention and institutional space needed to make change," while disability studies fosters a "critical consciousness," helping ensure that "the change serves the needs of disabled patients and patients in general."[44(p66)]

The emergent interdiscipline of writing in the health professions should not build toward a grand, unifying theory. But it should facilitate innovation and collaboration across specialties, drawing on the spirit of interprofessional education.

Methods

The chapters in the collection exhibited a range of quantitative and qualitative research methods, such as participant observations, interviews, surveys, content analysis, and narrative phenomenological analyses. Writing researchers should continue to refine these methods while seeking to expand their methodological repertoires. To these ends, big data and user experience (UX) seem particularly promising.

Big Data

The amount of writing produced in health-care workplaces and training programs is truly immense, and available data will continue to proliferate, spurred by technologies characteristic of the third and fourth industrial revolutions. In the field of education, researchers have used "big data" methods (such as data clustering, modeling, and prediction) to gauge the effectiveness of administrative' decisions, gain insights into students' self-regulated learning, deliver early warnings to students at risk of dropping out, and evaluate class assignments.[45] In the young discipline of writing analytics, researchers have used big data methods to analyze how students construct identities in writing,[46] gauge students' motivation and self-efficacy,[47] and assess writing programs.[48] As well, big data methods may identify more linguistic attributes that suggest a writer's growth;[49] help instructors reflect on their feedback practices,[50,51] which typically require them to "triage" between various concerns;[52] and clarify the features of genres that students and trainees need to produce, perhaps mixing statistical analysis with qualitative coding.[53] Big data methods have considerable potential to enrich writing instruction in the health professions.

UX

UX professionals strive to understand how users *experience* a particular product, service, interaction, environment, or piece of writing. They then work to minimize the "friction" between what users want to achieve and the tools they implement to complete that task.[54(p4)] In these efforts, UX professionals may deploy flexible, iterative methods, such as contextual inquiry, usability tests, A/B tests, listening tours, heuristic analyses, questionnaires, and black hat sessions.[54] An abundance of methodological resources are available online.

Researchers in the health professions have already adopted UX methods to a limited extent, with studies favoring technology development.[e.g.,55–58] Yet these methods have more expansive uses and may be particularly helpful in the design of patient education materials, paper or digital. For instance, researchers might survey patients to learn how satisfied they are with the current materials, identifying "pain points": specific problems that are arising. Based on these insights, the researchers can generate ideas for improvement, create prototypes of new materials, and return to the patients for feedback. To elicit feedback, they might record patients' first impressions of the new materials, observe how patients complete a series of key tasks, and ask patients more about their likes and dislikes in focus interviews. The researchers might then return to the drawing board, the cycle repeating until an optimal solution is reached. Since UX methods are cyclical and patient centered, they align well with quality improvement frameworks in health care,[59] such as Plan-Do-Study-Act.

Multidirectional Knowledge Transfer

Knowledge transfer should not be unidirectional, and as an emergent interdiscipline, writing in the health professions can contribute to other disciplines. As an example, Ariail and Smith adapted concept analysis, a method that is commonly assigned in nursing coursework and that, moreover, can appear in peer-reviewed journal articles. Following a similar procedure as their students, these authors extracted layers of meaning surrounding the concept *helping* in rhetoric and composition.[60]

Diversity, Equity, and Inclusion

Diversity, equity, and inclusion are vital in the health professions, helping providers meet the care needs of local patients and populations, promoting the success of early career colleagues, and fostering innovation across specialties.[61] In this collection, Cristina Reyes Smith discussed how reflective writing can contribute to cultural competence, supplying examples from an interprofessional elective course. Future studies should delve deeper into this area, identifying and validating more principles for best practice. In addition, future studies should explore how writing instruction can aid the study of complex, challenging issues, such as racial microaggressions, implicit bias, and health disparities,[61] as well as other systemic injustices. In these efforts, it may be helpful to consider both identity diversity (race, ethnicity, gender, ableness, sexual orientation, etc.) and cognitive diversity (biases, opinions, etc.).[62] The purpose should be to ensure the safety, dignity, and respect of all health professionals and those they serve. To these ends, Amayo et al. have proposed "twelve tips for inclusive teaching," which can be applied and analyzed in additional contexts.[63]

The areas above are only a few possibilities, and we hope that instructional scholarship on writing will advance in additional directions. Among other reasons, this work matters because it enables evidence-based practice, supporting health professions educators and writing specialists alike. We thus encourage a synergy of intraprofessional and interprofessional approaches, as contributors to this collection have modeled. That is, we should address the instructional needs in our own disciplines, as well as collaborate across institutional silos, adapt ideas from outside traditions, share results broadly, and work toward a culture of solidary in "writing in the health professions," which we have called an emergent interdiscipline: It is emergent because of its rapid expansion yet peripheral status. It is an interdiscipline because of its many connections to existing bodies of literature and associations of students, teachers, scholars, and clinicians. Ultimately, we hope this collection will lay foundation stones for future work, building, in time, not just knowledge and practices but also community.

References

1. US Bureau of Labor Statistics: Occupational Outlook Handbook. Healthcare occupations. https://www.bls.gov/ooh/healthcare/home.htm. Accessed April 18, 2021.
2. World Health Organization. Classifying health workers: mapping occupations to the international standard classification. https://www.who.int/hrh/statistics/Health_workers_classification.pdf. Accessed April 18, 2021.

3. Beard J, Monteiro R, Price-Oreyomi MB, Edouard VB, Murphy-Phillips M. Lessons learned from a peer writing coach program in a school of public health. *Public Health Rep.* 2020;135(5):700–7.

4. Valladares LM, Riegelman RK, Albertine S. Writing in public health: a new program from the Association of Schools and Programs of Public Health. *Public Health Rep.* 2019;134(1):94–97.

5. August E, Burke K, Fleischer C, Trostle JA. Writing assignments in epidemiology courses: how many and how good? *Public Health Reports.* 2019;134(4):441–446.

6. Mackenzie SL. Writing for public health: strategies for teaching writing in a school or program of public health. *Public Health Reports.* 2018;133(5):614–618.

7. Guerin C, Xafis V, Doda DV, Gillam MH, Larg AJ, Luckner H, Jahan N, Widayati A, Xu C. Diversity in collaborative research communities: a multicultural, multidisciplinary thesis writing group in public health. *Stud High Educ.* 2013;35(1):65–81.

8. Guerin C, Xafis V, Doda DV, Gillam MH, Larg AJ, Luckner H, Jahan N, Widayati A, Xu C. Diversity in collaborative research communities: a multicultural, multidisciplinary thesis writing group in public health. *Stud High Educ.* 2013;35(1):65–81.

9. Capous-Desyllas M, Bromfield NF, Nava A, Barnes B. Teaching note—strategies for enhancing writing among first-generation social work students: reflections on the use of peer writing mentors. *J Soc Work Educ.* 2021;57(1):189–196.

10. Chen X, Cheung M, Zhou S, Leung P, Glaude M. Reflections on social work doctoral pedagogy: a reciprocal approach to enhancing preparation for the academy. *J Teach Soc Work.* 2020;40(4):385–401.

11. Mirick RG. Teaching note—online peer review: students' experiences in a writing-intensive BSW course. *J Soc Work Educ.* 2020;56(2):394–400.

12. Mandell D, Shalan H, Stalker C, Caragata L. Writing for publication: assessment of a course for social work doctoral students. *J Teach Soc Work.* 2015;35(1–2):197–212.

13. Davis A. Journaling together: The antiracism project in social work doctoral education. *Smith College Studies in Social Work.* 2016;86(4):355–376.

14. Horton EG, Diaz N. Learning to write and writing to learn social work concepts: application of writing across the curriculum strategies and techniques to a course for undergraduate social work students. *J Teach Soc Work.* 2011;31(1):53–64.

15. Nazar H, Rathbone A, Husband A. The development of undergraduate pharmacy students as reflective thinkers for the evolving field of pharmacy. *Int J Pharm Pract.* 2021. https://doi.org/10.1093/ijpp/riab005

16. Kodweis K, Schimmelfing LC, Yang Y, Persky AM. Methods for optimizing student pharmacist learning of clinical note writing. *Am J Pharm Educ.* 2021;85(2):144–151.

17. Wale BD, Bogale YN. Using inquiry-based writing instruction to develop students' academic writing skills. *Asian-Pacific J Second Foreign Lang Educ.* 2021;6(1):1–6.

18. Hughes JA, Cleven AJ, Ross J, Fuentes DG, Elbarbry F, Suzuki M, Della Paolera M, Carter NS, Stamper B, Low P, Malhotra A. A comprehensive reflective journal-writing framework for pharmacy students to increase self-awareness and develop actionable goals. *Am J Pharm Educ.* 2019;83(3):312–322.

19. Andrus MR, McDonough SL, Kelley KW, Stamm PL, McCoy EK, Lisenby KM, Whitley HP, Slater N, Carroll DG, Hester EK, Helmer AM. Development and validation of a rubric to evaluate diabetes SOAP note writing in APPE. *Am J Pharm Educ.* 2018;82(9):1045–1050.

20. Sharif SI, Ibrahim R. Improving and assessing writing skills and practices of pharmacy students. *J Pharma Care Health Sys.* 2014;1:e105.

21. Bowman M. A framework for scaffolding academic reflective writing in dentistry. *Eur J Dent Educ.* 2021;25(1):35–49.

22. Gadbury-Amyot CC, Godley LW, Nelson Jr JW. Measuring the level of reflective ability of predoctoral dental students: early outcomes in an e-portfolio reflection. *J Dent Educ.* 2019;83(3):275–280.

23. Crosthwaite P, Cheung L, Jiang FK. Writing with attitude: stance expression in learner and professional dentistry research reports. *English for Specific Purposes.* 2017;46:107–123.

24. El Tantawi M, Sadaf S, AlHumaid J. Using gamification to develop academic writing skills in dental undergraduate students. *Eur J Dent Educ.* 2018;22(1):15–22.

25. Vergnes JN, Apelian N, Bedos C. What about narrative dentistry? *J Am Dent Assoi.* 2015;146(6):398–401.

26. Yanoff KL, Burg FD. Types of medical writing and teaching of writing in US medical schools. *J Med Educ.* 1988;63(1):30–37.

27. Wardle E. "Mutt genres" and the goal of FYC: can we help students write the genres of the university? *College Comp Commun.* 2009;60(4):765–789.

28. Tachino T. Theorizing uptake and knowledge mobilization: a case for intermediary genre. *Written Commun.* 2012;29(4):455–476.

29. Spinuzzi C. *Four ways to investigate assemblages of texts: Genre sets, systems, repertoires, and ecologies.* In: *Proceedings of the 22nd Annual International Conference on Design of Communication: The Engineering of Quality Documentation.* 2004 October 10: 110–116.

30. Vasconcelos SM, Wu W, Ivanis A, Hull E, Handjani F, Barron JP, Salager-Meyer F. Around the world: Teaching medical writing to doctors and scientists. *The Write Stuff.* 2007;16(1):12–15.

31. Salager-Meyer F. Origin and development of English for medical purposes. Part II: research on spoken medical English. *Med Writing.* 2014;23(2):129–131.

32. Laccourreye O, Maisonneuve H. French scientific medical journals confronted by developments in medical writing and the transformation of the medical press. *Eur Ann Otorhinolaryngol Head Neck Dis.* 2019;136(6):475–480.

33. Quality Matters. https://www.qualitymatters.org/. Accessed April 18, 2021.

34. Conference on College Composition and Communication. A position statement of principles and example effective practices for online writing instruction (OWI). https://cccc.ncte.org/cccc/resources/positions/owiprinciples. Accessed April 18, 2021.

35. Terry C, Cain J. The emerging issue of digital empathy. *Am J Pharm Educ.* 2016;80(4): Article 58.

36. Bleakley A. *Medical humanities and medical education: how the medical humanities can shape better doctors.* London: Routledge; 2015.

37. Schwab K. The fourth industrial revolution: what it means, how to respond. https://www.weforum.org/agenda/2016/01/the-fourth-industrial-revolution-what-it-means-and-how-to-respond/. Accessed April 17, 2021.

38. Parrish E. *An Introduction to Practical Pharmacy: Designed as a Text-book for the Student, and as a Guide to the Physician and Pharmaceutist, with Many Formulas and Prescriptions.* Blanchard & Lea; 1859.

39. Lingard L. The rhetorical 'turn' in medical education: what have we learned and where are we going? *Adv Health Sci Educ Theory Pract.* 2007;12(2):121–133.

40. Gorter D. Introduction: The study of the linguistic landscape as a new approach to multilingualism. *Int J Multiling.* 2006;3(1):1–6.

41. Gorter D, editor. *Linguistic Landscape: A New Approach to Multilingualism.* Multilingual Matters; 2006.

42. Shohamy E, Gorter D, editors. *Linguistic Landscape: Expanding the Scenery.* Routledge; May 15, 2008.

43. Scollon R, Scollon SW. *Discourses in Place: Language in the Material World.* Routledge; December 8, 2003.

44. Kenzie D, McCall M. Teaching writing for the health professions: disciplinary intersections and pedagogical practice. *Tech Commun Quart.* 2018;27(1):64–79.

45. Fischer C, Pardos ZA, Baker RS, Williams JJ, Smyth P, Yu R, Slater S, Baker R, Warschauer M. Mining big data in education: affordances and challenges. *Rev Res Educ.* 2020;44(1):130–160.

46. Anson CM, Greene B, Halm, M. Analyzing students' constructs of writing through reflections on their drafts. *JoWR.* 2020;4:140–158.

47. Tate TP, Warschauer M. Going beyond "that was fun;" measuring writing motivation. *JoWR.* 2018;2:257–279.

48. Householder M, Schaffer MW. Writing analytics and program assessment: how novice writers use rubric terminology in reflective essays. *JoWR.* 2020;4:104–139.

49. Crossley S. Linguistic features in writing quality and development: an overview. *JoWR.* 2020;11(3):415–443.

50. Alsop S., Gardner S. Understanding attainment disparity: the case for a corpus-driven analysis of the language used in written feedback information to students with different backgrounds. *JoWR.* 2019;3:38–68.

51. Lang S. Evolution of instructor response? Analysis of five years of feedback to students. *JoWR.* 2018;2:1–33.

52. Madson M. Five-canon eedback: Triaging errors in writing with classical rhetoric. *J Contin Educ Nurs.* 2018;49(2):57–59.

53. Graham SS, Kim SY, DeVasto DM, Keith W. Statistical genre analysis: Toward big data methodologies in technical communication. *Techn Commun Quart.* 2015;24(1):70–104.

54. Buley L. *The User Experience Team of One: A Research and Design Survival Guide*. Rosenfeld Media; 2013 July 9.

55. Stawarz K, Preist C, Tallon D, Wiles N, Coyle D. User experience of cognitive behavioral therapy apps for depression: an analysis of app functionality and user reviews. *J Med Internet Res*. 2018;20(6):e10120.

56. Borsci S, Buckle P, Walne S. Is the LITE version of the usability metric for user experience (UMUX-LITE) a reliable tool to support rapid assessment of new healthcare technology? *Appl Ergon*. 2020;84:103007.

57. Bitkina OV, Kim HK, Park J. Usability and user experience of medical devices: An overview of the current state, analysis methodologies, and future challenges. *Int J Ind Ergon*. 2020;76:102932.

58. Tutty MA, Carlasare LE, Lloyd S, Sinsky CA. The complex case of EHRs: examining the factors impacting the EHR user experience. *J Am Med Inform Assoc*. 2019;26(7):673–677.

59. Bate P, Robert G. *Bringing User Experience to Healthcare Improvement: The Concepts, Methods and Practices of Experience-Based Design*. Radcliffe Publishing; 2007.

60. Ariail J, Smith TG. Concept analysis: Using an academic nursing genre for writing instruction in nursing. In: Heifferon B, Brown SC, eds. *Rhetoric of Healthcare: Essays Toward a New Disciplinary Inquiry*. Hampton Press, 2008:243–263.

61. Roberts LW. Belonging, respectful inclusion, and diversity in medical education. *Acad Med*. 2020;95(5):661–664.

62. Yanchick VA, Baldwin JN, Bootman JL, Carter RA, Crabtree BL, Maine LL. Report of the 2013-2014 Argus Commission: diversity and inclusion in pharmacy education. *Am J Pharm Educ*. 2014;78(10): S21.

63. Amayo J, Heron S, Spell N, Gooding H. Twelve tips for inclusive teaching. *MedEdPublish*. 2021;10. https://doi.org/10.15694/mep.2021.000081.1

INDEX

Page numbers in **bold** indicate tables, page numbers in *italic* indicate figures.

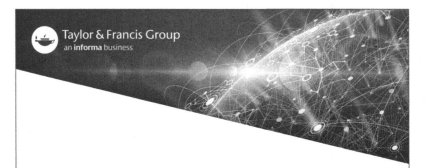

Printed in the United States
by Baker & Taylor Publisher Services